The Journey
from the Center
to the Page

THE JOURNEY FROM THE CENTER TO THE PAGE

YOGA PHILOSOPHIES & PRACTICES AS MUSE FOR AUTHENTIC WRITING

JEFF DAVIS

MONKFISH BOOK PUBLISHING COMPANY
RHINEBECK, NEW YORK

This revised second edition is published by MONKFISH BOOK PUBLISHING COMPANY 27 Lamoree Road Rhinebeck, New York 12572

Previously published in softcover in 2005 by Gotham Books, a division of Penguin Group (USA) Inc. and published as a Gotham Books hardcover edition in 2004.

Grateful acknowledgment is made for permission to reprint the following:

Excerpt from "That Lean and Hungry Look" by Suzanne Britt, Newsweek, October 9, 1978, reprinted by permission of the author

Excerpt from "Morning Swim" by Maxine Kumin, copyright © 1965 by Maxine Kumin, from Selected Poems 1960–1990 by Maxine Kumin. Used by permission of W. W. Norton & Company, Inc.

book and cover design: Georgia Dent
interior photos: Farley Crawford
author photo: Hillary Harvey

Library of Congress Cataloging-in-Publication Data

Davis, Jeff (Jeff Burgess), 1965-
  The journey from the center to the page : yoga philosophies & practices as muse for authentic writing / Jeff Davis. -- Rev. ed.
    p. cm.
  Includes bibliographical references.
  ISBN 978-0-9766843-8-1
  1. Authorship. 2. Authorship--Psychological aspects. 3. Hatha yoga. I. Title.
  PN145.D38 2008
  808'.02019--dc22
                                2008007047

Printed in the United States of America
Bulk purchase discounts for educational or promotional purposes are available.

10 9 8 7 6 5 4 3 2 1

Monkfish Book Publishing Company
27 Lamoree Road
Rhinebeck, New York 12572
www.monkfishpublishing.com

Publishers note: This book is not an instructional yoga book, but a series of suggestions concerning how yoga philosophies, principles, and practices can deepen writers' understanding of and experience of their writing process, writing style, and writing life. Any questions as to whether or not to proceed with particular poses or practices as well as any medical questions regarding contraindications should be referred either to a holistic health professional or to a qualified yoga teacher.

For my parents & teachers,
and for the one true thing, Hillary

CONTENTS

PREFACE FOR SECOND EDITION

A YOUNG AND MOSTLY UNKNOWN Ernest Hemingway met the newly celebrated F. Scott Fitzgerald allegedly in Paris's Dingo Bar, a common hang out for ex-pat writers. That year, 1925, Scribner's Sons had published *The Great Gatsby*, a book which helped make the young blond writer from Minnesota America's golden boy of literature. Hemingway recounts in a letter from the time as well as in his literary memoir *A Moveable Feast* how the literary boy wonder, so sloshed from booze, could barely balance on the bar stool. The account has been doubted, but the image has stuck.

Booze as muse—that's the idea perpetuated by images of hard-boiled American writers such as Faulkner, Fitzgerald, Hemingway, Capote, and a slew of others during the twentieth century. In fact, the book *Hemingway & Bailey's Bartending Guide to Great American Writers* (2006) details well-known writers' favorite cocktails and their habits for consuming them while composing. Carson McCullers, for instance, created her own Long Island Tea—a combination of iced tea and sherry she sipped throughout the day while at Yaddo, the renowned artists' community. Jonathan Miles, a reviewer from *The New York Times*, made this acute observation about the authors portrayed in the book: All are, well, dead, and only Hunter S. Thompson, who shot himself in 2005, could be considered "contemporary." *What's happened?*, Miles wonders. He half-jokingly bemoans, as if the good ol' days of boozing writers had vanished, that maybe most American writers in the twenty-first century no longer depend on the sauce to weather the vagaries of being a creative writer.

Something's happening here. Joyce Carol Oates, author of over 100 books, runs to revise. The more creative tangles her writing makes, the longer she must run. *Metta* (loving-kindness) meditation aided Alice Walker through a tricky divorce and gave her the compassion necessary to write novels such as *The Color Purple*.

Pulitzer Prize-winning author Ellen Gilchrist allegedly brought to a writers' conference her yoga teacher. Gilchrist said, in essence, "Here is the person responsible for my not self-destructing as a writer these past twenty-five years." Flamboyant novelist Tom Robbins recommended as early as 1988 to aspiring writers that they do something physical—hiking, swimming, yoga—to get out of their head. Even Papa Hemingway's actress grand-daughter Muriel wrote her memoir *Finding My Balance: A Memoir with Yoga* in 2003 with each chapter titled after a Yoga pose.

I'm not suggesting that all writers have dried out and replaced bourbon with breath work. But, despite our world's rampant problems and crises, many of us have figured out what yogis have been saying for a few thousand years: That it's all connected. More precisely, how the body functions and how the breath moves do alter our brain waves, which in turn affect whether or not we can concentrate and imagine. How the body functions and how the breath moves affect our intellect and those slew of obstacles that can block writers—fear and doubt, anger and envy, self-consciousness and self-criticism, depression and anxiety.

Granted, I know some writers hold onto their "stuff" like personalized luggage (or is it baggage?). I was heartened, though, when staff writer for *The New Yorker* Joan Acocella recently wrote that madness does not necessarily birth creative genius. In her collection of biographical essays *Twenty-Eight Artists and Two Saints* (2007), she writes "that what allows genius to flower is not neurosis, but its opposite, 'ego strength,' meaning (among other things) ordinary, Sunday-school virtues such as tenacity and above all the ability to survive disappointment."[1]

We're changing our view of the brain and creativity, which in turn is shifting how we view Yoga and creative writing. Around the same time in the 1980s that I was tracking Hemingway's favorite pubs in Montmarte, professors of neuropsychology also told me my adult brain could get no better and that all my willpower would not alter my brain's pathways nor reverse the damage done by my collegiate imitations of literary heroes.

Only new discoveries in the brain's hemispheric functions held any promise to me as a young idealistic writer. These discoveries suggested that the brain's two hemispheres, joined by the corpus callosum, accounted for separate functions. These discoveries quickly became co-opted by the then-vogue personality tests. Some of us used to take "brain personality" tests in the 1980s and '90s to explain away why we might be hyper-rational or overly dreamy. These "tests," oversimplifying the then-current brain science, suggested that creativity was mostly a right hemispheric function. "Creativity" on the right side, "rationality" on the left, the simplification went. During much of the ensuing twenty years, various forms of brain mapping aimed to pinpoint certain behaviors and traits to specific regions of the brain: The visual cortex governs sight, the auditory cortex accounts for hearing, the frontal cortex makes analytical decisions, and the almond-shaped amygdala in the hindbrain harbors our capacity for fear. This regional view of the brain, it turns out, is only part of the picture of how that throbbing cauliflower thrives.

Creativity actually involves the brain's neighborhoods talking to one another. When we're immersed in painting or writing or making music, the right hemisphere converses with the left; the rational frontal cortex speaks to the emotional hindbrain. Neurologist Kenneth M. Heilman speculates in his book *Creativity and the Brain* (Psychology Press 2005) that creative people might have more "connectivity" among their brain's various regions, or neighborhoods as it were. Creative endeavors are like the public local events that bring together the town's various citizens.

The old portrait of a stagnant gray blob that with age and abuse only degenerates has been revised. The brain is not a machine; it is alive and pliable. Thought changes gray matter, it turns out. Most neuroscientists now readily admit that neurons can change shape and that at least one part of the brain can generate new brain cells. This latter generally accepted discovery sparked a brush fire only a few years ago through the neuroscience community. Novelty and intentional actions, for instance, not only can arouse more of the brain's neighborhoods and encourage its neighbors to talk to one another; being alert to new situations also might even make more sidewalks for the brain's neighbors to saunter. That is, the brain's neurons can grow more connectors to stimulate more synaptic fire.

But more than science, more than theory, Yoga works its way with writers through experience. Since this book's first publication, I have worked with thousands of writers at conferences, festivals, and retreat centers. These places brim with serious, impassioned writers who intuit this journey does not have to be wrought with neuroses and addiction. They're right. My one-on-one experiences as mentor, coach, and editor with numerous established and aspiring writers have helped me refine these teachings and how to communicate them. Their experience confirms what yogis have known for centuries and what scientists are scurrying to validate: It works. I am grateful for what I have learned from these writers, and in this edition I share more of their examples.

In this edition I have also tightened, added to, and re-named almost every chapter from the first edition – especially chapters in Section II. This section more fully explores the connections between consciousness and craft. In that spirit, I also have added a new chapter, Chapter 5, that lays out the thrust of how Yoga alters and expands our creative faculties.

I have tightened some of the TAKE A BREATH exercises and I have replaced other exercises with new ones. I have since worked with visual artists and so have written a new chapter on how Yoga aids the artist's journey, and my work with students at Western Connecticut University also spawned a chapter with suggestions for teachers of writing.

Since 2004 classes and workshops in at least 15 states across the country have integrated Yoga with writing and art. I know a teacher at a high school for troubled and criminal teens in New York State who shows these teens how to weave Yoga with their writing process. It's an exciting moment for us to realize that we don't have to trade our life for our creativity — when we can replace booze with breath as our muse.

I doubt if the twentieth-century renegade writers were living today that Hemingway would have met Fitzgerald at Bliss Yoga Center striking Donward Facing Dog instead of Downward Facing Drunk, but isn't it pretty to think so?

ACKNOWLEDGMENTS

Numerous allies on this journey have helped me directly or indirectly to write this book. I am indebted to my first agent, Laureen Rowland, whose genuine enthusiasm, from our first conversation, helped make this book a reality. I appreciate the good people at Penguin/Gotham Books for their work with the first edition as well as my agent Linda Loewenthal for her patience and balanced perspective.

Thanks to those students who have contributed their examples and inspiration to this book. The good people at Byrdcliffe Artists Colony and Earthdance Retreat Center as well as many friends at various stages of this book's progress gave me a room of my own during my travels. Specifically, Yoga scholars Georg Feurstein and Trish Feurstein, neuroscientist Adam Zeman of the University of Edinburgh, and Frederick Turner of The University of Texas at Dallas responded thoughtfully to my pesky questions about Sanskrit and the brain.

And for this revised edition, I am grateful to Paul Cohen of Monkfish Publishing for recognizing how to improve an already good book that it might receive an extended life and to Georgia Dent of Monkfish Publishing for countless hours that have given this book a beautiful presentation. And thanks to my wife Hillary for providing an anchor for this journey and for her sensitive, honest reading of this new edition's manuscript.

INTRODUCTION :
REMEMBER YOUR BODY

THIS BOOK IS not about purity. If you smoke Marlboros, drink Jack Daniels, and cuss like my great-grandmother Mudder, that's your business. My Yoga teacher in South India, Sri T.K.V. Desikachar, sees tens of thousands of stressed-out, overworked, and overweight Indians a year. He never tells them to drop their bad habits. "Those things take care of themselves," he told me, "of their own time."

If the focus on Yoga intimidates or irritates as much as intrigues you, maybe you imagine svelte, self-righteous yogis sweating and twisting their bodies into impossible shapes. You need not worry, though, if your day's most physical act has been to walk to the corner shop for coffee and a bagel. Don't sweat. Really. Although sweating does loosen ligaments and prepare muscles for physically intense yoga sessions, your torso need not drop buckets of water to derive yoga's benefits for authentic writing. As this book will show you, being able to twist your imagination with a flexible spirit is more important for authentic writing than being able to secure your foot behind your head. Had anyone suggested when I was in my twenties to try Yoga to heighten my concentration and deepen my writing, I might have raised my eyebrows. But it happened. Yoga screwed up my life and my writing in beautiful ways.

This book stems in part from that experience and takes as its premise something simple yet potentially transformational: Yoga can aid your writing. Its non-dogmatic philosophy and its numerous tools can help you as a creative writer harness your faculties, immerse in your process, hone your craft, and above all else persevere this journey. My journey as a writer as well as my teaching and coaching experiences bear out that a wellspring for our creative writing is as close as our nose. Our breath and body—these in part can be the muses that help us navigate our fluttering mind, tricky imagination, and unpredictable heart as we write (and rewrite).

"Don't accept anything the speaker is saying. Test it out for yourself," the twentieth-century Indian philosopher J. Krishnamurti frequently said. This skeptical inquiry and this thrust of testing out things define the essential mindset for practicing Yoga. Part of what distinguishes Yoga from forms of exercise as well as from many other spiritual disciplines is its all-encompassing tools to understand *through the body's experience* what works and what does not work. So be ready to test things out. I had to.

As a writer, I've had a precarious relationship with my body. The summer after my freshman year in college, when I heaved stones under the hot Texas sun for my then brother-in-law's landscaping business, I wrote in a notebook one evening, my slight muscles throbbing, "I will be a writer." Anything to avoid that heat and backbreaking labor. That private declaration of independence came from more than pain avoidance, of course. After a few years spent under the tutelage of writers such as David Wevill, Thomas Whitbread, and Frederick Turner, I also realized that I wanted to be an extraordinary writing teacher as much as a writer. Those two pursuits I followed with fervor during my twenties, a fervor that exacted a cost on my body.

During my twenties and early thirties, I had become wedded to my writing and to teaching writing. At different times, I taught creative writing courses and poetry seminars at three colleges and at three high schools. I often traveled throughout the Southwest to teach hundreds of writing teachers the art of teaching writing. That was my life: writing and teaching writing.

I was a working head. Smug with my vegetarianism and a distorted asceticism, I had not made love in years, fell ill from stress at least three times a year, and by age twenty-eight had stress-induced bronchitis, chest pains, and a pinched nerve in my right trapezius muscle that often left me half-paralyzed flat on my back. With muscles aching chronically and a right arm shaking from too much writing and responding to students' writings, I'm surprised I didn't scribble in a notebook at the time, "I will become a stoneworker," which was starting to sound like more attractive work.

Not particularly athletic, I had intuited even at nineteen that more body awareness might help my taxed mind. As an undergraduate, I had sneaked off early one morning away from my roommates to take my first Yoga class. That was in 1985 in Texas, where Yoga among my friends was still relegated to one of the weird things people who wear funny beads and smoke funny weeds do. I knew it felt good. Unfortunately, for my body and my writing, for the next ten years I didn't stick with it consistently. No one in graduate school or in the numerous writing workshops and conferences I attended suggested I tap into the body or breath to alter my writing or to help me understand why sometimes, when I wrote, images and ideas flowed effortlessly and yet other times I sat and doodle-wrote for hours, sure that I was a fraud and hack. Would that someone had.

By the time I returned to Yoga regularly twelve or so years later, I was so wound up, balled up, and stressed that I had the tightest shoulders in my Yoga class. I had leapt into a high-pressure job as English department chair of a high-profile school. Around the same time, I also had abandoned a stagnating relationship to leave myself alone again with writing and teaching. My consistent, dogged, maniacal writing had dwindled into an Anaïs Nin–style cataloging of all-night excursions, and even when I could write a publishable creative essay or poem beyond my own foggy perspective, something in my writing process and style felt untrue, labored, dried-up. And as much as I understood elements of writing craft and process and style, I had no clue how the physical vehicle and subtle faculties that allowed me to write—in short, my body, mind, and imagination—functioned. I wrote from chin up, my shoulders clinched around my ears as if to block any awareness from seeping down to my torso.

Then it happened. In my first Yoga classes, I remembered (or is it re-membered?) my body, and my body re-membered my imagination. While gliding into Downward Facing Dog or Standing Forward Bend, I'd close my eyes and see my body, with no effort, as an ancient home with vast corridors, as a cottage in the Austrian mountains; aqueducts and rivulets with paper cups floating in them pulsed somewhere in my legs; a stranger's face, an old woman with braids and a scratchy scarf, rummaged around in my chest. A yoga class felt like an LSD trip.

Moving in Yoga poses felt like those few and increasingly rare moments I'd have at the desk that you might call "writer's flow" when self-consciousness and anxiety dissolve, when your imagination cooperates with your intellect and lets words unfold with few sputters, when time expands and you feel more alive than you ever have. Those visual experiences, the pleasurable pulsing in my brain, and the relief of the pinched nerve in my right shoulder were enough to keep me coming back to Yoga three times a week and then gradually impelled me to develop my own daily practice.

The "practice" became Yoga with a big "Y." Yoga triggered some shifts. I viewed myself differently as a writer. I could harness my energy and faculties for my writing rather than depend on their whim. I could work with deeply engrained obstacles—interior and exterior—that obstructed me from writing the kind of prose and poetry I intuited I needed to write. For a man in his early thirties, something else terrifying happened: Some of my chest's armor fell away, and I began feeling—for myself, for others. My writing, consequently, became richer, more authentic, more textured and nuanced.

Questions kept coming up: How could the body be a limitless yet immediate muse for writing? How does the practice of Yoga conduce an authentic writing life? Those questions have led me through a deeper study of Yoga's classical and post-classical texts of philosophy, through two yoga teacher-training programs, and to Greece and India to study with such generous yogis as Angela Farmer, Victor Van Kooten, and Sri T.K.V. Desikachar. These studies and my own experience confirm that Yoga is a philosophy and science for creative transformation. It's also a readily accessible practice that can address with openness our yearnings and needs as creative writers.

Each day Yoga and writing wed with one another at my desk, on the mat, and on the street. My mat in fact resides beside my desk. This journey has led me back to my body and to the faculties I embody—intuition, the unconscious imagination, intellect, emotion—a descent that has altered profoundly how I view, experience, and understand my writing practice and my writing life. This book shares with you my findings and provides you the guidance, the Yoga philosophies, and the Yoga practices to help you heed J. Krishnamurti's advice: Try things out for yourself.

Why yoga? Why not another form of meditation or some form of physical exercise such as running, aerobics, or lifting weights? Meditation alone certainly heightens concentration and relaxation, but focusing directly on our thoughts drives some people crazy. Their lower backs twitch, their noses itch, and their minds flutter. A writer friend I know took a six-week meditation class to help him quiet his jittery chatter. By the end of week one, he was ready to take literally the Zen saying, *When you meet the Buddha, kill him.* Stop trying to quiet your mind by saying, "Be quiet!" Instead, do as the fifteenth-century text *The Hatha-Yoga-Pradipika* recommends: Harness the breath and open the body, and thoughts will quiet.

Yoga reverses the feeling of being a victim to some mysterious muse whose erratic schedule rarely jibes with yours. With consistent Yoga practice, you can influence your concentration and imagination, your level of vigor, and your awareness of emotions—all beneficial attributes, as this book will explain, to writers. It's no secret, either, that we writers are given to depression, anxiety, and insomnia, too. Numerous current studies verify what the ancient yogis stated: Yoga helps the mind and its moods. And whereas physical forms of exercise such as aerobics and running do benefit the brain and body, Yoga's principles and tools offer a practical way that efficiently centers the "body-mind-imagination" and deepens self-understanding. Yoga is a way that emphasizes less how you look on the mat and more how you live in the world. Thankfully, it's a practice that also is invariably adaptable to any body, which is good news for most of us sedentary writers. To practice Yoga as muse for authentic writing involves the physical postures (*āsanas*), breath awareness (*prānāyāma*), concentration (*dharana*), meditation (*dhyana*), inner seeing (*bhavana*), and self-study (*svādhyāya*).

Why Yoga? Why not?

The word "authentic" is an adjective that stems from the Greek *authentes*, "one who acts on his own authority." So, we circle around to Krishnamurti's wisdom: Use this book to *test things out for yourself* and write from that space of experimentation. A number of writers report that they enjoy reading the book one chapter at a time as part of their morning practice. Then, they try the "TAKE A BREATH" exercise following almost each chapter.

For writers wishing to revive their practice, I usually suggest they begin with the first four chapters. These chapters lay out what I call The Four Preparations that can help you write with a deeper purpose, more discipline, more perseverance, and more concentrated immersion. Chapter One can help you explore what truly matters to you as a writer and remember your authentic intention as you draft, revise, and publish. Chapters Two through Four address some of the most common questions that writers ask me: "How do I find time to write?" and "How do I find the concentration and self-discipline to write consistently and effectively?" Yoga can strengthen your constitution and slow down your brain waves so you can endure intense writing projects with perseverance and concentration.

Yoga alters writers' consciousness. A shift in consciousness can hone craft as Section II explores. If you have an established writing practice, review Chapter One and then these chapters. Through simple Yoga tools you can heighten your senses to create what John Gardner called in *The Art of Fiction* the "fictional dream," the seamless web of redolent detail and sapid images a good writer often creates for readers. These chapters also explore how Yoga awakens in writers their most valuable faculty: wonder. And with yoga's tools for listening, you can regain your authentic voice, craft convincing dialogue, and write sentences whose music comes from the mix between brain and heart—literally.

Few creative writers have mastered the hazards of fear, anxiety, anger, and compassion—facets that, when witnessed, can lead to unforgettable writing. Section III explores how Yoga helps you handle that most primal emotion—fear—as well as transform its close cousin anger into satire. Complex characterization also confounds many writers. The challenge might have less to do with craft than with compassion (of the Faulkner variety, not of the doting grandmother variety). I'm not promising that Yoga will make you a better person, but because Yoga can help you practice compassion and truthfulness, you can learn to portray your subjects—yourself, other people, difficult fictional characters—with greater complexity and believability.

When it comes time to edit and revise, Yoga can also help writers let go of delusion and control. Section IV offers some tips. If you already have an advanced Yoga practice, you might review the chapter for advanced practitioners. Its ideas and generalizations may inform your reading of the other chapters. Another chapter encourages you to seek writing allies but not without a few warnings about writers' groups and writers' circles. Finally, I also have added a chapter addressing visual artists and musicians, based on my cross-over work with both, and I also have added a chapter expressly for teachers. This last chapter stems not only from my twenty years of teaching; it comes more directly from several teachers asking for such a chapter and for my deep sympathies and high regard for them.

Become a more versatile writer with Yoga's assistance—that's each chapter's thrust. Most chapters include "TAKE A BREATH" exercises to guide you through embodying your writing process. Several original Sanskrit terms—Sanskrit being Yoga's language—may deepen your knowledge and understanding of this sacred tongue.

Ancient Hatha-Yoga texts describe unique centers within the body that guide facets of our volition, personality, and imagination. Some texts describe seven, some eight, some more. You'll learn in this book, though, how some of these centers help you write from one center. Yours.

When an anthropologist asked a yogi, "Where is the center of the universe?" the yogi looked across the plain where they stood, pointed at a mountain, and said, "There." Then he said, "If that's where you're standing." Then he pointed to his left at a tree and said, "There. If that's where you're standing." Then he pointed to the place beneath the anthropologist's feet and said, "There is the center of the universe for you at this moment." He paused again.

"And there. It's always there," he said, pointing to the anthropologist's heart. He wasn't a relativist or a narcissist suggesting that the universe is simply a construct of a person's point of view, nor was he being clever or symbolic by pointing to the heart. The heart's location below our brain and in our torso can keep our awareness in our core, derived from the Latin word for heart, couer, from which we get courage. From that center, common to all of us, spirit and body and language align.

You know when you write from your center. You just know it. You write what your spirit, body, and language demand you write. It's a potentially hazardous path because your protective ego may no longer be in as much control, and this writing can shake you out of your comfortable habits by forcing you to write the truth—regardless of genre. With persistence, though, you learn you can persevere, that you can write no other way. You have no more excuses. And this curious work of engaging Yoga as muse brings us there, here, to the source of our creative impulse.

Writing *is* a journey. When Margaret Atwood asked several novelists a few years ago what it felt like to write, they repeatedly used words evoking a journey through a dark place. Many of them felt almost blind along the way, yet they sensed that movement forward would bring vision. Atwood writes, "I was reminded of something a medical student said to me about the interior of the human body, forty years ago: 'It's dark in there.'"[1] And perhaps this is how I've remembered to live and to write authentically: to make love to the darkness instead of trying to kick it out of bed. To make love to the darkness a writer moves toward doubts and doesn't try to repress them or let them control her. Such a writer finds ways to spelunker into the body's and the imagination's subtle caverns and to find hideous yet exquisite forms and names of oneself, of humanity, of God, and of whatever it is we call reality—the basic stuff of authentic writing and the basic stuff of Yoga.

This book encourages you to enter that darkness. It does not pretend to be Virgil to all of the Dantes in the writing world. Writing is difficult. This book, however, does suggest new ways for you to use Yoga's tools and live its philosophies, that you may find the courage, confidence, and skill to step into the darkness and so begin a journey from your center and then back to the page.

I

THE FOUR PREPARATIONS

INTENTION, TIME, PERSEVERANCE, CONCENTRATION

CHAPTER ONE

PUT ON THE ROBE:
WHAT ARE YOU WRITING FOR?

A N HOUR OR SO BEFORE DAWN, the congress in my head that years ago would wake me by trumpeting the day's debates seems this morning cooperative and sedate. I creep from bed across the hall's squeaking hardwoods to my study. On one side of my study, the window above my desk looks like a blank blackboard that complements my computer screen's white sky. On the study's other side, my yoga mat waits for me to step on it like a diving board. If my mat be a diving board, then that white screen must be the sky into which I dive. (I'm not one of those gonzo writers who actually leaps from downed planes flying over, say, war-torn Liberia and lives to write about it; metaphors placate my imagination just fine.) It's a precarious business, this writing life, one filled with little daily affirmation from other people that what you're spending your precious time and energy doing actually matters or is any good. No supervisor nods her head in approval. No customer survey rates your writing. No regular performance evaluation ranks you for writer of the month. Just the wide-open page and you, free-falling, twisting, teaching yourself how to shift your limbs to spin into airborne pirouettes, all with the faith that as you see some creative problem mounts and the brown ground zooms toward your face, your parachute cord will work. More often than not when you write, although it feels at times as if you get caught in trees or hurt your knees, you land upright on your two feet, your soles refastened to earth. The next day you can't wait to begin again with a new page.

Why on earth, of all the ways to spend the morning, do I choose to write? While I was a temporary resident at the Zen Mountain Monastery, Vice-Abbess Bonnie Myotai Treace, Sensei, raised a question about practicing Zen that reminds me of an essential question for writers: "Why, given the endless possibilities of a morning, given dawn, put on a robe at the sound of a bell".[1] Why put on your robe, indeed, and hobble to the desk? Why write? It seems like a good question for starters. Without a genuine motivation, we're possibly hobby writing, sky doodling. We got into this business of taking creative leaps for reasons other than an adrenaline rush.

Something I've learned from my yoga practice—to revisit a variation of the question "Why write?"—has changed the way I start things—my mornings, my classes and workshops, and my own writing sessions.   To begin each writing session, I've re-phrased the question "Why write?" to "What am I writing for?" "Why write?" is a question that begs defense. It's the question a father asks his teenager in college: "Don't you have anything better to do?" A more private question than its more direct sibling, "What are you writing for?" is to be asked of yourself. No other yogi, writer, or professor will hear you. That fact alone may make all the difference in the answer that surfaces. You may be surprised by what happens. Perhaps you'll feel more at ease about your writing as you connect what surfaces to your core identity as a writer. The phrasing "What am I writing for?" may even lead you to dedicate your writing practice to something or someone. In this way your writing may come from a source other than your ego. When successful, seasoned writers tell me "something is missing" from their writing practice, this simple gesture begins to satisfy some of their hunger. The response to this question becomes part of my intention for writing on any given morning.

What is an intention? An intention is not a goal. A goal is something you measure and check off when you have completed it. An intention is a conscious gesture to align your mind, heart, imagination, and body with whatever act you're about to begin. You attach yourself to a goal's outcomes and assess your success accordingly. You let go of an intention's outcome and let go of notions of success altogether. Goals guide business; intentions guide soul.

Intention can center the mind and imagination without restricting it. It also can deepen your connection to writing's purposefulness. An intention plants a seed, a suggestion that may manifest during that writing session or may not manifest until two weeks or a year later. Action with intention stimulates more portions of the brain and can lead to actual changes in our neuronal pathways[2], so we write with more mind and more brain, literally. Yoga without intention is exercise; writing without intention simply may be directionless.

What are you practicing Yoga for? Most of us take that first step onto the mat for personal reasons. An injury, the first signs of cellulite, loneliness, heartbreak, grief, addiction, or a gamut of physical and emotional ailments may propel us into Downward Dog Pose and Cobra Pose. In her classic book *Awakening the Spine*, Vanda Scaravelli lays out her poetic reflections for a natural, egoless practice: "Yoga should not be a training for body control; on the contrary, it must bring freedom to the body, all the freedom it needs."[3] The highest motive to practice Yoga may be liberation.

I don't know if writing will set us free, but I do know there's value in setting an intention as a writer. No need to expect grand or immediate answers to the question "What am I writing for?" Perhaps the answers that surface for you—today, tomorrow, next month—may reflect what other writers have said they write for. Jhumpa Lahiri, the youngest writer to receive the Pulitzer Prize, says she writes to confront and sort through the discrepancy between her Indian parents' worldview and her more American worldview with which she has grown up.[4] Sindiwe Magona, a novelist from South Africa and now working for the United Nations, says writing is therapeutic for her and for others.[5] Essayist Jean Bernstein says she must write because questions, voices, images, surface in her like "splinters," and writing essays is the best way she has found to pull out the really irritating ones.[6] These motives sustain writers and propel them to the desk each day.

What are you writing for? Perhaps, like many writers, you write to make sense of the world. If lucky, you can form some order out of chaotic human experience. For now, what you write for may be nothing more than the pleasure or wonder you've experienced when wielding words. Something related to a core principle also may stir you to write. If you hunger to make sense of how the taco-chain owner who migrated from Mexico twenty years ago is filthy rich and yet pays his illegal immigrant employees thirty-five dollars for fourteen-hour shifts, then exploring justice's complexities may be what you write for. Sometimes what we write for seems as fleeting as the hidden blue jay cawing among the birches, but these more remote, at times ineffable, motives help us write from our center.

When checking in with this question, watch your ego. A thirty-year-old writer, Elise, recently asked me to help her figure out her first novel's focus. She had almost finished the first draft of the story, which follows a young woman's emotional and political entanglements as she avoids marriage to pursue her dreams of opening an animal sanctuary, but Elise felt that the story, and she as a writer, had started to lose direction. "What stirs you to write this book?" I asked. She responded almost without hesitation: "To prove to my mother I've accomplished something. I have three degrees in languages and have nothing to show for it." Oh, the mother motive. I'd heard about it, although thankfully I've never had to wrestle with this one myself. Elise's ego, I sensed, still clung too tightly to her manuscript. She didn't trust her own authority. I suggested she let the project rest for a while and instead explore a deeper motivation that leads her to write even when her mother's not approving or disapproving; otherwise, she not only may censor herself when drafting and rewriting, but she also may be sorely disappointed when the book's completed, and her mother still doesn't nod her head. Will the book, then, be a failure? Two months later she hadn't taken my advice. Her mother's judgmental air still hovered over her shoulder. I took her through a simple process to slow down her thoughts, to ground her body, and to help her locate an authentic drive that would both sustain and focus her writing. Within a few minutes, she realized she wrote to satisfy an insatiable hunger to figure out what it means to be a woman in this country, to live an ethical livelihood, and to have conflicting loyalties between having a family and following a personal dream. These issues mattered to Elise. The next day she centered herself and kept in her heart some of these intentions. The results? She finished a second rewrite of the manuscript within six weeks and submitted it to her agent.

Many writers appreciate admiration and approval, but that motivation can consume us. Nonfiction writer Michael Stephens has admitted how, as a young writer trying to prove himself, spite and competition in his writing group fueled his young blood at St. Marks Poetry Project. Whether green or seasoned, we seek it. Nothing wrong with a little praise or ego drive, except that it can become an addiction that can steer us away from a more sustaining path. "Stop trying to get your audience to like you," writer Gerald Burns once told me and a group of other writers. Writing mainly to please someone—even an imagined audience—may sustain a writer for a while, but those exposed roots only extend so far. Fiction writer Ellen Gilchrist says there is next to "... nothing the outside world gives me in exchange for my writing that is of value to me. I do not take pleasure in other people's praise, and I don't believe their criticism."[7] Would that I could always be that clear. Gilchrist knows why she writes: She loves language. For some writers, it's as good of a reason as any.

When you privately ask "What am I writing for?" the ego can rest (and it's rare for our writers' egos to rest). You don't have to impress anyone. In this space, you can be more honest with yourself about what leads you to write. A few years ago, my former father-in-law (a retired stockbroker) and I were talking about books and writers. He said, "Well, you know, most writers publish books for one reason: to make money." I disagreed. He looked at me and said, "Well, all right, Jeff, why do you write? When you're writing, aren't you thinking about making money?" I grinned and told him that I ask myself every morning what I am writing for and never does "to make money" surface; otherwise, I would've stopped writing long ago. He smiled back and said, "You know, you'd make a lousy stockbroker." I didn't detail to him exactly what I write for, because sometimes the reasons are difficult to articulate, but I should have told him about my father's journal.

When I was five, my father gave me possibly the most important gift he's ever given me: one of my grandfather's datebooks that my father had used as his own daybook. It contains my father's scribbled boyhood descriptions of mowing the lawn and walking to the lake with his friends *as well as such sketchy observations* of my own as *I saw a hobo by the tracks today. I wonder where he goes. What he sees. I want to ride a train someday.* I've been riding the train of language and imagination ever since. With that journal, my father gave me the writing bug that never left my system.

So, before I write, I stand before my desk, hold my hands at my heart, close my eyes, take at least two full breaths, and quietly ask, "What am I writing for?" This gesture is not to be precious but to give myself all the help I can get. This gesture prepares my body, mind, and imagination before I take a leap. The answer's content and nature often depend upon my writing project. Sometimes an answer wells up in fragments and phrases: "to help others," "to tell the truth," "to hold myself together," "to figure out what I think I think and what I think I know," or often even something as vague as "to follow language's currents." Sometimes, I have to wait for several minutes, and, granted, some mornings give me little more than faint images. Yet lately, voices more urgent have surfaced in the morning: "Fight the tide of complacency" and "Do something for peace." Words may not save us, but it's worth reminding ourselves of our words' intention. Doing so gives me hope.

I take students through two important parts to setting a writing intention. Once we've listened for a few breaths to whatever rises in response to this question (the first part), we clarify the simple topic or specific focus for the day's writing session (the second part). Maybe this clarification is something direct like "I intend to write with clarity" or something juicier like "I intend to receive wild images for a new essay." This second part does not take away from writing's magic; it gives the magic direction. Sometimes, writers choose to keep this part general and say, "I'm open to the moment."

Other writers tell me that making a simple twofold intention grants them more ease while writing, and one writer in Portland, Oregon, says that setting this two-part intention lifts her out of what she calls her "morning neuroses" so she can promptly move on to "writing that matters." As a writer who can get lost in distractions and digressions, I enjoy the hazardous interplay between having an intention and not knowing where the train's taking me; the intention gives my wanderings some slight direction, like the pull of my mother's voice calling years ago whenever I had strayed miles away into the woods. Remembering both my larger intention of what I'm writing for, morning after morning, and the more specific intention of a single morning's session often brings me home.

Many of the exercises in the rest of this book will offer you possible specific intentions. Take them or leave them. They're there to help you focus your imagination and your mind.

Two last words about intentions, though: First, let go of outcome. If after one session or if after a week or a month, you still haven't written what you set out to write, don't fret. The writing likely took you somewhere you wouldn't have arrived at had you avoided the desk altogether. On the other hand, if you do accomplish precisely what you had intended, relish it and move on. And this: Sometimes the answer about what you're writing for is right in front of you. One writer I met in a workshop in California last year said that one morning no answer was surfacing until she heard her four-year-old son's laughter in the next room. "To sustain that laughter," she said, "—that's what I'm writing my stories and essays for."

It's a little past dawn, the mountain mist rising with the sun. From the window above my desk I spot a wild turkey walking across my lawn, then two, three, soon eight baby turkeys with one adult leading and a second adult following. Like schoolchildren lined up on a field trip, the chicks are being led near the garden and beneath the oak to find their morning feed. This, I think, is as good a reason as any to rise early, put on my tattered robe, and sit at my desk: to watch hope manifested in ten awkward bodies hobbling across my lawn like words in a sentence in search of some small seeds of reassurance.

TAKE A BREATH

It can be just this simple: Do what you need to do to settle some of your inner chatter. Sit comfortably in a chair or on the floor near your desk, or stand in front of 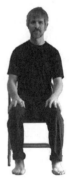 *your desk. I usually prefer to stand in* **MOUNTAIN POSE** *(tādāsana), my feet hip-width apart, my spine long, my hands at my heart. Try it. As you breathe, focus on your lower body and feet to help ground yourself literally in your physical connection to the earth and to draw attention away from your chatty head. Chuang Tzu noted, after all, that the venerable teacher breathes with her heels.*

Just breathe. Stand or sit for a few minutes, listening to your breath. Inhale from your belly, and exhale. Let your thoughts drop to your heart.

Then, ask yourself, "What am I writing for?" Listen. Wait for a word, a phrase, or image.

Second, clarify a more immediate focus for your 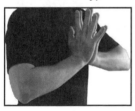 *writing, such as a subject or an intention to receive insight. Then, while writing, remind your body of those intentions.*

Keep it simple.

CHAPTER TWO

SHOW UP & SHAPE TIME

IN 1944, MIKLOS RADNOTI KNEW the Nazis would shoot him and the other Jews marching across Hungary any day, any hour. When his wife later had his body exumed from a mass grave, they would find a notebook of poems tucked in his field jacket's pocket. Somehow, he stealthed out a pen, the sound of gunfire rattling like bones, and wrote a series of poems.

Radnoti's actions are a haunting reminder of my mortality, of this odyssey's limited time.

Writers cannot wait until their kids go off to college or until retirement or until divorce or until they quit a job to begin writing. Writers with packed lives write before the family wakes up. They write on the subway, on lunch break, in the forty-eight minutes between when their children have fallen asleep and before they fall asleep. They write knowing they are mortal.

One way or another, we make peace with time, stop fighting it, and avoid bemoaning its apparent scarcity. There's plenty of time to be had, and if we can't change the way time works, then we can change the way we work with it.

To transform conditioned habits of how we live in time, some of us need jolts to startle our whole being—mind, spirit, body. Yoga shook me up. Then Zen. During my residency at the Zen Mountain Monastery in the Catskills, the monks tossed me into the liturgy, the rituals, with little explanation. In the predawn haze, bells of different pitches rang on cue, a bass drum boomed on cue, and we bowed and prostrated on cue. As I fumbled and sweated in my new monastic robe, my skeptical mind's radar set off several red beeps: What are we bowing to? Why doesn't anyone explain the purpose of these movements and chants? Isn't all of this ritual meaningless routine?

The monastery worked on me from the outside in. With no psychobabble or sweet talking, but instead with bells and sticks, with structures and strictures, the monastic experience helped me develop more of the discipline I needed at that time in my life. Although my life before then was fulfilling and spiritually grounded, many of my days had lacked authentic form; no genuine daily rituals anchored my awareness. Not so at the monastery. Every day had a distinct structure that varied occasionally: Awaken at 5:00 a.m. and walk in silence to the zendo, meditate, chant and bow at the dining hall, eat breakfast, chant in preparation for work, practice, work, chant and bow at the dining hall, eat lunch, rest, meditate, engage in art practice, study, rest, and so on until sleep. We slept for maybe six hours. The schedule exhausted me. Being awake is hard work.

The monastic experience hooked up well with my Yoga practice to give me tools to hone my writing life: namely, structured days and rituals to mark transitions between activities. I have met too many writers to know that despite our well-defined goals to pursue projects, we often let other less inspiring projects assume priority. Then we delay, we excuse, we neglect, and ultimately we forget the original idea.

I hear some variation of the following almost each week. You choose this path as a writer that resists the status quo, that says of this day "I will meet it full-faced and open-eared," that lets an hour shape a looping phrase into a poem or song or essay. And still you flounder. Errands and cleaning, shuttling soccer players and attending board meetings consume the space you had set aside to meet your muse as if another part of you conspired against too much wonder and ecstasy, against too much Truth.

What to do? What to do about the dogged beast called Discipline that has eluded writers and artists and musicians alike for centuries? How long will your muse wait?

Discipline. There it is. Some of us lug baggage with that word stitched on it. A friend of mine in marketing recommended that I not mention or highlight the word "discipline" in my pieces about writing because this baggage would block the message. But discipline is the message. So, let's unload the baggage. The word "discipline," like disciple, stems from the Latin *discere*, "to teach." A writing practice, like any practice, requires self-discipline. When we cultivate self-discipline, we teach ourselves of our capabilities, of our body and imagination's inherent relationship, and of what external and internal tools work best to enact a personal and artistic alchemy. Without self-discipline, we'll only make half the journey, if that far.

Re-imagine self-discipline. One great thing about being an adult writer or artist is you get to choose discipline, make it your own. No parent or teacher imposes it. Self-discipline need not be rigid and unbendable.

To re-imagine self-discipline, consider your relationship to time. My writer friends and students usually fall into one of these two extremes: Either their days fill up quickly—with other work, errands, familial duties, social engagements—or their days have wide-open space bounded only by light and dark. Time Crunchers hunger for an hour or two every other day simply to sit with their thoughts and their laptop. They're busy and important people at their jobs who keep companies functioning; they're busy and important parents who keep their children fed and clothed and sheltered. They snarl and secretly envy my other friends whose lives fall into the latter category: the Time Stretchers. These few writers and aspiring writers, who either by wealth or by wit succeed in leading a simple life, are privileged to wake up when they wish, write when they wish, and sleep when they wish (with some regular exceptions, of course). On the other hand, these same writers, who avoid penciling in their activities like monks bowing on the hour to the bells on Wall Street and who have time to write, may be the more frustrated at deciding what to do with themselves and their days.

Such a writer recently asked me to help her. "I have all the time I need," she said, "but I won't write anything unless I have a deadline." As a masseuse with a few private clients, Brandice had hours each day to visit friends, read the mounds of books that lined her small apartment, and comb her imagination for her own book ideas. She had written for years for local and prominent national magazines, but she wanted to finish her first book proposal (something she had tried three times before). Every time she had started her book project in the past, something else headed the muse off at the pass. After I helped her sort through her manuscripts and determine her book's unique focus, I had her do two things: We cleared a space in her cluttered work area to "sanctify" her project, so to speak, and we pulled out her daybook. "Make an appointment with your writing," I suggested. In her near-blank daybook, she wrote in two-hour blocks for the Tuesday, Wednesday, and Friday of the following week. Six hours was a good start. "Keep these appointments," I suggested. "During these allotted times, refrain from checking e-mail. Don't go on a fall foliage tour. Don't even schedule a massage client. Don't write any articles. Write your book proposal." She did so—with some occasional "falls from the page," of course. But in a month she had shifted her habit of distraction into a habit of discipline.

Successful writers can be time crunchers or time stretchers, but both require some form of voluntary structure. One writer and well-known writing professor, Donald Murray, has composed most of his books ten or fifteen minutes at a time. Between classes and conferences, between errands and meetings, he writes in patches until gradually he has gathered enough material to stitch a book. He then makes more time to sit for longer stretches to weave the pieces together. How much less intimidating to pen a good paragraph for thirty minutes than to wrestle with twenty pages for eight hours.

Other writers, of course, have months each year to wrap themselves in words. Truman Capote wrote while lying down in bed or on a couch, always ready to assuage his appetite with cigarette and coffee (which, he claimed, turned later in the day to "mint tea to sherry to martinis"). He always wrote drafts longhand in pencil. Then he wrote another revision in pencil. And a third draft on a very special kind of yellow paper. Very disciplined. (But then, who knows? The lovely, froggy writer, who pioneered the popularity of "creative nonfiction," was known to fib and exaggerate.) Some writers float for days in that luscious write-space. While writing *Pilgrim at Tinker Creek*, Annie Dillard said she slept until noon, then would write at one sitting in the afternoon and then another sitting after dinner and a walk until midnight or later. Tales of such nights of the living imaginations sometimes feed our romantic notions of the writer's life. Living without regard for nutrition or respite or the rest of the whirling world sometimes is the writer's equivalent of living in a personal monastery or ashram—a *satsanga* of one.

SCHEDULES AND A REGULAR "PRACTICE"

An artist came to me. "I don't know if writers have this problem," she said seriously, "but I can't seem to get myself to paint regularly." I assured her we do. She had talent. She had even had a few shows in New York, including her first solo. Still, when time was hers, she putzed around with graphic design work or straightened up her brushes and paint tubes for the fifth time in a day.

Working with her, I realized something: Time and space desire shape. Imagine if no object had form. Earth and the 10,000 things—walnuts in a boy's palm, raindrops on a pond, a kiss in autumn—simply would not exist. Imagine self-discipline as giving form to the gifts of days and hours. Then imagine the form that writing and art give mind and spirit.

To work on cue—whether we have a stint of fifteen minutes or a stretch of fifteen weeks to write—we need creative structure in our lives not unlike our body's creative structure. External structure, especially self-designed structure, can liberate our muse.

"More than half of the practice is just showing up to the zafu," Abbot Daido Loori was fond of saying at the monastery. How many times had I heard that? Sri T.K.V. Desikachar talks about showing up at the yoga mat, and we writers must "show up" at the desk. To make time to show up, most writers will tell you the same thing: Sacrifice something. Not a virgin or a goat. Not your husband. Not your friendships. Forgo a movie here and there. A lunch here and there. Hide your television. How about starting with that voice that keeps telling you, "You can start on your own writing with more discipline as soon as ..." As soon as what? As soon as you quit your job? As soon as you move to the Virgin Islands? As soon as your kids leave home? Put that voice on the altar today and relish slaying it.

To assist you with the sacrifice, make appointments with your writing. It's that simple, and yet I'm amazed by how many aspiring writers resist this simple fact: Writers write regularly and despite their lives' busy-ness. They "schedule" time to write. If long chunks of time intimidate you, think short and frequent. This suggestion may be this chapter's single most important one to heed. If you keep appointments with your hairstylist or with that friend who hounds you to have lunch each Wednesday, then why not keep regular weekly, if not daily, appointments with your muse? (She's probably more fun and less gossipy. Maybe.) I learned this simple fact from my Yoga practice. It became a "practice" once I started practicing at home at least three afternoons a week. Soon, I was engaged in Yoga on my own six or seven mornings a week and started tuning into what my body needed, how to use āsanas to relieve tension in my neck or to help me relax; the āsanas became assimilated into my own body and imagination instead of remaining forms that a teacher called out to me to execute. This regularity transferred to my writing habits.

Years ago, I would jot a page or two in the morning and sometimes write three pages madly into the night and every once in a while squeeze in twenty minutes in the afternoons. My writing practice suffered from the irregularity, and if a deadline wasn't pressing, weeks might pass without my writing at all. I changed my erratic ways. I started finding the joy and authenticity of meeting my muse at the same time of day at least four times a week—despite my then cluttered schedule. As a result, my body and mind calmed down on cue when I arrived at the desk each morning so my imagination could come out to play. Even when I didn't think I had anything to say or to write, I sat at the desk and wrote. My productivity has increased tenfold, and my muse appears far more regularly.

My daily schedule includes setting an intention and practicing from thirty minutes to two hours of Yoga and meditation, usually first thing in the morning (after, that is, I've fed my twelve-year-old arthritic and demanding cat Miklos). Typically, I pencil in chunks of four to eight hours for five days out of the week to write (sometimes with notes about which pieces I intend to work on) as well as times to prepare for my writing classes and miscellaneous business. I usually write for three hours in the early morning, break for breakfast, and write until noon. Then, depending on the rest of my life, either another two to three hours carries me into the afternoon or I conduct other business. I don't always write with such time constraints, but for someone who has made his life deliberately unstructured from a conventional point of view, such constructions help me work well.

Be flexible but regular. If developing a regular schedule is new to you, even if you've been writing for years, you might use this simple formula: 3-60-15. Write three times a week for sixty minutes each session for fifteen days (that is, three days a week for five weeks). Or this formula: 7-60-15. Seven days a week for sixty minutes for fifteen days. The fifteen days is a marker to see if this changed habit will stay; it provides a reachable end. If your schedule allows it, it's probably better to write for less time on several days each week (for example, one or two hours on three days a week) than to write for several hours only once a day each week. When you sit, just write. Recognize you have to wade through a lot of crap to locate the clear springs, but you'll benefit from scheduling appointments for the wading. When I suggested to one aspiring writer that she take only thirty minutes three times a week—that's all—to start her book and to do so diligently, she did. Thirty minutes became an hour. Then, she could not not write her book. Less than six months later she came to a workshop and told me, "That simple suggestion has changed my life. I'm almost through with the first draft of my book." She's not the only one.

And once you sit, stay put. You might be happily writing for thirty minutes or so and, suddenly, without your noticing it, you're out of your chair and filing your *New Yorkers* according to cultural era. What happened? The ego loves to sabotage your efforts. If you've given yourself an hour to write, refrain from answering the phone, getting a snack, checking e-mails, or whatever other sneaky obstacles might try to keep you from your soul's work. If you have something on your desk to stabilize you—a stone works for some writers—gaze at it and remind yourself of your own ability to stay anchored in your seat and intention. A stick of incense helped one student I know. Three evenings a week when he came home from work, he'd turn on his computer and light a stick of incense on his desk. While the incense burned, he continued to write. When it extinguished, he could leave his desk (although he often stayed for more). Most incense sticks burn for an hour or ninety minutes, so try it.

Schedule breaks if you need to. During my breaks in the middle of long writing sessions, I regularly saunter along the nearby roads or through the woods, or I work lightly on the paths I forge in the woods, and without fail the walk or the work produces something in my imagination that wouldn't have surfaced if I had stayed at my desk. Philosopher Immanuel Kant was renowned for walking the same route every day at precisely the same time in his small town. The locals allegedly could keep time according to when he strolled past their homes or shops. Poet and director of creative writing at Brandeis University Olga Broumas wrote three books while walking, she once told me in an interview. Scheduling a break, as opposed to taking one at whim, often keeps my body and mind alert and my imagination fertile for another thirty, forty minutes until it's time to saunter.

SLOW VINYASA AND WRITERS' RITUALS

We could use a little slowing down. We speed-read, gobbling our words only to forget most of what we've consumed. As we read, so we live. The alarm clock rattles before dawn, and you're up and off to wake the kids, shower, shave, grab some toast, prod the kids to eat and dress, drop the kids off, dash to work, make your calls, pick up the the kids and shuttle them to soccer practice, and you have forty-five minutes to yourself to eat or catch your breath before you pick them up again, feed them, help them with their homework, and put them to bed. You didn't spend the day's allotted time; clearly, it spent you. And you and your days feel cheaper and cheaper by the week. With the world too much with you, you wonder how you ever thought you could manage the time to write.

I know of few more decent pleasures than when time stretches like the back of a hammock on a summer afternoon. My Yoga practice of *vinyasa* has helped me not so much to manage time but to stretch it. Some people refer to vinyasa as a physical Yoga system characterized by a quick yet artful sequence from one yoga pose to the next, as in Sri K. Pattabbi Jois's *Ashtanga Yoga* (headquartered in Mysore, India) and David Life and Sharon Gannon's *Jivamukti Yoga* (headquartered in New York City). Practicing vinyasa authentically, as these teachers would tell you, has less to do with speed and quantity of poses than with awareness and intention. *Vinyasa* is to flow with a body-mindful awareness from one situation (another translation of āsanas) or activity to the next.[1]

I used to find myself shuttling from one thing to another, oblivious as to when lunch stopped and work resumed. Now, I try to make more time to taste waking up; to prepare breakfast and give thanks and to bow out when finished; to acknowledge the beginning, middle, and end of my writing time; to look someone in the eyes as I speak to her, notice her breath, and say a genuine good-bye before we part. Yoga does indeed calm the mind's whirling fluctuations; it also, though, calms our actions' whirls.

Practicing *vinyasa* by tending to the point when one activity, like a poem's line, ends and the next one begins can help us stretch time for our writing. Awareness frames a writing session from beginning to end. When we discipline ourselves to tend to our days' and our writing sessions' transitions, then our writing doesn't just pass us by. We move toward writing from our center.

One way to tend to these transitions is to create very simple rituals. Rituals, however small and personal, align our intention and attention with our body's action and open the barn door to our imagination. It's no secret that writers are ritualistic creatures. Margaret Atwood wrote of writing as a venture into utter darkness where a writer encounters the dead. No surprise, then, that, as Atwood tells it, writers create their own rituals before making their dangerous descents where they'll meet darkness, the dead, their demons. Isabel Allende, for instance, once lit a candle before each writing session to honor her deceased ancestors.

In addition to setting a twofold writing intention, I also do a couple of other things to open the gate. I pay homage to Ganesha, the potbellied, elephant-headed god of writers and of auspicious beginnings. Ganesha embodies the wisdom of maneuvering successfully in this world with courage, grace, kindness, and resolve. I'm not Hindu, but this big-eared, four-armed figure so enchants me that I cannot help but have a simple place for him by my desk and in my heart. Ganesha at once removes obstacles for me and places them in my way; plus, he's the scribe of Yoga. No wonder writers like him. If distraction is your biggest block, Ganesha helps you haul this stone out of your path. Author Diane Johnson said when she was blocked while writing her latest novel, *L'Affaire*, she sought out a guru who gave her a mantra—a simple but charged chant—to help her. She still uses it as a prewriting ritual. If you don't favor Ganesha or a chant, you might do as several of my students have done and acknowledge your own talisman, divinity, or good luck charm. Keep it simple but meaningful.

I also bow to my laptop. Well, not exactly. Ganesha sits next to my laptop, and before I write I bow to that quality to remove obstacles, so it looks as if I'm stooping to my laptop (an idea Michael Dell might like). I bow before I begin to write, invoke a brief chant that asks for the removal of obstacles, and bow as I end each session. You might do similarly. When you've finished your writing session, acknowledge the end. Let your computer or notebook hibernate while you incubate. Place a cover over your computer, or put your notebook away in a regular spot. Stack your papers. Put your books back. Polish your lucky stone. "To really complete work practice," abbot of Zen Mountain Monastery John Daido Loori writes, "requires cleaning up, putting the tools away, picking up the loose ends, 'leaving no trace.'"[2] Then, bow again, say something, or with your thoughts acknowledge whatever you invoked to begin your session. Blow out the candle. Once you've noticed at least two full breaths, then flow into your next activity.

Some of this talk of tending to the details may seem too precious for you. As I used to, you may feel at home not knowing when your writing stops and when checking e-mails begins. You may think you work best by keeping manuscripts smeared with peanut butter stains from six months ago stacked or splayed out on your desk. Yet, if you feel spent with your writing, and if you feel your writing no longer stems from an authentic space, try something different. One man in Portland, Oregon, has been a writer for thirty years and yet had been recently discouraged. After trying some of these suggestions, he wrote me to say that the simple ritual of moving through some simple yoga poses before his writing session "helps me form a boundary of good energy around my writing time." To write mindfully, some of us need creative boundaries.

Keep unattached to the forms. That is, avoid spending so much time constructing elaborate structures and rituals that you neglect the most important reason you may be reading this book: to write. Second, be flexible. I don't live a monk's life of absolute regularity. Surprises happen, and as with any enduring structure, I must bend. Once you set schedules and construct structures, keep them voluntarily and without feeling enslaved by them.

Wield words into shape because you have to. With no big advance, no promise of an audience except earth and thou, do it with the same necessity that rain and skyscrapers eventually fall, that leaves and personalities change coats. You have no choice. Be your own disciple. Shape your days with discipline the way waning sunlight hones dusk.

Center yourself. Set your intention. Embody your intention. Write. Start with fifteen, thirty minutes a day. Soon, space and time expand.

Being aware of time means we can choose not how to spend it, as if time were currency, but how to shape it. And if we shape time, we can shape where our minds and imaginations and hearts reside most of our days.

Consider a gardener's wisdom. My old poet friend Bob Trammell lived in a conventional middle-class neighborhood, in Dallas no less, where he shaped his front yard and back yard into mini-prairies. With wild buffalo grass and wild peonies teeming over the curb, his neighbors at first thought he was creating a health hazard even though he was creating a much healthier lawn than that of his pesticide-laden neighbors. I wondered how he had the time to tend to it. He told me once that fifteen minutes a day in the garden led to a garden more likely to flourish than four hours every two weeks or three weeks. If he made a ritual of tending to the garden for fifteen minutes a day, too, then while he worked on other projects or cooked or drove his son to school he would have in his imagination images of sunflowers and chamomile florets. In a way, that fifteen minutes a day was an investment in the quality of how he imagined the rest of the day.

Bob contracted liver cancer a few years ago. The doctors at Baylor and in Houston told him he had six months tops to live. They told him, too, it didn't really matter what he ate or what his habits were: he would die in six months, they said. In the next two years, though, as the blood slowly withdrew from the surface of his skin, as his skin started to sag around his once sharply defined cheeks and arms, and as his once distinct rugged twang started to fade, in between tending to his son and his wife and to the literary non-profit organization he founded, in that two years, he jogged, took all kinds of herbs, smoked a few joints to kill the pain, re-gained his practice of Yoga and meditation, and he wrote. In his last two years—18 months longer than the doctors doomed him for—he wrote and published short stories, drafted most of his first novel, and completed two volumes of poetry, one about dis-ease.

We all have responsibilities. We all have hardships. We all suf-fer. Sorrow excludes no one. And we're all going to die – at last and too soon.

Several years ago, Bob and I each were reading a lot of Chinese poets together and were each committed to writing one poem a morning to prepare for a mutual reading we were to give. I'd rise early before going to teach and sit in my chair and wait for a poem. And one always came. But sometimes, around 6:30 a.m. or so, the phone would ring. It'd be Bob. "What are you doing?" he'd ask sort of mischievously. "Are you writing?" Yes, Bob, I'm writing.

TAKE A BREATH

Keep your writing sessions simple but meaningful. Record in your daily planner three appointments with your muse this week. Show up. Align your mind and body with your imagination by setting a twofold intention. Then, enact a simple ritual that will invite your muse to open a gate. Before the ritual, tend to your breath's rhythms and notice how you feel in your body. Aim to give each part of your body—from your crown to your soles (not just your thoughts)—to the ritual. A simple bow after two full breaths may suffice before you sit. Lighting a candle—with attention to the match and box, to the wick and flame—may help to frame your writing session. Stay with your appointment to write until the end. Then, with the same attention you gave your opening ritual, put away your things so you can begin the next session with openness and clarity. And bow out. Give thanks. Appreciate where you've been going during this session and where you're going next.

CHAPTER THREE

STOKE YOUR WRITER'S FIRE

ONCE YOU MAKE YOUR SACRIFICES to create and stretch time for your writing, your body may not want to cooperate. When a writing problem persists, an image won't surface, or words scurry like mice away from your mind's light, your body may decide it's time to take a nap. Or maybe after you eat another row of Chips Ahoy!, your body reasons, you'll have more food for thought. This journey isn't easy, you realize. It requires work, if not a lot of knowledge about craft and skill. More to the point, writing requires persistence and perseverance.

I met perseverance while driving through East Texas. On one of my wayward excursions when I lived in the big state, I stopped to eat in a small town. The cook, a woman with rough and sweet eyes and big frosted hair tucked in a net, rustled for me a plate suitable for a Southern vegetarian—thick mashed potatoes swimming in butter, cornbread drenched in butter, green beans, cooked carrots, and squash all awash in butter. The man sitting on the diner barstool next to me introduced himself as Walter. A farmer. Now a widower, he was prompt to tell me.

"I'm sorry."

"No, don't be sorry. Etta was a great woman. One of a kind. Hardworking. And a pistol too. We had a good life," he said with the rhythm of hammering nails and with a slight smile and heavy eyes.

I asked him how he had kept going during the past year.

"Work. Work saves me." He had been building a fence around his entire farm from the best wood around. For the next fifteen minutes he detailed how he had chopped the wood, hauled the trees, shaved the posts, dug the holes, and wedged the limbs together. He still had miles to go, though, he said in so many words, and I was sensing he wanted me to help him build it if I had the time and inclination. "Wanna see it?"

I had nowhere in particular to go. Once I finished the last bite of melting mashed potatoes and tipped the big-haired waitress, I followed Walter in his old blue Ford pickup for about five miles outside of town to his farm. Four hundred acres, and for four months he persistently had been replacing the collapsing wooden fence with a new oak one. Transformed from trees with ax and hand, sweat and grief, each log, wedged and secured like the cedar logs of a homegrown cabin, gave the landscape shape. Every morning, he told me, he awoke before dawn, gathered his materials and tools, and raised the fence one limb at a time. By noon, he'd have a significant line of fence in place; then he could spend the rest of the day tending to his farm. From his porch, I took in the vertical lines of pines, oaks, and elms that reached from earth to sky sliced and defined by Walter's oak fence. When Etta died, he could've rolled over and pulled the sheets over his head. He could've said, "To hell with it," dropped his tools, and walked away from what he'd started. But he didn't. What Walter had for fences and barns and porches, writers have for writing: namely fire.

Heat in Sanskrit is called *tapas*, possibly the singular most important quality for Yoga and for authentic writing. *Tapas*, the earliest recorded yogic concept,[1] which translates also to "ardor" and "austerity," describes yogis' practices of burying their heads in the sand, or sitting nude in subzero weather to cultivate their "inner heat" that they may attain transformational powers. To each his own, but I'm not into that sort of thing. Luckily for us, Patanjali's *Yoga-Sutra* (c. 200 c.e.) and other yoga texts denounce these extreme measures as being ironically driven by pride and as destructive to the body—not Yoga's aim. So, gladly, I take a more benign approach to *tapas* as perseverance.

Tapas describes the fire in the belly that propels us to work well and to persevere in the world. It is the burning enthusiasm that excites us when we discover a blue-sky idea, a delicious image, a tapestry woven plotline. We stay up an hour later concocting the story, or we may madly record in a notebook that vital detail, such as a dream we don't want to—or cannot—forget. The electric rush from our imagination gives our days an extra kick, and we may ramble like a daft man to strangers on the bus about our fantastic new idea. Some of us live and write for that rush. The problem is, the flame wanes. The novelty wears thin. Maybe what we thought was a startling, innovative story idea turns out to be a rehash of plotlines stretching from Dante to Dostoyevsky. The sustained fire that lets us write day after day even when our head hurts or even when we meet rejection upon rejection is also *tapas*. Once we've tapped into our fire, how do we keep it burning? How do we avoid this intellectual, imaginative, spiritual burnout? Or if we're burnt already, how do we rise from the ashes?

We can begin practicing *tapas* by tending to how we talk about our writing. One student recently complained that she had been writing short stories for ten years but that recently every time she sat down to write she felt no spark. "I already know what's going to happen in my stories, so I'm not excited anymore to write," she said. I asked if she spent too much time thinking about how her stories would unfold before writing them—thus squelching the joy of being surprised as she wrote. "Maybe," she said, "but I think most about my stories as I talk them out with a friend of mine. We both share story ideas." There might be the problem, I suggested: talking. The *Bhagavad Gita* (17.15) describes a type of *tapas* and control of speech called *van-maya-tapas*. The passage advises the yogi to speak the truth with kindness and with nonharmful honesty. I offered her a variation of how as a writer you can speak without harming your writing and to speak honestly about your writing: Speak about what you've written, not what you're going to write. A former acquaintance of mine used to spend each night at a coffee shop telling me and others about the fantastic novel he was going to write. For a few weeks, his eyes would open wide and his voice would grow animated as he described this marvelous plot about an escaped prisoner and an aide to the President of the United States. I loved to hear him talk about it. Yet, after a year, he hadn't budged beyond outlining some ideas. When I asked him when he was going to write the novel, he said, "Well, I think I've already written it by talking to everybody. It doesn't excite me so much anymore." Let the surprise simmer and surface while you write, not while you talk.

Still, some of us must transform our constitution at a subtler level. We can change all of our external circumstances to help our writing: We can rearrange our schedules to write for an hour or more a day, we can change jobs, we can move to the Bahamas, we can build a studio in our backyard, but all of this changing and rearranging will come to nothing for most of us if we lack some inner heat.

A student of mine several years ago said he used to flounder whenever he realized that a short story would require several more revisions to "get it right." After writing for seven years, he had expected it to get easier. When he still struggled, he often lacked the will to persist. Another student in the same class complained, "My last story has been rejected ten times." She lacked zeal as well. How do you keep writing? At the time, I could offer little other solace than to advise them to keep writing and to build resolve. I told the student frustrated with rejection to hold out for twenty rejections. When I had started sending off work to be published over sixteen years ago, the twentieth one was accepted. One in twenty is a fair ratio.

I realize now, though, that both of these students, both good writers, might have benefited not just from a reality check about the hardships of writing but also from some yogic tools (*upaya*) to alter their internal heat—tools that I now share with my students. Although lack of perseverance may be in part psychological, Yoga also works on the psyche in part via the body—the physical body and the subtle body. These labels of "physical body" and "subtle body" come from how the ancient *Taittiraya-Upanishad* (Part II, 2.1–5.1), as well as some later Yoga texts, describe our bodies as having three core layers: the physical (gross) body, the subtle body, and the causal body. For now, we'll consider only the first two. The most obvious body is the physical body of blood, bones, organs. Yoga poses most directly moderate the physical body's circulation, metabolism, cell production, organ function, and sensory stimulation. Beyond the physical body is the subtle body, the body of breath, emotion, intelligence, and knowledge. The subtle body, accessed by breath control and other yoga tools, helps yoga practitioners shift their energy—their physical, mental, and emotional energy. Several ancient yoga texts describe specific energy centers and energy channels in the physical body that can be manipulated and controlled. As "woo-woo" as it may sound to talk about energy outside the context of petrol, electricity, solar, or wind, biologists' and neurobiologists' recent research, as well as studies in acupuncture, are confirming the existence of some such energy conduits.[2]

Our inner fire simmers most pronouncedly in an energy center located approximately, but not literally, in our belly. Most of us have heard of the solar plexus, our inner sun, located near our navel, that can burn bright within throughout the day. To Hatha-Yogis and Tantra-Yogis, this region of the subtle body, called the center of our city of jewels (*manipura cakra*), stores our ability to manifest will into action. Our English tongue's metaphors reinforce the idea: We must have "the guts" to walk across hot coals, or we must have a "strong stomach" to withstand hardship, or we might have "fire in the belly" that lets us act upon our deepest desires. Dead metaphors, like yogic symbols, suggest our ancestors had some intuition about how the body and psyche relate.

From just above your navel to your waist's left side, right next to the upper portion of your small intestine, resides your pancreas gland. Working in harmony with the pancreas and the liver, the pancreas's endocrine cells secrete the protein hormones insulin and glucagon, which together moderate blood sugar content. Healthy doses of insulin especially boost our energy by shuttling glucose across the livers' and muscles' cell membranes. To avoid energy stagnation, the pancreas's exocrine cells produce enzymes that aid the small intestine's digestion.

One ancient cleansing process called **SHINING SKULL CLEANSING** *(kapāla-bhāti-kriya)* efficiently clears some of the body's passages to give you instant vigor and energy, like drinking a double espresso without the erratic brain activity or the caffeine letdown two hours later. Involving rapid, forceful exhalations and passive inhalations, this process also fires up the liver, spleen, and pancreas—all working for your digestion—so again the digestive tract can be restful to boost your stamina.

Then, try sucking in your gut. A practice that involves sucking in your abdominal walls is called **SOARING LOCK** (*uddīyāna bandha*)—loosely translated as "a lock that lets energy fly up."[3] The subtle body contains over a hundred energy circuits called nadis that maintain the physical body. Since many of these energy circuits originate in or near the belly region, this practice can quickly rouse a dormant, sluggish body and a resistant psyche. In **SOARING LOCK**, the energy flows from the lower abdomen up to the brain. When this region, then, is active and fluent, we have the stomach to confront what we avoid, to follow through on promises to ourselves and to our muse, and to transform wispy wishes and base dreams into elegant phrases, sentences, poems, stories, and books. We have heat to write what we need to write.

Give these practices time. Don't expect to breathe rapidly or to suck in your gut for one morning and miraculously be able to endure the slew of rejection letters, cure your anxiety, and write to the finish line. But these practices work. They work if you let them, and they work if you practice them repeatedly. Persistence requires patience, not a panacea.

It was 4:30 the other morning, and I had been writing for three hours. When I can't sleep, I sense what my body and mind need to do. That morning, it was walking and writing, writing and walking. It's autumn, a season that often heightens my focus. The predawn autumn air's crispness collects the skin between my brows as it collects the energy in tree limbs. Chlorophyll-deprived, the birch and maple sleeves of our road have slowly grown golden and amber. In autumn my body feels as if its leaves change hue and gradually fall to a cold floor, forcing my mind and body to focus upon its remaining nutrients. Maybe the shortened daylight makes me fear, unconsciously, that time may be falling away and that I, thus, must work with more awareness and persistence.

In this melancholy season, I welcome an internal heat. While walking toward town, I saw a glow from behind the local glassmaker's house, so I mothed my way toward it and found the young glassmaker in his shed blowing his torch. From the metal pipe, blue, orange, and yellow flames licked the liquid he kept in a vat. He looked up, nodded, and continued, concentrating on his work. I thought for a moment of Heraclitus, that pre-Socratic mountain dweller obsessed with flames, whose fragments on fire remain: "Lightning is the lord of everything" and "Everything becomes fire, and from fire everything is born." Within fifteen minutes, from his hands a vase with pecan-colored and goldenrod-tinted swirls was born.

So it is with writing. The *Shiva-Samhita* says that if you keep a sustained focus upon your belly center, you can make gold. The best writers I know are alchemists who make treasure from base words. What's alchemy's source? Heat.

TAKE A BREATH #1: SHINE YOUR SKULL

Intention:
Try this practice when you need to muster the resolve to write with vigor and perseverance.

A Friendly Warning:
Anyone with high blood pressure, poor lung capacity, ulcers, or eye or ear irritations should avoid this process. If pregnant, avoid these practices because of their pressure on the abdomen.

SHINING SKULL CLEANSING BREATH (kapāla-bhāti-kriya) *gives you back your luster. Here's a way to practice: Before your writing session, sit quietly for at least two full breaths, lengthening your spine in both directions. Set your twofold writing intention. Then, when ready, exhale vigorously through both nostrils, allowing the inhalation to take care of itself. Vigorous exhale, passive inhale, vigorous exhale, passive inhale. The exhalation should draw up your abdominal walls, which warms up the belly's sun and shoots rays of light, so to speak, to your skull. Then, relax your body and stomach as you begin your writing session. As you encounter challenging parts of your writing or as your energy wanes, redirect your focus to your inner sun. Try another round. After a week try three rounds of forty. Gradually build to three rounds of sixty and then one hundred and twenty.*

TAKE A BREATH #2:
STOKE YOUR WRITER'S FIRE

Shandor Remete, a remarkable yogi and teacher from Australia, calls his Yoga forms "Shadow of Yoga" (www.shadowyoga.com), a name he draws principally from the ancient text Shiva-Svarodaya. *The following practice marks the very beginning of one of his forms he taught me in Boston. It's a variation of a traditional practice. You might review the illustrations for* **SOARING LOCK** *(uddīyāna bandha).*

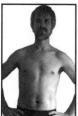

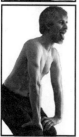

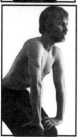

Stand in **MOUNTAIN POSE** *(tādāsana) next to your desk, feet a foot apart. Set your twofold writing intention. Then when ready, place your hands on your hips. Keep your soles and heels rooted. Take a full inhale. Then on the exhalation make the following simultaneous movements: As you bend your knees and slide your hands, arms straight, down your thighs with your fingers facing inward, exhale all of the air out of your lungs with your mouth open and your tongue stretched toward your chin as far as it will go. Drawing your tongue out naturally lifts the abdominal walls. Then, holding your breath, draw back your belly and lift it up or suck it in so your abdominal region will be slightly or significantly concave. Retain your breath for three seconds. Holding the abdominal lock and your breath, return slowly to mountain pose. Release the lock and inhale deeply and gracefully. Repeat at least three to five times. This process takes some getting used to. Be patient. Within a week or less, most writers adapt. While stimulating*

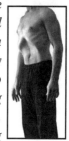

the abdominal walls as well as the internal organs of digestion, it also warms the belly's sun—the gastric glands.

Then, move from your mat to your desk to write what needs to be written from your belly. With each word unfolding on the screen or page, imagine the heat flowing from your belly through your limbs to keep you stoked even when the day and the practice get dark.

CHAPTER FOUR

RIDE THE WAVE OF CONCENTRATION

"I HAVE ATTENTION DEFICIT DISORDER," a writer told me. We were discussing writing habits, and she—a writer and English professor for over twenty years—said she recently hasn't been able to sit still for over thirty minutes. Not that she doesn't want to: She has plenty of willpower. Not that her schedule won't allow it: She has lots of free time. Her mind, she said, won't allow it. When I asked her when she was diagnosed with ADD, she said she labeled herself. She had accepted, I think, this label as a valid excuse for her not being able to concentrate anymore.

I've met other writers like her. I've been her.

One Sunday afternoon, I realized I could no longer read. I picked up my copy of Italo Calvino's story collection, *cosmiccomics*. The words on the page seemed like mass lumps, familiar yet incomputable as if I were staring at a wall of stones and waiting for them to speak. I was 32 years old. I had been writing seriously and teaching a bit too seriously for ten years, and that afternoon I realized a terrifying secret: I could not compute words on the page. The disconnect had nothing to do with Calvino's magical charms he wields with words; it had everything to do, I understand now, with my over-worked brain and stressed body. I had tried that same week to sit and meditate and, hearing the jumble my once-clear mind had become, I wanted to scream. My writing suffered a series of slow deaths.

Victims of our own minds and possibly of our own self-definition, we buy into the idea that we live in "the Age of Distraction." A book by that name came out a few years ago, a politician recently gave a speech called "Politics in the Age of Distraction," and another writer recently published a book titled *The Zen of Listening: Mindful Communication in the Age of Distraction.* When I tell other writers about this tag for our era, they nod their heads in recognition of lives cluttered with Palm Pilots, faxes, Blackberries with a hundred programmed numbers, televisions with five hundred channels, and e-mail boxes with twenty Listserv messages coming every few hours. Who has time, someone might wonder, to contemplate world peace, much less personal peace to write a novel?

But we writers are not special in our challenges to concentrate. The Age of Distraction has been going on since well before this era of gadgetry. The mind, a microcosm of the universe's perennial dance of change, naturally shifts and wanders as it reflects nature's inherent tendencies to be in flux. It's comforting for me to know so, since my mind still pings and pongs on some days from writing a paragraph to wanting to paint the barn to alphabetizing my novels by their first line. Still, to sustain this journey, we'd do well to find ways that keep our body-minds centered on the task at hand.

Concentration, simply put, may be the gateway to transformation and to authentic writing. With faculties focused on one thing, to-do lists and yesterday's frets slip away, the mind's wheels slow down, and its little demons of distraction disappear. Imagination opens through your eyes that work in tandem with your fingers' grooves on the keyboard. Nothing comes between you and the page. You are connected. You are immersed.

Such steady concentration seems a mystery to some writers. A writer I know can write for six hours straight on the same subject without budging from the screen. When I asked him how he does it, he said, "Oh, it's simple." Then he took a deep breath and held it. Is having concentration as easy as holding your breath? Not exactly. But he is onto something.

When I consider my own experience, my work with other writers, the ancient texts, and current brain science, I must admit one simple facet that directly influences our ability to concentrate: breathing.

I often return to a popular yoga text, the *Yoga-Sutra*, comprised of 195 aphorisms penned by yoga scholar Patanjali probably sometime around 200 c.e. Consider the second sutra, which translates loosely as "Yoga is the cessation of the mind's fluctuations" *("Yogah-cittavrtti-nirodhah").* One of Yoga's aims for over two thousand years has been to quiet and to harness our thoughts and inner chatter through a form of concentration called *dharana.* *Dharana* describes a sophisticated form of concentration that advanced yogis achieve after several years of intricate practice.[1] I'm less interested in this vital practice's esoteric dimensions, however, than I am in its practical application to help writers be at ease with a deliberate focus on word upon word. What I call joyful concentration is a way to be authentically centered upon our writing. As breath and body befriend a writer's mind, joyful concentration comes from openness and ease more than from force or will and is, dare I say it, inspiring.

Most experienced writers glare, if not sneer, when someone mentions inspiration. There's a certain truth to not being smug about the ease of one's writing, for often when I've thought my writing has gone swimmingly, I've in fact come close to drowning in delusion. Speak of inspiration among writers, and you're likely to hear some variation of the formula, "Writing is 95% perspiration and 5% inspiration." These wizened scribes know that their work is toilsome, sweat wrenching, Sisyphean. Even when they have the flu or a migraine, they must push their monolithic manuscripts up the inclines of their personal underworlds. Only neophytes, they say, speak of and wait for chubby cherubs or dancing pixies or sword-wielding goddesses to visit before writing. I concede the labor part. But these inspiring visitations may not be sexy matters of magic; they may be simple matters of breath and body.

In Anne Lamott's *Bird by Bird*, a delightful book on writing, the author mentions the importance of breathing to her writing practice: When she deliberately deepens and slows down her breathing, that incessant internal chatter that wants her to color-code her clothes or deep-clean the microwave dissipates, or at least quiets long enough for her to begin the necessary work of writing. In her simple breath work, the author has stumbled upon one of the most fundamental principles underlying the practice of Hatha-Yoga and the attempt to gain some control over the mind's fluctuations. Yet she almost apologizes for even mentioning breathing in the context of writing for fear she might sound like her flighty New Age friends. To focus upon our breathing, however, need not lead to crystal healing and channeling Oscar Wilde; it can move us toward the center, concentration.

I have a simple theory about the bards who sang to the muses to inspire them. Homer asks the muse to "sing" to him of Odysseus, Ovid prays the gods "breathe" upon him the tales of the world's metamorphosis, and the Puritan poet Milton doesn't call upon God to sing of humanity's fall from Paradise but upon "Thou O Spirit." These bards—as they call for song, breath, Spirit—may be praying to have what every writer deeply desires and needs to write well and long: the song of joyful concentration. Song is a wielding of words with heart-centered breath that praises and celebrates the human condition as well as informs our soul of reality's darker regions. These bards ask for this breath. When Milton called upon the Spirit instead of God, he must have sensed the root of "spirit," the same as the root of "inspiration": the Latin *spirare*, to breathe, and the Latin *spiritus*, the breath of life, soul. "To breathe," incidentally, is the root as well of "perspiration." So, perhaps, the more accurate formula for creative toil is, "Writing is 95% perspiration plus 5% inspiration, which equals 100% breathing."

When yogis speak of breath, they often speak of *prāna*. *Prāna* in Sanskrit is sort of the *chi* of Yoga, the *spiritus*. What makes breath possible, *prāna* is that creative element that let Prometheus mix water and breath into clay and so create human beings, that births lotus flowers from muddy waters, that lets images and memories and words combust into epics or memoirs or novels. In short, prāna is creation, the in-breath of the gods and goddesses. To be inspired is to breathe in. *Pranāyāma* is the art of becoming aware of and harnessing breath to vitalize the body, to alter space within the body, and to increase concentration and awareness. To engage in *prāna* is to part the clouds—the clouds in your lungs and mind.

Most of us forget the art of breathing.

This is your brain on erratic breath: My friend Helen will begin a story about how her daughter landed a new job with a consulting firm, but before she can finish that story she's telling me another about the mouse she saw last night scurry across her kitchen floor and before she finishes telling me what her languid cat did in response she starts another story about the time her older sister tried to bury her in the backyard. I love trying to follow Helen's stories within stories, but she rarely gets to the punch line. Although she writes more coherent short stories, she often complains about how long they take her to write.

Erratic, shallow breathing correlates to a distracted, agitated mind and to rapid brain wave patterns in the brain's front portion (the frontal cortex). These "beta" brain waves bounce and flip at about thirteen to thirty oscillations per second. On an EEG (an electroencephalograph, or machine that maps the brain's electricity), beta waves look like jagged flames. When we're in "beta brain," we can multitask, chat to three people at once, or navigate busy sidewalks or streets to get to our next meeting. Beta brain is busy brain, and it's where many of our minds live much of the time. If we could measure New York City's brain wave patterns, they'd likely be off the beta chart.

Multi-tasking worsens performance. One recent study demonstrated that multi-tasking mathematics students, for instance, not only performed less efficiently and less accurately, but they also performed with what neuroscientist Richard Restak calls less fluency and less grace. "The brain is designed to work most efficiently," Restak concludes, "when it works on a single task and for a sustained rather than intermittent and alternating periods of time."[2]

This is your brain on easeful, harnessed breathing: Brain wave oscillations slow down by half. A predominance of alpha brain waves in the frontal cortex correlates to focus, to the state we call "flow" that high achievers, runners, and writers describe. It is one-pointedness. Such one-pointedness distinguishes mastery from competency. According to Restak, what dinstinguishes chess players, musicians, and mathematicians who advance in their respective fields is the capacity for sustained concentration.[3]

This brain business in part explains how I regained my concentration. Soon after that fateful Sunday afternoon with Calvino and my private terror, I found my way to a Yoga studio. Soon, I was coming to class three times a week, and after a few months I figured out how to practice a few poses on my own at home. The movements, the harnessed breath, the inner focus, each contributed to centering my erratic thoughts and lining up my faculties. My thinking cleared up. The capacity to read carefully and to write well returned, only this time with a spacious consciousness I had never experienced.

That experience prompted more experimentation. I developed a sequence of poses, harnessed breathing, and inner focus to instill concentration and perseverance when I write. In my notebook I drew stick figures and made notes to help me remember what I was discovering. I have practiced some variation of this same sequence every morning of every week for several years. This sequence also has become the basis for how I work with many writers one-on-one, and it also formed the foundation for my studies with MFA in Creative Writing students.

Fourteen graduate students sat around a seminar table, notebooks out, pens ready, their required readings splayed for all to see. I had just been hired at a university to mentor one or two students a semester in a course we each would design together, and the director had asked me to lead a residency seminar related to Yoga and writing. One student walked in, looked at me, and said, "Oh, shit. You're the teacher."

I smiled and said, "Yes, that's how it goes."

An hour before the seminar had started, I had been eating breakfast incognito among some of the students. This particular student had sat down next to me. The guy across from him asked which seminar he was signed up for.

"Oh, some yoga thing," he had said. "I don't know. Sounds kinda whacky."

I couldn't have orchestrated better the grad student response I had expected. And now the posturing cynic sat again beside me and among what seemed in retrospect some highly self-conscious students. They fidgeted. They seemed to be sizing each other up and wondering how they each were being sized up. Some of them knew each other from the previous year; many of them were brand new to the program.

Rather than begin with a lecture, which is what they expected, I started with a concentration exercise that included harnessed breathing and a focused gaze. Most of them tried to comply, but one young woman especially could not stop giggling. She'd clear the long brown hair from her eyes, perk up her spine, widen her eyes, pinch her lips, but no matter how many times I tried to re-direct her and others to forget being self-conscious and to try to concentrate, she would begin to fidget with her pen and then begin giggling again, at one point almost uncontrollably. The rest of the seminar actually went well. Three hours later, the students, includ-ing the cynic who had put his proverbial foot in mouth, ended up mostly fascinated and hungry for more.

Since then, I have worked with some of these students to track Yoga's effect on their concentration, persistence, and confidence. One such student was 24, newly married, trying to carve a free-lance writer career, and soon would begin raising a family. At 24, already she knew she had a hard time concentrating. "I get really anxious," she said. I could see it in her hands and eyes and hear it in her voice.

Carolyn and I worked together that semester as well as the following year in a special study. Over time, she learned to inte-grate Yoga as muse into her writing practice and process a few times a week. The Writer's Concentration Sequence, as I call my regular sequence now, steered her through her second year—with family matters to complicate her writing life. She reported to me her writing intentions, how long she practiced the sequence, and the results in her writing and in her writing mind. Although not everyday brought some unheralded victory on the page, Carolyn repeatedly reported that working with the sequence helped her calm her nervousness and boost her self-confidence—facets that helped her focus steadily on her writing. This MFA in Creative Writing student became thrilled when she could write for a consistent hour without distraction and had her first "writer's moment" — an experience of receiving insight from her unconscious..

Katie came to me with a book idea. Encumbered with bags of four-inch three-ring notebooks that tried to contain her mounds of notes and drafts and transcriptions, she sat down and for ninety minutes talked nonstop about her book idea, her work, her experiences leading up to the book, her marriage, her child, her sister-in-law—all ostensibly related to her book idea and why she sought my guidance. When I read a draft of a story for Katie's book, the pace flustered me like her speech: The story was speaking *at* me, scenes were left incomplete, characters undeveloped, transitions almost invisible. "Any suggestions?" she asked. After I commended her on what was truly a compelling book topic, I said, "Let's practice breathing." She grinned and grimaced simultaneously ("grinnaced"?). I tactfully explained to Katie what I observed in her writing and recommended we focus upon her breathing patterns as a way to help her slow down her white-rapid thoughts. Luckily, she was open to the idea (or at least was open to humoring me). After introducing her to some breathing exercises, I suggested she practice them at home before and even as she wrote and revised her stories. For the next four weeks, at the beginning of our writing sessions we practiced breathing exercises for ten minutes.

The changes were subtle, yet significant. As she spoke, she caught and redirected her thoughts before they spiraled out of control. The pace of her writing allowed readers to dwell richly in key places. Images became fuller and more precise so the texture of her baby's moist hand versus her husband's coarse knuckles could enter her readers' imaginations. Katie told me, too, she felt more focused as she wrote and checked herself when she seemed to be speeding ahead to get finished. Heeding her breath, she said, helped her slow down and appreciate her writing as she wrote. She was, in essence, learning the tunes to her own song of concentration.

To re-learn the song of breath is not difficult. Just remember two things: direction and rate. Direction involves guiding the flow of breath by engaging certain muscles. Many of us learn to breathe in, suck in our bellies, and feel the breath in our chest. This type of breathing—now called paradoxical breathing—has been correlated with several stress-induced and coronary problems. Instead, when you breathe in, let your stomach relax (Really—stop holding it in.). When you breathe particularly from the belly region's abdomen and diaphragm, located within your lower rib cage, brain patterns are more likely to slow do an alpha rhythm, those waves that induce more artistic surfing as stress floats out to tide.[4]

Rate refers to the speed at which you breathe in and breathe out. Let the song last a little longer than normal. You can learn to breathe in the same volume at the same number of seconds as you breathe out, for instance—a quick way to calm the chatter. Later, you also can extend the rate you can breathe in for five seconds instead of two. With sustained mindful practice, your breathing will deepen and lengthen of its own accord.

As you write, keep breathing. Many of us get so caught up in the tension of writing that we're not aware how erratic—or non-existent—is our breathing. Instead, write and let your breath be easeful and deep. Unconscious tension held in your neck and shoulders might dissipate. You keep your eye on the bouncing breath, so to speak, and before you know it, an hour has passed and five pages have been written.

We can tap into this inner spring of joyful concentration by making slight readjustments not only to how we breathe but also to how we ground our thoughts in our lower bodies—instead of in our heads. Distraction may stem partially from blocked energy in our lower body. Near our sacrum and our tailbone is a plexus (system of nerves) that helps moderate our basic functions of urinating, defecating, and having sex. The perineum—our torso's base, located between our anus and genitals—along with this system of nerves comprises our root clearing or center, our *mūladhāra cakra*. *Mūla* means "root" in Sanskrit as well as "firmly fixed, source or cause, basis, the foot, lowest part or bottom, foundation."[5] When we contract the perineum, we ground the lower body's energy in a lock called *mūla-bandha* (root lock). By engaging *mūla-bandha*, we also contract not only the pudendal nerves located near our genitals and the perineum but also a series of energy channels that in turn stimulate and moderate our liver, gall bladder, stomach, and spleen. When irritated or compressed, these passages affect how other parts of our body function. Consider the obvious: If food, that potential source of physical nourishment, does not run through us easily and does not provide our bodies with optimum energy, then our torso and brain's little helpers will scurry around, unable to focus clearly upon our writing afoot. Awakening this area can help us write from a steady place of sustenance instead of distraction.

Gradually, you might work your way up to practicing a simple sequence of breathing and yoga poses. Repeating a simple form aids concentration, too. With this sequence, some writers seek to change old habits. Such change is difficult. A neuroscientist might say that changing an engrained habit is a matter of repatterning engrained pathways in the brain. Repeated actions, again accompanied with attention, do help create new brain patterns. A sequence's simplicity helps the body to remember it, which helps the analytical part of the brain—active when learning new material—to quiet. The regularity of the same simple sequence establishes a routine that aligns intention with imagination, intellect, and heart and that also aligns these faculties with physical energy. With frequent practice, we can teach our mind to work for, not against, our writing.

All this said, every day is a surprise. On some mornings, I flow through this sequence, intending to anchor my mind on my writing at hand, and a flood of thoughts carries me away. Sometimes, I start over. Sometimes, I just hobble to the desk and hope the keyboard clicking will grow louder than those wheels churning. So be it.

With the four preparations—intention, time, perseverance, concentration—accept where you are. Admittedly, writing often has its own agenda and might rage, rage against your trying to harness it. But a harness is not a shackle. With the right intention and spirit, it's simply a way to give a bronco loving guidance. Maybe you become a body whisperer.

TAKE A BREATH #1: RIDE THE ALPHA WAVES

This practice helps you use the **ROOT LOCK** (mūla-bandha) *and* **EQUAL MOVEMENT BREATHING** (sama-vrtti prāṇāyāma) *to heighten concentration for your writing.*

Intention:

Engage this practice when you need extended concentration to write on a single subject for long periods of time.

Sit firm yet soft, grounded with the earth. Take one of four seated positions. If you can do so, sit comfortably in a kneeling position with your buttocks resting on your heels. You can place a pillow between your thighs and calves if you wish. This pose—called **ADAMANTINE POSE/KNEELING POSE** (vajrāsana)—*opens the perineum and pelvic floor as well as piques the feet and legs. In this pose you may feel adamantine, glowing and stalwart. Or try to sit on a cushion with your knees out to the sides, your right heel tucked firmly beneath your perineum (the muscle at your torso's spine between your genitals), and your left heel resting in front of your right foot or ankle. This pose, a variation of* **ADEPT'S POSE** (siddhāsana), *also rouses the root area. Otherwise, sit either in an* **EASY CROSSED-LEGGED POSE** (sukhāsana) *or on the edge of a chair in* **WRITER'S FRIENDSHIP POSE** (maitrīyāsana)—*the latter being a perfect preparation for writing. Review the illustrations and captions for seated poses if you wish. Close your eyes and focus on your breath. If you're comfortable doing so, on each of the* *next five exhalations, direct the flow of your breath upward as you contract and draw up your perineum. You may have difficulty doing so without contracting your anus at first, which is a common way to start. This contraction is the root lock,* mūla-bandha. *Once you're comfortable with this lock, just focus again on your breath, and set your twofold intention. Once you remind yourself what you are writing for, you might set a specific intention such as "I need to recall and follow the sequential details of that horrific first date for my memoir" or "I need to give this central scene my best concentration for at least three hours." Let this intention matter to you. Feel its pleasurable weight in your body like a natural root extending from your torso's base that will keep you anchored so you can write what you need to write.*

Doing nothing special with your breath, for a few minutes keep your eyes closed as you try to follow the stream of images—sights and sounds and associations and stories and voices—that float through your consciousness. Try not to impede the mighty stream's flow. Take a few minutes to observe their random movement. Don't edit.

Now, let's try to shift the rhythm from beta brain to alpha brain waves. Keeping alert yet relaxed, breathe deeply. To a slow count of four, let your inhalation expand your diaphragm and belly like a balloon that floats up to your chest. Then, as you contract your perineum, to a count of four slowly let the breath's inner force float out your nose and down your torso as you imagine it massaging your organs. That inhalation and exhalation is one round. Keep this stream's motion between your root center and your chest moving steadily for ten full rounds. Anytime you sense the stream wishes to flow off course with a thought about your kids' supper or a deadline, return your attention to the breath. As you heed your breath, feel this stream deeply in your body.

When you open your eyes, keep your thoughts in that stream as you return to your writing intention. Begin then with that intention and write one breath at a time, steady from your body's base to your heart region, calmly, deliberately. When your thoughts flow off your pen's or word processor's course, focus on your breath and your root area, and guide your mind back to your page. Feel that your lower body befriends your mind to give your writing the concentration it deserves.

TAKE A BREATH #2: A SEQUENCE FOR A WRITER'S CONCENTRATION

Intention:

Establish a simple regular routine that will allow you to manifest your writing intention, stoke your fire, and concentrate.

This sequence, the one I practice each morning, has become the staple for many of the workshops and retreats I teach. It's endlessly adaptable. Writers who, because of physical ailments and aging bodies, are restricted to chairs have learned its variations. Writers with more physically vigorous practices use it as a skeleton for designing their own sequences.

Try it. But try it not once or twice or thrice. Try it five times a week for three weeks or three times a week for five weeks. Give it fifteen sessions. Then, decide whether or not it works.

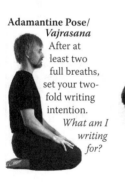

Adamantine Pose/ **Vajrasana**
After at least two full breaths, set your two-fold writing intention. *What am I writing for?*

Half-Camel Pose/Ardha Ustrasasana:
Keep your mind focused on your intention and your heart region. Rise to your knees, interlace your hands...

Adamantine Pose Variation
As you inhale, curl your toes under, and as you exhale lower your hips, on your heels. Let the spine, jaw, & breath relax.

Standing Forward Bend / *Uttanasana* to
Standing Mountain Pose / *Tadasana*

Let your mind focus on your intention and your lower body. On an inhalation, bring your hands forward, lift your hips, and fold into a forward bend, knees bent if you wish. With arms and neck relaxed, slowly lift into a standing position. Bring your hands to your lower belly and step toward your mat's front.

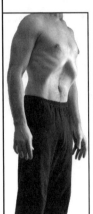

Shining Skull Cleanse / *Kapalabhati Kriya*

Bring your intention and attention to your lower belly below your navel. Use your abdominal muscles to pump exhalations vigorously while inhalations are passive. Begin with 10 cycles, and graduate to a higher number If unfamiliar with this practice and its cautions, please refer to Chapter 3 for details.

Standing Mountain Pose in Balance

Hands at heart, lift right knee for one breath.

Wide Legged Forward Bend / *Prasatrita Paddotanasana*

Exhale and bring your right foot back three to four feet (or wide enough for your comfort) and face your mat's right side. Inhale as you lift your arms and gaze above you. Exhale and bend forward (knees bent if you wish). Fingers face forward, elbows draw in. Wrists, elbows, and shoulders align to protect joints. Close your eyes and stay here for a few breaths as you keep your faculties focused on your intention. This is a good place to 'check in' with receiving any insights or images.

Transition Pose to Warrior II

Open your eyes, and inhale as you lift your torso, arms to the sides.

Warrior II / *Virabhadrasana*

Exhale as you turn your right foot out ninety degrees and your left foot forty-five degrees. Inhale deeply. Exhale as you bend your right knee and face over your right arm. With spine vertical, drop your torso back slightly to assure you are not lunging forward. Anchor weight in both heels as well as in your perineum, and keep your chest open. Align the knee over the heel, being sure not to let it drop inward. Gaze stays just beyond the front middle finger. Observe a grounded confidence, clarity, and focus. Stay here for 2-5 breaths.

Side Angle Pose / *utthita parsvokanasana*

Right foot forward, exhale as you rest your right forearm across your right thigh. Open your torso by rotating your left hip and then your chest and your left shoulder toward the ceiling. Either keep your left hand on your hip or extend it diagonally so that the forearm comes near the ear. If your chest is open, you can gaze underneath your extended arm and toward the ceiling. If you feel pressure in your neck, gaze to the side or floor. Keep your intention and attention in your heart space. In this pose, observe the mutual groundedness in your feet and aspiration as a writer. Stay here for 2-5 breaths.

"Inhale back to **Transition Pose**, face the front of your mat, and repeat on the other side."

Transition to Downward Dog
Inhale as you pivot your right hip forward and your right heel up, and place your hands at the front of your mat. Glide your right foot back three or so feet into a lunge.

Downward Facing Dog
Exhale as you – moving from your lower belly –draw your left foot beside your right and your hips. Keep weight of hands on the finger knuckles and on each hand's not on the wrists. Close your eyes and your intention as well as for potential lift index outer pads – check in with insight and imagery.

Child's Pose
Bring your knees to the mat as you draw your hips to your heels, and lay the tops of your feet flat, your forehead to the mat, and your arms to the sides. With eyes closed, stay here as long as you need., and observe any clarity of inner space.

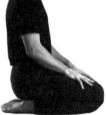

Stalwart Pose /
Inhale and lift your torso so your sitz bones press again on your heels. You may take a folded blanket between your calves and hips, or come into a comfortable seated pose of your choice. Observe in your body and mind any increased vitality and alertness.

Alternate Nostril Breathing
/*Nadi Shadona Pranayama***
Eyes can be closed or opened at a half gaze. Fold your right hand's index and middle fingers into your thumb pad. Rest the thumb tip on the outside of the right nostril or near the bridge.

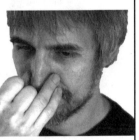

Rest the ring finger tip on the outside of the left nostril or near the bridge. Here is a variation of a breathing cycle: Close the right nostril, and breathe in through the left nostril. Open the right and close the left nostril as you exhale through the left. Breathe in through the left. Shift nostril openings, and exhale through the right. Repeat at least 2-4 more cycles. IN: Left. OUT: Right. IN: Right. OUT: Left. Breathing normally, sit for a few moments to observe how you feel and to observe any potential insight or imagery related to your intention and writer's focus.

Then, move from your center to the page. Write with the same embodied, full-breathed presence and focus. Once, your body remembers this sequence, it won't let you forget it, and you can use it as a framework for several of the other TAKE A BREATH exercises that follow in the next section.

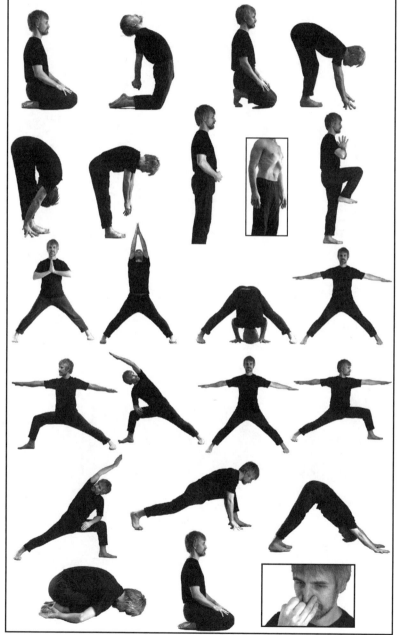

II

SETTING OUT

Consciousness & Craft

CHAPTER FIVE

FROM PEA TO GARDEN: CONSCIOUSNESS & CRAFT

EACH OCTOBER, MY BACKYARD gets bigger. At least, so it seems. The rows of maple, pin oak, and willow that line our one-acre pond disrobe and expose not only their bare limbs. They inevitably show off as well a bushy squirrel's nest or a tighter hawk's nest that have been hiding all spring and summer. And as if space itself expands, the naked leaves reveal what else they have been keeping from view—namely a wide open field of some thirty golden acres once farmed, and several miles beyond it a ridge of craggy mountains that line the horizon called the Shawangunks. The nests have been there all along. So have the mountains. And still, each autumn and winter I'm slightly dumbfounded that nature can be so coy and clever in what she conceals and reveals on cue. "Nature loves to hide itself," Heraclitus, that hermetic Greek, once chiseled on stone. Indeed.

I think of those trees like a writer's mind. Our minds sometimes cling to the urgent and hide from view a manic cycle of fret, obsession, and compulsion. Of the urgent, I do not mean the real potential catastrophes—the failing relationship, the troubled teenage son, the aging mother with a broken hip, the leaking roof. Those matters need tending to (although they do not necessarily need obsessing over). I mean the general riff-raff of self-consciousness that sabotages any creative endeavor.

Writers pay attention, so the adage goes. But to what? We notice how just as the mind loves to hide itself so it also loves to clear the clutter. We glimpse among the limbs an animal hole that leads to a memory that might be worth pursuing. A story of a baker and his wife keeps returning like a swallow. A melodic line tinged with melancholy from a cicada in our head darts to the surface and then scurries away. Something happens, the mind's space expands, and you see as if for the first time a sixty-eight-year-old woman in a pink bikini who has been nesting there for months. Can you catch her? Or at least follow her?

Consciousness is slippery. To many contemporary thinkers, it's the last frontier that still defies our understanding. Still, consciousness shapes craft. That is, if we writers can refine our awareness of how our faculties work, then this awareness in turn can affect what we call writing craft. The chapters in this book's second section set out to explore specific facets of that very tenet—how intuition shapes drafting, how imagination shapes imagery, how deep listening shapes prosody. This chapter attempts, or hazards, a few thoughts not only of how our consciousness as writers can expand but also of how a Yoga practice can facilitate that expansion.

FACULTY MEETING

In 1901, William James, ever the purveyor of the mind's wily ways, delivered a series of lectures on religion and neurology at the University of Edinburgh. He shared in one of those lectures what he called an unshakable realization:

> [O]ur normal waking consciousness, rational consciousness as well call it, is but one special type of consciousness, whilst all about it, parted from it by the filmiest of screens, there lie potential forms of consciousness entirely different. We may go through life without suspecting their existence; but apply the requisite stimulus, and at a touch they are there in all their completeness, definite types of mentality which probably somewhere have their field of application and adaptation.[1]

That "rational consciousness" James describes feels like—once it dominates all other "types of consciousness"—the size of a pea to me. That feeling reminds me of being 22 years old at my first faculty meeting ever at a high school. *A faculty meeting!* I thought.

Eager to leap into the classroom, I was equally excited to talk with my colleagues about the best ways to engage our students in reading all the great books. The first meeting's focus, a full two hours, was to hash out the new tardy policy, dress code, and disciplinary procedures. Some teachers argued that three tardies should merit an infraction while other teachers rose to the occasion with their best thinking to say that one tardy should send students directly to the office. Another teacher, a more pragmatic sort, said that when the tardy bell rang he preferred simply to lock the door. The dress code raised even more volatile "rational" discourse as if over summer vacation these teachers had been developing their arguments and couldn't wait, like good Athenian citizens, to take a stance in the school polis. In defense of my former colleagues, most of them were quite dedicated and effective teachers, but that first faculty meeting made an impression. My mind shrank that morning, I'm certain of it, and I walked out feeling like what my father called a "pea brain."

We writers have our own faculty meetings in our minds. Rationality, and a petty, nervous rationality at that, often prevails. Of course, we writers must cultivate a critical consciousness. We must be able to discern the riff from the raff and know how best to craft a story, poem, paragraph. We must learn our craft, and learning our craft mostly requires that rational consciousness. But there are other faculty members in attendance—imagination, intuition, emotion, lucidity, intellect.

And reason and the rest of them, it turns out, are a sinewy part of the rest of consciousness's body. Cognitive scientists have been poking around human consciousness for decades. They claim, rather certainly, that reason is mostly unconscious. In fact, Mark Johnson and George Lakoff note that cognitive scientists "as a rule of thumb" say that most consciousness is unconscious. "Most" meaning 95% on the conservative side. Not only that, but this 95% shapes and structures the paltry 5% of which we are aware.[2] It makes my head hurt to think of that.

I stand out back beyond the row of trees that line our pond at a stone wall where my woods meet the farmer's field. Around my scuffed boots are the typical autumn debris of lichened twigs, blue stone chips, leafy carpet. What I can see of earth in any given square foot is but a fraction of its mass. Most of it remains invisible. Dampness in the air, the frequency of the mourning doves' chortle, and the gray streaks forming in the east indicate, to me, rain will come by dusk. Still, most of what is happening at this very moment at this very spot remains far beyond my purview.

And there's so much more under foot. Since I awoke three hours ago, my sense organs have taken in a swirl of sensations never to be registered in long-term memory, and in this short time as I've practiced and written and made tea, rivers of thoughts have passed by unnoticed. 42 years mixed of memories in woods, of reading Thoreau and Dillard and Bass, of sitting in zazen, of inherited constructs of "nature" and "self" shape what and how my eyes see, how my ears hear at this moment at the stone wall. And even more buzzes at the autonomic level. The way light hits my retinas, the quivers on my skin, the shifts in heart beat and blood circulation all contribute, too, to how my mind frames everything to make sense and meaning.

5%? I'd be lucky to be aware of 5% of what's going on at this faculty meeting.

How do we, then, put aside our mind's nervous dress code concerns and bring out those other faculty members?

NERVOUS WRITERS, ALL OF US?

Part of this journey takes us into that dark space called the body. Dylan was right, almost. You've got a lotta nerve, or nerves to be exact. We're nervous creatures, or rather we're neuronal beings. The brain has 100 billion of these miniscule specialized cells who, in various combinations, shape what we choose to pay attention to, how we concentrate, how we imagine, how we intuit, how we rationalize. How well our nervous systems function also might influence how well our creative faculties function. Take the somatic system. It governs conscious sensations—hearing, seeing, touching—as well as the muscles that hug our bony skeleton. It also governs the body's habitual and willful movements primarily via motor neurons. The axons of these motor neurons send impulses from the central nervous system to the skeletal muscles and, voila, your fingers wipe your nose or scratch your mustache, and your larynx kicks in when you call out to your teenage son, "Please use your iPod headset!" These conscious movements, external and internal, engage the brain's cerebral cortex, the part of the brain responsible for much conscious sensory perception, intellectual thought, and decision-making.

Typical human consciousness simply cannot penetrate most layers of the body's nerves. Luckily for us. Can you imagine if your body's systems relied on your being aware of and making decisions each nano-second for your blood to circulate, your liver to function, your endocrine system to release the appropriate amounts of hormones? One of the body's small wonders is the autonomic nervous system. It works somewhat though not completely *autonomously* (and not automatically) from the somatic system. Like the somatic system, the autonomic system works by relaying signals between the central nervous system and motor neurons. It does so, though, mostly without your conscious choice. When a stranger pops out from around a corner or when you hike up Nepal's tall peaks where oxygen is more scarce, the autonomic sympathetic nervous system receives signals to speed up blood circulation, your heart beat, and your breathing rate—all without your having to think about blood and breath.

But in this fight-or-flight system is where things get tricky for us writers. We don't *have* to be aware of this system in order for it to operate. Yet, after years of unconscious and shallow chest breathing and a general disregard for the physical body, for instance, your sympathetic nervous system can become over-stimulated, perennially preparing your body for fight-or-flight. In this state, it constantly releases excessive adrenaline and cortisol (which over the long haul can shorten cell life), fatigues your motor neurons (which leads to aching muscles), and makes you cranky and cloudy. It's as if your body is working in a state of emergency, and you're not even aware of it. Most human bodies can get by with their renter's general abuse for twenty-five, even thirty-five years. But after forty, forty-five years of such physical wear and tear, consciousness can constrict if not collapse.

So, damned if anxiety doesn't push petty rationality out of the way and start to rule your faculty meetings. We're not talking tardy policies anymore. We're talking now about how the whole school is going to pot, how the world's going to end anyway so why get up, how back in the day things were brighter. Most of your faculty threaten to quit or at least go on strike. Anxiety, after all, does not always inspire creative immersion, imagination, or intuition to work full force. When the world is ending soon, who the hell wants to write anyway?

WRITER'S BLOCK BETWEEN BODY & MIND

Yoga won't fire anxiety. But a Yoga practice might shut anxiety up long enough to put another faculty member in charge.

This cold October morning, my hamstrings feel tighter and more wound up than my drunken great-uncle on New Year's Eve. Come into a standing forward bend, and most of us meet our humility. Still, with a bit of attention and harnessed breathing all moving in tandem with my torso's motion up and down, my hamstrings unwind an iota. I consciously breathe in through my nose and engage my diaphragm as I consciously lift my torso and lift my kneecaps, and I consciously breathe out as I draw my torso down. After years of practice, my attention centers upon my hamstrings for the moment, but my marginal awareness extends simultaneously to include parts of my inner body from my foot up to my hips along my belly and back to my shoulders. And there it is—my awareness, breath, and physical motion all working toward the same end. So it is with each Yoga pose I move through.

Any time you consciously slow down or speed up your breath, that choice sends signals to the cerebral cortex which then sends signals along the appropriate neuronal pathways. Conscious breathing, in other words, stimulates the cerebral cortex. When we breathe consciously while engaged in creative activity, we're inviting more clarity and more intellect to our writing. With practiced conscious breathing, we also might increase the chances of heightening our senses, a process essential we will discover in a later chapter for inviting imagination.

If over several months, you were to move through a series of simple Yoga poses and breathe consciously as well as stretch and strengthen the skeletal muscles consciously, your somatic system likely would strengthen the motor neuronal pathway to the cerebral cortex. A strengthened somatic system simply means that the nerve pathways that link, in the crudest sense, "body and mind," are integrated. As your autonomic system begins to moderate itself, your body's unconscious would begin to calm down, and your mind's consciousness would follow. You can even learn to inhibit your motor neurons, which leads to a state of alert relaxation. With such an alert yet relaxed state, consciousness opens to other faculties, in part, because your awareness is no longer cut off from your inner and outer body.

Then you add creative intention to your practice. You learn to move and breathe from one Yoga pose to the next with a writing intention guiding the poses, so to speak. As you're breathing in a standing pose, you learn to pay attention to what your intuition signals to your consciousness regarding your writing intention. As you're leaning over in a forward bend with eyes closed, you learn to pay attention to what your imagination proffers your consciousness related to your writing project. You learn to follow your faculties' subtle movements as carefully as your body's movements so that your mind no longer feels so alien. On this journey, you learn to navigate that other dark space, the mind. More pathways open among the various facets of this consciousness. More open passages, less blocks.

Creative blocks, many of them, dissolve. And when new ones surface, you learn how your Yoga practice carries you through them as well. With this practice, your consciousness can expand. You bring just a bit more light to that otherwise dark cave and become more aware of what's going on in there. Really.

When I was in college, I had a book called *Maps of the Mind*. It was an illustrated guide to the great Western thinkers' constructs of our psyche. Darwin had a page. Nietzsche, Freud, Jung, Rogers each had theirs. Each page illustrated the same basic human skull outline and was filled in according to the respective thinker's theories. The Freud skull had three neat divisions marked from top to bottom, Superego-Ego-Id (this latter division was illustrated, I'm sure, as some dark dungeon with dancing demons). Other than being astoundingly reductive, these maps had one major problem, I realize now: They suggest the mind is restricted to the head.

Mind pervades the body. I couldn't have said that several years ago with any degree of confidence, but I can now. The more you train awareness to navigate the body's hidden terrains, the more you recognize and experience the mind we embody. Again, George Lakoff and Mark Johnson, in *Philosophy in the Flesh*, challenge the entire Cartesian project of dividing body and mind in Western thought by, in part, demonstrating that our physiology shapes and gives form to our very capacity for reasoning. Hence, they describe and map "the embodied mind."

We cannot with one breath pooh-pooh poor Descartes for suggesting mind and body are separate and then with another breath scoff at the idea that Yoga's systems of body, breath, and mind could possibly alter our creative consciousness.

With the body in an alert yet relaxed state, we can write with less fret and with more easeful clarity, immersion, imagination, intuition, and discernment. The pea becomes a peach or possibly a bean stalk.

DOUBLE-MIND: WITNESSING THE UNCONSCIOUS

At some point, while writing, the unconscious and conscious do this strange dance. A world unfolds. It begins with a floor made of pocked hardwood planks, hewn from oak 200 years ago. Then two boots, farmer's boots, walk across it and past a boy of all of four-years-old sprawled on the same floor crashing a baby blue plastic plane into a toy metal truck as the television glowing over his small form crackles that Clinton has approved NATO bombing in Yugoslavia. And over the next several days and weeks as the boots lead you to a character named Walter who walks outdoors to his old barn and into the hardships of farming in 1995 and to questions you have been wrestling with yourself about agriculture in this country and our nation's troubled foreign policy, part of your mind completely immerses itself in Walter's world and another part of your mind observes the immersed mind, and somehow you're able, with no small feat of a miracle, to maintain this state of double-mind as if hovering in a lucid dream for hours, for days.

We can access double-mind any number of ways, but a Hatha-Yoga practice and meditation get me there. Yoga poses draw the mind inward, notes David Coulter who authored *Anatomy of Hatha Yoga*, whereas physical exercises scatter the mind. And Yogic meditation especially teaches us how to witness consciousness. As I sit in meditation and count my breaths or center my inner gaze, a veritable aquarium of strange fish pass by my awareness's light. In other sittings, or later in the same sitting, it must be feeding time as all the little fishies dart to the surface. Usually, at least now after years of practicing meditation, one fish—call him Walter—might swim by. Or another one—call her Walter's dead wife—darts to the surface. In meditation, I observe them one by one and let them go. In some sittings, the aquarium seems delightfully empty and dark. Not a fish stirs. Water quivers in darkness. *Stillness*, I hear my peanut gallery voice comment, and still all remains still. I can be in stillness while observing stillness. And at the page I can be immersed in the imaginative worlds that unfold while observing that immersion.

Leaves fall away, your backyard expands, and you witness it happening. The bean stalk becomes a garden. Immersion, imagination, emotion and intuition—all witnessed—attend the meeting on the page.

CHAPTER SIX

THE ART OF FIRST DRAFTS

SOMETHING, AN IMAGE, A BREADCRUMB, a glass shard, slips into awareness, and you wonder whether or not to follow it. You do, and it takes you down an alley until you wind up at a backyard fence overgrown with ragged trumpet vine. You find yourself suddenly immersed in studying the creeping plant's botany and its growing patterns in the South. Days pass. You're still entangled in the trumpet vines. You hadn't planned this. You had set out to write a simple story placed in Georgia in which a gorgeous but dangerous wealthy woman—call her Helen—cons her gardener lover Doug into becoming her hit man. He crept down an alley one evening as part of his recognizance, and now the trumpet vines have spread across five pages. One morning you come across a passage in a garden book that describes the ubiquitous *Campsis radicans* as a "monster of merit." The deep cups with tender lips painted in sunset orange and honey yellow must show its merit. Its roots and vines, its ability to drop a child seed at the very moment it's ripped from the ground, her incessant desire to spread and control and dominate must make her a monster. You're onto something. Trumpet creepers, you realize, cover Helen's gardens. You don't know where it will take you, but the writing seems to thrive on the not-knowing. There will be pruning and cutting back to do, but that can come later. For now, get lost.

The white page, the blank screen, the dark, blank mind—these need not be moments for the writer's neuroses to open its chatty mouth. What do I write? How do I begin? Which path do I follow?

What if I have nothing to say? Maybe, just maybe the blank page is an opportunity for the writer's confidence to emerge. The first draft is little more than an exercise in re-discovering your own writing process and learning to trust it. When you trust your own process and your own faculties, then you might become more versatile as a writer. With this versatility, you develop—or re-capture—your authenticity. By definition, you act upon your own authority. And you act in the moment of writing itself.

To draft in the moment, with our minds primed with craft, we let go of knowing too much about our subject and instead learn to trust especially that oft-misunderstood faculty, our own intuition.

"Get lost," I told a young writer. He had asked me for tips to start his novel. "Get lost," I said again, "in your drafting."

We have a stigma about getting lost. Some people view it as a sign of weakness. Parents dread the thought of their children getting lost. Some of our religions and fables teach us the hazards of straying from the path. One definition of *wander* is, after all, "to deviate in conduct or belief; to err; go astray." Rooted in wind, to "wander" sounds like being "wanton," to have no discipline. Yet, there is a discipline and an art to being able to wander well as writers.

If we fear getting lost, we might draft like an overscheduled tourist. I used to meet once a week with a writer to help him with his first novel. Although the storyline was potentially complex with intricate subplots and ideas about time bending, the characters felt flat and the scenes, sketchy. Reading the draft unnerved me, as if I were taking an hour-long tour that shuttled me through Manhattan's highlights. "What do you enjoy about writing itself?" I asked. He squirmed and said he liked the ideas, getting the ideas out, but he didn't like wasting time with a lot of description, character development, or subtle suspense. He just wanted to get "through" the story, he said. There's the rub.

When we draft like taskmasters, we're prone to stay "on track" and "on schedule." We know where we want to get to—the story's ending or punch line, the points we want to make—and we use language to "get there" as efficiently as possible. Staying safely on subject while drafting can be helpful for report makers and journalists on deadline but hazardous for novelists, poets, or creative nonfiction writers. We often remember surprises, novelty, revelation, and we encounter such things more often not when staying on schedule but when taking time to stray.

Instead, we can be open to the moment of writing, to the moment of something swirling in the peripheries of consciousness. Scottish novelist James Kelman drafts blindly. "I hear a character speaking," he once told me. "I often don't know who he is or even where he is. I just hear his voice say something, so I write it down and respond to him with another voice. Soon, I have two characters." While drafting one novel, Kelman knew on page one or two that the narrator Sammie was a drunk. Several more pages into the first draft, he realized Sammie had been beaten blind by the police. What was he going to do with a blind drunk for a narrator? He went with it. The novel, *How Late It Was How Late*, earned him the Booker Prize.

Drafting is a time for journeying, for uncovering your story's unexpected plot twists, for delving more deeply into an image that keeps bugging your imagination, for discovering a character's disturbing yet telling blemish. When you get lost in the draft, you often realize something essential you might not have found had you stuck with a writing "plan."

Dawdling isn't what I'm getting at, but slowing down is. We can "slow draft." Most of us have enough speed in our way of life; drafting can be a subversive act of sorts that resists our speed-driven culture. Slow draft. Slow drafting calms the taskmaster mind and awakens the fertile, intuitive reservoir of images stored in our embodied imagination.

In Yoga, we understand intuition as "inborn knowledge" (*sahaja-jnāna*) or "inner knowledge" (*antar-jnāna*). Its knowledge arrives in flashes like goldfish bypassing analysis and darting past consciousness's periphery. Its trigger point might be in the third eye. The third eye, when awakened, leads us. It is often called the *ājnā-cakra*. The word a⁻jnā means "command," hence *ājnā-cakra* translates as "command center" or "command wheel." Granted, my analytical mind and worrisome mind often pull all the levers and flip all the switches. A big patch covers the third eye. The challenge for me is to recognize who's in charge while I'm drafting.

This third eye opens when the pituitary gland and the pineal gland are stimulated. The pea-sized pituitary gland, located at the base of the brain and connected to the hypothalamus, is made up of two lobes with complementary functions. Because its posterior lobe is thought to regulate intuitive and emotional thoughts while the anterior lobe is thought to help us form concrete thoughts and abstract concepts, it's often called "the seat of the mind." The pituitary gland secretes hormones that in turn moderate several of our other glands and organs' functions. It is captain of our endocrine system and co-captain of our subtle body and imagination, that realm of the unconscious accessed by breath, emotion, and intellect.

Situated just behind the pituitary is the cone-shaped pineal gland. It can inhibit thoughts trying to assert themselves into action, thus encouraging our thoughts' inward turn. The pineal gland, then, is what helps the goldfish shoot past analysis and distracting thoughts.

When you close your eyes and direct your eyeballs up and toward one another, your eyeballs' nerves may feel tense. But if you can relax and hold this position for ten slow breaths, you may be able to direct and pay attention to inner images. By breath four, stray lines of light may appear in that dark space, and you can see with your eyes closed.

It is possible to access the unconscious, the intuitive, the imaginative with your eyes open and focused on the page.

LET THE MIND FOLLOW THE BODY'S DRAFT

The body makes a draft. The body's draft is the current, stimulated by intentional movement, that opens the mind to that more-than-5% of typical quotidian conscious thought. It doesn't take much to let a writer's mind slip-stream behind the body's draft. Engage in a few simple movements, and consciousness quickly shifts to being in writing's moment. Intentional movement becomes part of a writing process, the body making a wake for more mind to awaken.

One morning I stood on my mat, sensing it was time to write a fresh short story. I centered myself with a few breaths and inquired, "What am I writing for?" "To connect" was the simple response. Then I clarified a simple writing intention: To be open to whatever character, whatever voice surfaces while I move. I would let a voice and image carry me.

I stood in Standing Pose (usually called Mountain Pose), which involves rooting the feet with matter beneath them and following with the third eye the breath's current through the body and bloodstream. I closed my eyes and shifted the eyeballs toward the third eye. This practice (*shimbhava*) can help you slow down some of the brain activity aroused when eyes are in their normal outward position—even with closed eyelids—to receive sensory input. It also helps you direct your thoughts toward the pituitary and pineal glands and may alter your inner vision temporarily. Almost instantly I saw nails and then a hand hammering. With eyes still closed, I took a few more simple movements—I bowed into Standing Forward Bend and then brought my feet back to Downward Facing Dog so that my body formed an upside-down "V." Eyes still closed, I heard the timbres of the character's craggly voice and glimpsed faint traces of his creviced face. And then the first line. That was enough to begin. I moved to my desk and followed that line and wrote into the shadows the imagination made on the page. A story started to unfold.

Don't fret about holding on to each intuitive insight that surfaces in the body's draft. Trust the words, their associations and sounds, that unfold phrase by phrase. Recall what needs recalling. Trust your faculties. Don't wait for angels to tap their feet to keep the beat of your sentences. Do enjoy creating new paths, one word at a time, and the angels may appear. Don't worry how you look on the page because you're the only one watching: overwrite, digress, strike the wrong chord with a word choice. You will know later what you must return to and clean up.

WRITE *INTO*, NOT *ABOUT*

Aspiring writers of memoir and personal essay often have difficulty with all of this getting lost business. They have a memory to write about, they say. Something happened, and they want to get that experience into words. Other writers of creative non-fiction often tell me they are writing a book about a subject: I'm writing a book about Isadora Duncan, they say, or about happiness or about permaculture.

This about-ness is rout with problems. It makes a clear divide between subject and writing. It suggests that a memory or an idea looms wholly intact somewhere in consciousness, and that the writer's job is to translate this Memory or Idea from this World of Memories or the World of Ideas onto the page. So we plod on, trying to dig in with memory's shovel and analysis's pickax, certain that with enough will power we will excavate and bring to the surface the sweet gem of what happened or of what we're thinking. This digging also presumes that we already know what we need to write before we begin. Writing, this line of thinking goes, is simply memory's manual tool.

Memories don't stay still. Neither do ideas. They change shape in our consciousness each fleeting moment, and to pretend that we are archaeologists or translators of past experiences not only can frustrate us with an impossible task; it also robs us of the vital experience of the writing moment itself. It robs writers of the very making of memories and the making of ideas that happen as words unfold on the page. Joel Agee says that as he wrote his last memoir, "I learned that to remember is, at least in part, to imagine, and that the act of transposing memory into written words is a creative act that transforms the memory itself."[1] When we admit imagination and intuition into the creative act, then writing involves more than transposing some past experience onto the page. Writing becomes an experience.

When you draft, change your preposition. Write into not about a memory. Write into a subject. Write into a character, even if the character is someone you think you know. Start off with a glimmer, a trace, a hiccup of space. Move deftly sentence by sentence.

When you let space surround each sentence, you possibly engage intuition and imagination as you write.

BEGIN WITH THE CONCRETE

Begin with the concrete detail or sensory image, and you're less likely to stray into distancing analysis. Images anchor the imagination in the virtual physical world your words create. Writing description also stimulates the brain's more intuitive visual cortex and parietal lobe, so drafting in the concrete often bypasses the more abstract and analytical voice that wants to figure things out and explain them away for writer and reader.

Take an image. Maybe it's one that haunts you, a woman pacing a room. Describe the red chiffon dress with an orange leather belt she wore or the fresh scratch on the side of her cheek. See where describing that image's surfaces in detail takes you. Or describe a character's quirky action. A story draft might start with "Alison reads dictionaries backwards. She tries to read a letter's worth of words a week. This afternoon, she's on 'u.' Umbilical." If intrigued enough, you'll ask about your own character, "Why does she read dictionaries backwards? Why this discipline? Why is she reading the definition of umbilical when this story starts?"

The same process works when writing nonfiction. I have worked with a client named Becky for over two years using these practices. She lives across the country, but we "meet" by telephone every two weeks. Initially, she just wanted to see if she could develop a writing practice again. A counselor and therapist by trade, she remembered enjoying the process of thinking and imagining that writing instilled when in college almost twenty years earlier.

"I wonder if I have anything to say," she confessed. I suggested we focus less on what she has to say and more on what images might need to be written into. Her background in therapeutic practices opened her to the suggestion.

We began with some over-the-telephone exercises that led her through paying attention to certain images that swam by and following them. For a while, her writing often led to dead ends, but her passion was in the path work. She didn't worry that she didn't know exactly what she had to say before she drafted.

Together, we intuitively heeded key images that arise in her writing, which signal potential topics for essays and articles related to counseling. During our two years in working together, she has cultivated working habits of being a writer and of trusting her own writing process. After the first year, she started taking the image-driven scraps and crafting articles for her clients. A health magazine recently published the first article she submitted, and an editor of another magazine has solicited an article from her.

Now, Becky trusts the not-knowing.

Some writers, like James Kleman, begin in the middle of a conversation. "What's the story with your obsession with red pansies?" Benny asked his sister-in-law. Indeed, you say to yourself and to your character. What is her obsession with pansies? Who is Benny? You won't know until you draft some more.

Sometimes writers begin with a tango of topics. A novelist might start with an itch to explore the relationship between botany and desire. An essayist may wonder how myths of goats relate to notions of masculinity. A poet might set out to see in a series of couplets how the idea of origins and eggs relate. Characters, situations, anecdotes, and images—all the concrete aspects of writing imaginatively—become intuitive ways to explore these ideas.

HEED YOUR BREATH & DETOUR

As you draft, breathe. Most of us hold our breath when we write. Intentionally holding the breath is an advanced Yoga practice, but doing so unconsciously can create tension in our bodies and arouse the sympathetic nervous system, which may induce unconscious anxiety. Periodically noting your breath while writing, on the other hand, helps you draft with a bit more ease (although it won't make writing easy). Your slow exhalations dissipate the chatter while you write, and breath awareness reminds you, too, that your source of drafting encompasses other parts of your body besides your head. You release physical tension so you can be open to imaginative tension.

If compelled, detour. As in "un-tour." For instance, listen to a word's sound and let it rebound throughout your inner ear until by association another word suggests another path of words to take. Let's say you're writing about a time when you picked apples. The word apple in the first line of poetry or the first scene of a story might tickle the word garden or Eden or Snow White. Recurring images and sounds not only thread a series of lines or scenes together. An impression of a word—its connotation, its music—may prompt a memory, an analogy to a film or anecdote, another word, image, or metaphor. When we let our inner ear and eye follow these feathery associations, we let each word and sentence guide the next word and sentence. The piece's inner logic of interrelated words guides you as much as the outer logic of ideas and plot.

I'm not suggesting a random, disjointed stream-of-consciousness. Instead, you follow a thread and follow your breath and at some point, any point, an image or word may beckon you to digress. Keith Abbott describes his writing process as a jazz improvisation: In the moment of writing itself, you let the music play you. Either way, you'll have perhaps a new, even richer story to tell. Read Arundhati Roy's *The God of Small Things* or a novel by Milan Kundera, Salman Rushdie, or Tom Robbins to sense how prose's current can charge fiction.

But cut yourself a little slack, because not all sounds are musical and not all ideas are worth keeping and sharing, just as not all food is piquant. Permit yourself to write crap. Pull out the leftovers, old worn-out drafts from ten years ago, if reworking them gives your imagination something palpable to sink its teeth into. Even if what you write sounds as if you've been writing the same thing for years, write it. Some writers have only one idea their whole life, on which each novel or set of poems they publish simply plays a variation. If you insist on drafting only when you feel each word must be recherché to avoid your words tasting like a rechauffé, then your muse might starve. You'll have time later to clean up the mess—the excesses, the creative indulgences—that you made. For now, enjoy the trek. Drafting, like cooking, can be messy.

Writer Kent Haruf pulls the wool over his eyes—literally a wool cap—when he dives into his first drafts so he won't be worried about hitting the right keys on his keyboard. He explains in the essay "To See Your Story Clearly, Start by Pulling the Wool Over Your Eyes" that he writes sections of stories loosely to quell his analytical mind and "to stay in touch with subliminal, subconscious impulses and to get the story down in some spontaneous way."[2] He's following his third eye. It can work. I've tried it. My imagination's engine, with this newfound freedom, chugs along on and off the track. This practice works best, though, if you can type comfortably (although I've had writers try it hand writing in their notebooks too). You might close your eyes or turn out the lights, clarify an intention that is no more specific than to receive whatever your intuition has to give you and, with your eyes still closed, let go and write in the dark.

It's early but dark this late November day. Sunlight has another hour's worth of orange stripe, but already the ochre moon almost full has risen above her barren peach trees. From her garden chair, the two lights somehow fill out the trees with more promise than they had last summer when in full bloom and when she first hired Doug to prune them and the trumpet vines, when she saw in him an end to that other dredge who could not let go, who would not vanish. She cannot see now how the scheme will close. She cannot see the garden from the trumpet vines. But that's okay. She sips her brandy and closes her eyes, and with her other hand fingers the sheer's blades, steely and warm, and waits for an answer.

TAKE A BREATH #1: UNBOX YOUR THIRD EYE

Intention:
The following practice can help you access your third eye center as you venture on a new piece of writing. You also can try it when you're stuck in the middle of a piece and need a way to get "off-track."

Open your laptop to a blank screen or your notebook to a blank sheet. The whiteness, vast and endless like sky, daunts some people.

Rather than willing your way through the clouds, step back and unbox your third eye.

Come into a comfortable seated position with your sitting bones evenly planted on a blanket, floor, or chair's edge. As your spine extends in both directions, close your eyes and focus on your breath. Let the inhalation inflate the belly and the exhalation draw in the belly. After at least two full breaths, remind yourself, "What am I writing for?" Once you've heard a subtle response, recall the subject of the piece you wish to draft. Maybe it's a story idea. Perhaps you have a title or character. That's all you need. If you have no subject and instead wish to keep the sky completely open, so be it. Your intention is to trust some other faculty besides your will and analytical mind to help you start a piece.

Imagine your breath's movement to your third eye. With each of the next five exhalations, contract your perineum—the muscle at your torso's base between your anus and your genitals. The lock you're creating in your perineum naturally directs your exhalation's energy back up your spine to your third eye. On the inhalation, follow a path from your third eye down your spine to your perineum. The exhalation reverses the direction back up to your third eye.

Then, with your writing subject circling within your breath and with eyes closed, gaze up and between your eyes toward your third eye. You may be able to hold this gaze for a minute or two. If you feel a headache surface, return your eyes to a normal position, close them for a moment, and try again.

On the next exhalation imagine that a lid on your third eye opens. Either it's a dominant image, expected or not, large or small, that relates to your subject, or it's a piece of dialogue germane to your story or idea. Heed whatever it is for only a few seconds, a minute at most, once it surfaces.

Then begin drafting. Don't worry where it's taking you. Heed your breath. Trust your wits and words to lay out a gravel path. Later, you can always retrace your steps. For now, the journey's the thing.

TAKE A BREATH #2:
FOLLOW THE BODY'S DRAFT

Intention:
The following practice can help you integrate intentional movement into your writing process—a seminal part of engaging Yoga as your muse and in trusting your body and your faculties.

First, practice the few Yoga poses illustrated here— **STANDING POSE, STANDING FORWARD BEND, DOWNWARD FACING DOG,** *and* **CHILD'S POSE.** *Get comfortable not in striking the "right" pose but in feeling both steady and soft in your own variation of the pose. Move through the poses in sequence. Repeat the sequence enough times that you can do them with your eyes closed. Trust your body to remember.*

Then, come back to **STANDING POSE.** *Close your eyes and just breathe a few times. Ask yourself gently, "What am I writing for?" Listen, and connect that feeling to your specific writing intention—to follow the body's draft and to be open to an image, a character, or insight that will begin your draft.*

With eyes still closed, sense if something is brewing—an image, a voice, a rhythm. If not, don't fret. If so, let your third eye keep witnessing it. With eyes still closed, inhale and bring arms overhead, and exhale as you bend forward into **STANDING FORWARD BEND.**

An existing image or voice or shred of dialogue might change. Something new but related might surface. Move intuitively if you're comfortable doing so; otherwise, continue with this sequence by stepping your feet back into **DOWNWARD FACING DOG** *and then gradually into* **CHILD'S POSE,** *your third eye pressed upon your mat or blanket.*

All you need is a glimmer. Trust it, and move to your notebook or computer. When you need more insight or surprise while drafting, repeat this sequence or some variation of it.

CHAPTER SEVEN

UNSPOKEN WORDS, UNSTRUCK SOUNDS: TO THROW AN AUTHENTIC VOICE

H OW DID BILLIE HOLIDAY cultivate a voice that conjures in one moment the image of an auto mechanic's oil mixed with whiskey and in the next the image of a sleek black panther moving at midnight along a baobab branch? As a young lady, did Bessie Smith notice the way her voice romped with the spirit of a robust bull gliding upon a river's lip? Did teachers tell little Janis Joplin that her voice vibrated people's sinews like a wild bird's caw? So I wondered one night as these vocalists' serenades haunted me. What distinguishes Smith, Holiday, and Joplin as vocalists, and not just singers, rests less with the songs they wrote or were given than with how their voices could mix the matter—words on sheet music. A vocalist's voice is will, spirit, and soul stirring breath's rhythms. So, too, in the lines of a fortunate writer who can mix the stuff that makes a writer's voice and gives it a timbre.

No facet of writing seems as fleeting and strange to attain as that ephemeral quality we call "voice." Voice animates otherwise stagnant written words. It charges written words with personality and verve, or with reservation and gravitas. It is a writer's near-invisible signature on a page like a watermark. But if you hold a novel's page up to the light, you still won't find the secret traces of a writer's voice. So, how do writers, without the resources of vocalists, create distinct and authentic voices? Since writers can't whisper directly on the page like Marlene Dietrich or sneer like Ani di Franco, some rhetoricians suggest that we "write in the language of intelligent conversation" and that a writer's voice should sound "natural." But how do we sound "natural" with the written word? And who is to determine whether the speaking voice of William F. Buckley, Jr., Howie Mandel, or Snoop Doggy Dogg is the better model for sounding "natural"?

The ear's the thing. We learn to listen. We do not find a voice as much as we find our way with the cadence of unspoken words, a combination of movements with favorite images, ways of thinking and finagling sentences and that might in part distinguish one writing voice from another. Such listening requires stillness. We grow up, after all, hearing so many other voices of authority—parents, professors, mentors, bosses—that no wonder it's a challenge for some writers to hear a voice they might deem as their authentic one, that voice of their own authority. When you dwell in stillness, though, your inner ear opens.

When we read something written with an authentic voice, it often strikes some chord deep within us. Perhaps since most reading and writing occurs in silence we would say such a voice strikes an unstruck sound. An unstruck sound, *anāhata* in Sanskrit, originates from the heart region, a region that yogis have realized for centuries is a source of authentic language. So the over-used phrase "to write from the heart" might have substance. Something in an attuned ear that hears an "unstruck sound" can help writers fashion a distinct, authentic voice on the page. Careful study coupled with steady listening might lead to writing with confidence and courage that manifest's a writer's deepest intentions.

You set off on this journey to "find" your voice only to realize several years and mountaintops later that all along your voice has been residing in the home of your heart.

This journey towards stillness, toward opening the inner ear, invites us to move into the self without becoming self-absorbed. "Moving into one's self" is an essential practice within numerous Yogic traditions. It often involves studying, memorizing, chanting, and reciting passages from sacred texts to deepen one's understanding of the self's nature. Through this practice, we honor those teachers who have gone before us and have laid stepping-stones for us that we may eventually add our own stones. By memorizing and reciting passages, we also honor language's sacred capacity to inform our hearts. These modes of what is called *svādhyāya* ("moving into the self") also work on the self the way being absorbed in good writing does: We dissolve our ego needs into another text that something greater than the ego might be aroused to reflection and action.

I read provocative books and poems not to reinforce my tightly constructed notion of reality or of humanity—something I did when a teenager. I read to allow my sense of self to expand, to be inclusive of far more than my defensive ego might want. Similarly, some of us read ancient Yoga texts to reflect upon what the "self" is or is not. This practice of self-study for yogis has two turns: a turn toward texts and a turn toward one's own mind and heart, both to explore the nature of the authentic self. So, too, this practice for writers has two turns: a turn toward texts and a turn toward the mind and heart.

Writers learn to read with their ears. Most writers who have mustered an authentic voice study or have studied certain texts that have preceded them—the sacred and the profane. On my bookshelves, the *Bhagavad-Gita* rests next to George Bernard Shaw's plays. The *Yoga-Sutra* informs my reading of *Crime and Punishment* and vice-versa. Both texts can move you into uncomfortable parts of the self. Writers study writers whose voices they admire and texts whose rhythms they wish to emulate. While Steinbeck, an atheist, rewrote *The Grapes of Wrath*, he immersed himself in the cadences of the King James' version of the Bible. Read some rolling passages from Exodus and then read Steinbeck's rolling passages about migrant farmers, and you'll hear what struck the compassionate novelist. When we read with the pace of a summer afternoon sentences deftly crafted, voices of the dead and of the present might mesh with what voice we deem our own. Such a way of reading with the inner ear is more likely to lead a writer to developing a memorable voice on the page than listening solely to the way she speaks in "intelligent conversation." I converse with the printed word. I converse with dead writers. And, I admit, they shape my voice.

Like trying on personas to see which one fits for an identity, we try out other writers' voices to see which ones sound right. True, Emerson wrote that "imitation is suicide." Yet, the then-self-reliant zealot already had spent years imitating and emulating Carlyle and Lamb until the point that he at last developed a nearly inimitable voice as orator and essayist, a voice we now admiringly—or usually so—call "Emersonian." Eliot also wrote some of his best poems while immersed in reading the rhythms of Donne's poems, of Ovid's tales, of St. John's Gospel. Nobel Prize recipient Seamus Heaney has written about his "Hopkins ventriloquism," how Gerard Manley Hopkins's voice shaped young Heaney's ear.[1] Just as our identities are unique composites of other elements, so are most writers' voices. An authentic writer's voice, then, does not come *ex nihilo* from some ideal plane of originality; it is in part a voice influenced by a mentor or even the butcher down the road.

Stylized strings of words influence our own inner ears. When we put ourselves in this river of influence, we might admit that a voice, certainly a writing voice, is not ours. That is, I don't have or own my writing voice. So as soon as I can let go of trying to own my writing voice, let alone find it, ironically my authentic voice might emerge.

We don't find our voice. We throw our voice. Heaney mentions his ventriloquism. Emerson called essayists ventriloquists. They let other voices resonate within their inner ear, that ear in the heart perhaps, to hear and feel what strikes them right.

I started to find my voice through ventriloquism. My grandfather had told me all about Edgar Bergen, the renowned ventriloquist who set his dummies, the gentlemanly and monocled Charlie McCarthy and the dimwitted and bucktoothed Mortimer Snerd, on his knees and breathed life into wood. After I saw television footage of Bergen doing his thing, I thought at age ten he could perform the most magical act: He could throw his voice.

The texts you study aren't dummies, but they can work like Charlie McCarthys. I've encouraged writers for years to seek out either a remote mentor or a dead mentor. A remote mentor is a writer still living, yet who advises a writer solely via the mentor's texts. A dead mentor is the same, of course, just dead. So Scott

Russell Sanders could be a remote mentor; Virginia Woolf, a dead one. Most of us love the writing of certain authors. You sense in that voice something kindred that kindles your heart, that may even register a visceral response. With this view of writers, you realize you exist in a huge community with boundaries far superseding your home's space and your biographical age's time. Through such study, your writer's heart may never be alone.

Imagine you've found a mentor. Find a passage—fifty words, a hundred, may suffice. Then read and heed—slowly—the syllables, the twists in syntax, the edgy wit or bawdy humor, or the saturnine gravitas that drums through the paragraphs. Let the passage wash over you. Then begin to record, word by word, this passage. Notice how your body feels as you handwrite these sentences' rhythms. Your inner ear cannot help but tune in. Numerous writers keep notebooks full of such passages, not just for the passage's message but also for the qualities I've just noted: the cadences, the images, the twists, the tones.

Commit a few lines to memory. Choose something that you feel expands your sense of who you are as a writer, something that informs your own writer's voice. *Committed to Memory: 100 Best Poems to Memorize*, edited by John Hollander, is a good source. Although poetry with regular meter, sound, and form is easier for the brain to retain, some fiction and nonfiction merits memorization, if not recitation as well. You don't have to chant Molly Bloom's reveries or Raskolnikov's observations, as yogis do with sacred texts. Still, the process of memorization can bring a passage's essence inside of you, so to speak. You'll feel and hear those rhythms creeping into your writing. (So be careful what you choose to memorize.)

Imitation might kill the self, but emulation might revive the self. Michael Cunningham's novel *The Hours* is an extended study of emulation and an homage to one of his dead mentors, Virginia Woolf. You can read by heeding another writer's sensibilities to language, to experience, to humanity. What about the writer's work reveals truths about our complex emotions? How does this writing allow you to descend into the questions that keep you awake at night? Why, with this author's book in your hands, do you tremble with self-recognition and self-realization? How is your sense of self altered or challenged? On what subjects does the writer often focus? What types of characters? Themes? Are the writer's sentences typically long or short? How are they varied for effect? Is the writer's vocabulary typically lifted from the streets or borrowed from literary dens? Do images and metaphors pepper the writing, or is it seemingly plain-spoken? You're not demystifying the magic of that mentor's voice. You're discovering how to honor that voice via emulation—the highest compliment.

A few years ago I mentored an MFA student in creative nonfiction. We designed a course to help her understand this fluid genre and to help her develop – or hear – her own voice. First, she read the texts of Chesteron, Lopate, Tom Wolfe, Capote, Didion, and others. Then, she chose six passages from these texts to copy. After reviewing some of the questions above, she centered on subjects important to her writing—her relationship to her father, her awkward relationship with another twenty-something guy, and so forth—and wrote into those subjects in the style and voice of Capote, Didion, and the like. For the first time, she said, she began to hear how a writer's voice emerges on the page.

She threw her voice. And in the process, she began to let her own unfold.

Moving into the self by emulating another voice increases a writer's versatility. The other writer's voice becomes an intelligent dummy, so to speak, for your self to fill out, for your voice to breathe into without fear of too much self-disclosure. You can hide behind your mentor's voice like a ventriloquist. And such hiding is fine, as long as you know you're doing so. One student chose Annie Proulx as a mentor, and then wrote a fictional piece about sex—its mishaps and disappointments, some exquisite fantasies—as if Proulx had written it. If you've feared exploring some dreadful feelings about your existence or your work's illusory nature, and if your mentor is Barbara Kingsolver, then write a piece from a desperate character's point of view as if it were in a Kingsolver novel. You'll know you're finished when you reread the piece and can't believe you wrote it.

At some point, though, on this journey toward stillness we make the second turn of self-study. We learn to listen to that still, small voice within, that source of our own authenticity unmediated by mentors.

I first heard that voice when I was eight and taught my cousin Donna how to pray. I attended church; she never had.

"How do you pray?" she asked. We got on our knees beside her bed, bowed our heads, cupped our hands.

"Don't speak out loud," I said. "Just talk in your head without speaking and say whatever you want to say to God." I concentrated and waited. I don't recall what I tried to discuss with the Almighty, but I did hear a voice, confident and kind, knowledgeable and unassuming. "Yep," I said to Donna, "I can hear God speak." She didn't believe me. "Listen, just keep your eyes shut, and listen," I said.

Smirking, she tried it. Perhaps not to be one-upped, or possibly blessed with a window opening within, she said, "Yeah! I hear Him." For the first time I had become aware of a steady, guiding voice that later became part of my writing voice.

Pat Conroy said he first heard his voice when eighteen years old. Conroy's father ruled his house with a domineering, abusive voice, and then his high school basketball coach's similar voice tore talented young men's confidence into pulp. While the coach was blowing out one of his tirades, Conroy recalls hearing a strong voice within him say, in essence, "Don't listen to that voice. You have your own voice that will guide you." Listening to that voice, Conroy said, would later serve him well as a writer. I suspect it helped him later listen to what his heart needed to say, not to what his ego wanted and not, when he wrote the novel *The Great Santini*, largely based on his father, what his father's ego would've wanted. To hear and to distinguish one authentic voice among the chorus that fills most of our thoughts is not schizophrenic; it is an essential part of unfolding your writer's voice.

We must speak to ourselves, for writing is largely a solitary art. Only if I can hear myself think can I muster the courage and clarity to write one decent sentence after another. The rhythm and pace, the hesitation and repetition, of how an inner voice stitches phrases and clauses is different from those qualities of an outer voice.

Many of us might be terrified to sit with ourselves for too long. It's noisy in there. Yet it's a habit that can allow our minds to discern when we're writing from our ego or when we're writing from the unstruck sound. Writing habitually from this source allows our body's natural rhythms to guide our subjects, word choices, metaphors, sounds, and sentences. Gradually a style ensues that we feel pumps from our cells and fits our skin; gradually an authentic voice emerges.

As our voices change and assume so many textures over the years, we may wonder if any of us writes with what we call our own voice. But don't fret. We can find pleasure and authenticity not so much in refining some fixed singular voice but in plunging into our own dark ponds' bottoms where thoughts and images mix in the silt with voices of the dead, spawn words, and surface as a voice. Just try not to hang on to any one voice for too long or even to call it your "own." Listen. Respond. Hook it and reel it in, playing it for all it has to give. Then let it go. Throw it back to the river.

TAKE A BREATH:
STRIKE YOUR UNSTRUCK AUTHENTIC VOICE

Intention:

This practice can help you hear and feel your authentic writer's voice coming from your heart.

Come into a comfortable seated position. Any seated pose or even sitting in a chair is fine. Lengthen your spine in both directions as your body becomes alert, yet at ease. With eyelids softened or closed, draw your inhalation to your heart region as your chest expands. After at least two full breaths, ask yourself, "What am I writing for?" Tune your ear to your heart to hear whatever inner voice or image bubbles up. When you feel the response sufficiently sink into your heart, clarify your specific writing intention for this session. You might acknowledge that you wish to write with your authentic voice for a specific subject or scene—either one you've been writing into or   a new one.

Bring your palms together, slightly cupped, at your chest's center. This mudrā, *or hand gesture, is called* anjali-mudrā, *a common gesture of respect. Close your eyes, and again let your in-breath fill your heart space. On the exhalation, imagine your breath pushing your palms apart as you draw your bent elbows behind your torso toward one another so your palms face forward on either side of your shoulders* (**EVEN-HEARTED POSE**). *You will feel your chest and neck open. Let the next inhalation naturally draw your palms back together at your heart region. Continue this movement between your palms and your breath until you're comfortable with the rhythm.*

Then, imagine in your heart you have a second mouth, ear, and eye. Imagine that with each inhalation your hands are drawing into your heart's mouth whatever you or a character deeply need to say—images, sounds, stories, words. With each exhalation, imagine your heart guides that movement outward. Repeat this rhythm until you feel you've brought sufficient energy into your heart space before writing. Then, sit for a few minutes and listen to what your heart says for you to write. What does it need you to write? Notice how the voice sounds. Its tenor and tone may even register a visual image. Honor what you hear or see.

If nothing surfaces, relax.

Then begin to write. As you write, imagine a line of communication extending between your heart and your hands. Continue with each breath to write with the interplay between taking something in and giving something out. Ease into the words and sentences, the images and metaphors, that naturally unfold.

When you've finished drafting, you might revise anything that seems forced or not quite the language of the unstruck sound. Then read it aloud. Notice if it registers the same texture that you felt, heard, or saw when you listened to your heart while sitting still. Try this practice for at least fifteen consecutive sessions. You might find within a few weeks or months that how you write stems from another, richer source than before, a source that may be best described as your heart center. Anāhata. And so continues the journey from the center to the page.

CHAPTER EIGHT

PRESENCE & THE WRITER'S RESERVOIR OF IMAGES

T HOREAU, that perpetual present-moment monger and chanticleer to the blind and busy, wrote perhaps the most beautiful and influential ode to the life-altering benefits of heeding the present. In the chapter "Where I Lived and What I Lived For" of *Walden*, after taking note of the woods' vital sounds and sights about him, he writes that in comparison with sculpting clay or carving statues "it is far more glorious to carve and paint the very atmosphere and medium through which we look, which morally we can do. To affect the quality of the day, that is the highest of the arts."

Still, I think every writer would be wise to try it. Why? Existentially, so you can live in such a way that no day slips past your imagination. Pragmatically, so you can create a world of words your readers' imagination can enter. To be able to write about the cracks in a basketball player's knuckles or the patches of dirt beneath a gardener's fingernails might require having a useful imagination and memory that can store and then recall images in the moment of writing.

But how do we develop a useful imagination and memory? Why not begin with reassessing how you spend each day, or, rather, how each day spends you? How much of the bird talk or office chatter do you hear? How much of the asparagus tips do you taste? Perhaps, we need to pay more attention to the phenomenological world of hiccups and paper cups and paper cuts. We don't have to sweat the small stuff. We just need to heed it.

We write from the center by grounding ourselves where we are: here in our bodies, in our minds, in this world. Heeding this world's physical currency can help you not only to reembrace and explore your intricately physical existence; it may give you the sensibilities to create virtual worlds of words that stem from an authentic source.

Much of this journey involves becoming more aware of how your own creative faculties function. If in drafting we learn to heed intuition, in cultivating presence we hone perception and imagination. The three faculties of perception, memory, and imagination, it turns out, influence one another to create for a writer a rich reservoir.

When we get lost in our mental machinations, our words tend to float into ephemeral abstractions and analysis. We talk and talk on the page instead of write. I know someone who each morning writes whatever she's thinking to help clear the clutter. The problem with this practice, she says, is she gets caught up in her own "stuff," in her own spinning wheels and soon spends three hours psychoanalyzing herself. It feels good, she says, for a while, but then she feels spent like her time and cannot write her novel.

Writing that reverberates with others' deep imagination strikes me as authentic. It's authentic because it comes from a source beyond the ego mind's spinning wheels. Much authentic writing then is sensuous and sensual. Verbs lick us. Images ignite our imaginations. Suggestive diction caresses us. An image in writing does not merely appeal to our senses. An image triggers our inner senses and often impresses upon our reader's imagination. By inviting themselves into the imagination's inner sanctum, images dissolve some of the distance among writer, reader, and language. They connect.

Get outside of yourself if you want to find yourself. That's the advice writer Marvin Bell gives to his students. He's right. The core self that helps writers craft exquisite worlds for others to enter is not locked up inside some personally embroidered baggage or inside those whirling ego thoughts.

What is the way out? Luckily, our bodies come equipped with numerous passageways: the senses. Senses—all five or six or one hundred of them—are our body's tentacles to the physical world of lightbulbs and sunlight. Sense receptors connect parts of the body with the brain and, like breath, to the natural world. Senses shape our perception of reality, so no wonder yogis often learn first to experience fully and then to harness reactions to the core five sense organs (in Sanskrit, *jñāna-indriya* or the cognitive senses).

No doubt the world's distractions numb, deafen, and blind us. After staring at a computer for four hours, I can step outdoors and feel my eyes relax and widen. After being in a rancorous town hall meeting or being on Union Square for a few hours, my ears close. The senses lead us, according to one Yoga text, to heaven or hell: heaven if we can harness them, hell if not. If harnessed, they fill the writer's reservoir.

The writer's imagination is a reservoir, an organic and fluid space that holds images retrieved over the years from paying attention to the small stuff. Presence in this physical world fills that reservoir. And when that reservoir brims with images from broken leaves or the cruel lines of a little girl's mouth, then a writer has resources, months or years later, for the particularity and sensuousness that round out a virtual world of words.

Life's details—a mother's goofy patchwork dress that she wore to her child's elementary school's open house, a dog's distinct chlorine-cedar odor—matter in embodied writing. Ezra Pound implored a young writer in essence, Don't write "red." Write "rose" or "rust" or "ruddy." Toni Morrison's character Milkman in *Song of Solomon* remains with me in part because of how he earned his nickname (a man saw him being nursed by his mother—when the boy was ten years old). Barbara Kingsolver's fictional Africa in *The Poisonwood Bible* remains in my memory for the unique, subjective way she transformed it through five distinct female perspectives. The novel revolves around a missionary family from Georgia that travels to the Congo. The first daughter to narrate the story says in her first sentence, "We came from Bethlehem, Georgia, bearing Betty Crocker cake mixes into the jungle." That detail says a mouthful about the family and especially the mother.

We learn that the mother also packs "a dozen cans of Underwood deviled ham; Rachel's ivory plastic hand mirror with powdered-wig ladies on the back; a stainless-steel thimble; a good pair of scissors; a dozen number-2 pencils; a world of Band-Aids, Anacin, Absorbine Jr.; and a fever thermometer."[1] These intimate details are the particularities, the details of a narrator's or a character's unique experience and identity. They invite readers into the rich textures of a singular world of words.

"No ideas but in things," William Carlos Williams said decades ago. Although the quotation has been misappropriated frequently from this author of poems about red wheelbarrows and broken glass to mean that one should simply describe things and not think about ideas, he was onto something that cognitive scientists now recognize: Ideas, like language, stem from our physical reality.[2] I'm curious then to explore this intricately wired vehicle that shapes so much of my experience, for our bodies are made to proffer us the particular details and images that establish an authentic style. We might rewrite Williams's quotation as "No ideas but in the body."

Becoming aware of the body and journeying into the imagination's layers can be tricky. When I started practicing Yoga, I had next to no idea what went on below my shoulders. It is dark in there. The imagination also remained a mystery. Some days it flourished with images and insight. Most other days, work and a consuming intellect shut down the reservoir. I remember sitting in my friend Bob's living room one day, my head so busy I could barely hear what he had to say about Li Po. "Just stop thinking," I mourned to myself. "Just for one minute, stop thinking."

Yoga gradually softened my eye muscles and opened my pupils. One day, after practicing, I took a walk down the city road where I lived. On my many walks and bicycle rides before, I had seen the neighborhood in clumps—houses, bushes, trees, buildings. But on this day, for no apparent reason, I suddenly stopped to stare at a plastic bus bench. The planks and nuts and bolts, the simple engineered curves, the peeling advertisement for El Centro College pasted to the back, became animated as if I could see the hands that made them and the thousand bodies that had come and gone. My mind, typically spinning, was relatively still. I was sensing more than thinking.

Your senses impress themselves upon your imagination. And your imagination has layers that correlate to what in Yoga are called the physical body and the subtle body. The physical body is the gross body of organs, muscles, and bones. Some of us are not even in touch with the body's or the imagination's physical layer because our mental wheels spin out of control. To play with how your physical imagination works, look at something in the room where you're presently reading this book: a picture frame, a lamp base. Gaze at it, taking in a few details—dust particles or dents. Close your eyes, and see the object with your inner eye. This ability to recast an image with our inner senses comes from our physical imagination. The more clear our sense organs, then, the more likely a perception becomes a stored image for later retrieval while writing.

Take that same image in your inner eye and change its hues and let it transform into something else. You're playing consciously with the subtle imagination. The subtle imagination grants us not only the capacity to invent images based on our sensory experience; it also grants us other visual images, inner sounds, and smells without clear reference to a memory. Whereas an image from the physical imagination stems almost solely from impressions made by outer senses, an image from the subtle imagination can be influenced more directly by the mixing of a writer's breath, intellect, emotions, and unconscious. These images surface in dreams and often appear like ghosts on our consciousness's periphery.

Imagine you're talking to the woman who sells you flowers and herbs down the road. Without your knowing why, the sound of a baby crying to the tune of a bullfrog or an image of a man sprouting from a water lily surfaces in your subtle imagination. You continue talking to the woman about azaleas and marigolds, but as soon as you get in your car, you pen a note to yourself on your receipt: "baby bullfrog" or "water lily man." Maybe the image won't amount to anything worth writing about, but the habit of heeding these peripheral images keeps you in frequent contact with your unconscious. Writers—as do most creative people in their fields—pay more attention than other people to the images on the margins of awareness.

Yoga helps writers do the same thing by exploring the subtle body and the subtle imagination. The subtle body is comprised of emotion, intellect, breath, and energy. We begin this journey by paying attention to sensations and tensions within the physical and subtle bodies. You can imagine an ache or sensation richly. Maybe you're weary of feeling tired and achy, broken and bruised. But rather than reach for the aspirin, ignore it, or complain to your partner, try a fourth option: become increasingly aware of the ache and sensation. When you increase awareness of your body's subtle aches and sensations, you can not only improve your yoga practice; you also can tap into a whole new source of writing.

Proprioceptors are specialized receptors that note what's happening with tendons, muscles, and joints. Thanks to these receptors we have that touchy sense. Heeding their subtle signals, what is called proprioception, activates our brain's cerebrum in conjunction with the imagination, which lets us see in our mind's eye what might be happening and where within our body.

This subtle work also trains the inner senses. The mix between the physical and subtle imaginations may be the basis for enduring fiction writing, as well as for the memorable imagery rife in so much creative nonfiction and poetry.

"Not to live in the physical world is the greatest poverty," Wallace Stevens also wrote. The Nobel Prize winner spent most of his adult days as an executive for Hartford Insurance. His days were busy, his mind preoccupied with claims and legalities, the otherwise trivialities of the insurance world. And still, his reservoir filleth over.

The world's minutiae—the hues of the sun as it bleeds behind clouds, the melody of a child's whine—awaits to ignite your imagination. The world of physical stuff can hold your imagination captive until you heed whatever is calling you. Just practice paying attention and simply sensing without too much thinking. With a relaxed body, render subtle textures and tints with vivid verbs and images.

Or follow your nose. In a notebook, track what you smell from the moment you awaken to the moment you drift to sleep. From your lover's hair to the cilantro in your omelet to your wet cedar deck, sniff out those hidden smells and similes, and record the images. Take note of what sounds, what ditty bells, you enjoy versus what sounds, what clamorous bells, you despise. Be particular, personal, quirky. Celebrate and censor. If logging sounds sounds dull, try tastes or touches.

Mix it up. Our sense organs don't always comply to delineated categories. That is, what we see and smell shapes our taste. Some people see numbers in colors. Nabokov saw the number "5" as red, and others might hear the color purple trumpet. In *Musicophilia*, Oliver Sacks describes how certain musical melodies register distinct visual images. This sensory overlap or "cross-firing" is called "synesthesia," something scientists once scoffed at as anomalous or fictional. But the brain's sensory compartments, neuroscientists are acknowledging, aren't so compartmentalized. The visual, auditory, and motor cortexes communicate so intimately in some instances that some form of sensory overlap may be more the rule than the exception.

So practice experiencing a day like a Picasso model. Picasso's Cubist and post-Cubist portraits placed ears where we'd expect a nose and mouths where we'd expect an eye. We can smell sounds and taste color. We can feel a smell's texture. So try to see the colors and shapes of cardinal clicks. Listen to the pitch and tone of morning light upon tree leaves. Stroke the skin of midnight air. Most of us must force our brains to re-experience the world this way. So, if it helps you, first note a sense in its typical category (sight, sound, et cetera), then try to shift categories. How would this taste sound? How would this sound look? Write at least ten a day for the next fifteen days.

All of these practices are just that: practice. They're ways to retrain your senses to be alert and to fill your physical and subtle imaginations' reservoir with material, so when you're writing you can retrieve readily the appropriate image or detail. Your words and phrases may have a texture more akin to a homemade cup of hyssop than of Lipton. Practicing presence can help you remember the splendor of your outer senses and rediscover the mystery of your inner ones, for words can work magic upon our intellects, imaginations, and emotions in ways that enlarge our inner senses and our sense of an embodied self.

TAKE A BREATH:
LET YOUR IMAGINATION GET ON YOUR NERVES

If you're not familiar with the following four simple yoga poses— **MOUNTAIN POSE, STANDING FORWARD BEND POSE, KNEELING POSE,** *and* **LYING RELEASE POSE**—*I suggest you review the illustrations so you're not caught up in getting poses "right." You might try the poses twice without regard to the prompts, and on the third time* t r y *the sequence with your eyes closed. Treat the poses as catalysts to awaken your physical and subtle imaginations.*

Intention:
Generate fresh ideas and enrich your writing's par-ticularity and sensuousness by heightening your outer and inner senses.

Come into a comfortable **MOUNTAIN/STANDING POSE** (tādāsana). *Anchor your body in both feet, close your eyes, and focus on your breath for at least two full inhalations and exhalations. When ready, set your twofold intention first by asking yourself, "What am I writing for?" Then, specify this session's writing intention. Perhaps you want to be open to the present and see what happens with your embodied physical and subtle imaginations. Perhaps you want to project and transfer what you experience into the body of one of your characters. Or if you write personal essays,* *this practice can offer surprises about the stories latent in your body's pages.*

Once comfortable with your intention, tend to each sense organ. Look around your room and notice what's happening with your sight at this very moment. With eyes fixed on something, notice how your body feels as you appreciate how light transfers data through your eyes and registers signals in your brain, which in turn sends signals scurrying throughout your body's cells and nerves. Then, close your eyes and notice how you can, if you wish, recall images of the room's objects. With eyes still shut, open your ears and hear what's rustling outside of you. Then, try to hear what's stirring inside your body: breath, heartbeat, something subtler. As you breathe, take in scents, however distinct or faint, and appreciate how smells and breath constantly energize your body down to your soles. Notice your tongue and how the residue of taste lingers in the back of your throat or, like lost words, on the tip of your tongue. And heed some of the millions of touch receptors from your head to your toes, your body an electric vibration of constant sensory information. Stand and embrace that fact for a few breaths.

Then, when ready, begin to notice any slight sensations at the muscular level or at the nerve level, and let one sensation direct your imagination's focus. Perhaps there's a sensation in the back of your neck or something on your left foot. Or in your right hip. Let your imagination go there. How would you describe this sensation? Does it have a hue, a rhythm, a voice all its own? Be with it for a few breaths. Then, with your inner focus still on that sensation, inhale, and exhale as you bend from your waist down into **STANDING FORWARD BEND** *(uttanāsana). Bend your knees, if needed, to avoid strain. Stay here for a few breaths, and notice if the sensation changes, moves, transforms. Breathe with it. As you're in this pose, notice what related image might surface. Avoid forcing anything. It might come from your physical imagination of memory or from a subtler and as yet inexplicable source. A person's face or body. A scene. A building. Something moving. Absorb its particular textures and shapes.*

When ready, take a full exhalation, bend your knees, and come onto your shins, tops of feet on the mat, into **ADMANTINE POSE /**

KNEELING POSE (vajrāsana) *or another seated position. Keep your eyes closed. Is the sensation the same? Has the image developed, moved, or become something else? Can you stay with the image and let it unfold, move, shift shapes if need be? Try to stay with it for several breaths and let it soak your body.*

When ready, rest on your back in **LYING RELEASE POSE / CORPSE POSE** (savāsana). *As you release your back body into the ground, try to feel the images residing in the physical space of your specific bodily sensation. How do these images feel? Then, explore how your original physical sensation and these images might relate. These might form part of your story, your character, your self. There may be a cause-and-effect relationship, a symbolic relationship, or something as of yet undisclosed that only drafting can reveal.*

When ready, open your eyes, and write a piece of fiction, nonfiction, or poetry that explores the feelings and significance of a physical sensation. Assume your own point of view or another person's or a character's point of view. You could begin by describing a character—or yourself—in an imagined or actual situation or by describing the physical sensation. Gradually honor and explore the bridges, the connections, between the physical sensation and the imagery.

CHAPTER NINE

THE GENIUS OF WONDER
IN WAKING DREAM

E ACH MORNING BEFORE DAWN, novelist Nicholson Baker
would slip out of bed without waking his wife, creep down-
stairs without stirring his kids, make a pot of coffee, light a
fire in his wood-burning stove, flip on his laptop—the only other
light besides the flames—and write. In that dark twilight space
between wake and dream, Baker created a quirky novella that celebrates the extraordinary of the ordinary: *A Box of Matches*. His
naïve narrator, a medical textbook editor who lives in Maine with
wife, kids, and duck Greta, riffs on everything from the pleasure of
how a dishwasher's top rack rolls out to the exhilaration of scrub-
bing first thing in the morning a dish left out overnight ("smiling
with the clenched-teeth smile of the joyful scrubber").[1]

What Baker and his narrator embody are what novelist Jonathan
Rosen says every writer he admires embodies: wonder.

Wonder is genius. In her journals published as *Falling Through
Space*, Ellen Gilchrist writes, "I know a lot of two-year-olds who
have genius. They are terribly observant, absolutely curious, willing to take risks....How to hold on to that native genius and also
learn the things we need to survive." Poet Charles Baudeliare, a
hundred years earlier in an essay about modern art, similarly wrote
that, "Genius is the capacity to retrieve childhood at will." Both
Gilchrist's comment about "how to hold on to" and Baudelaire's
reference "to retrieve...at will" imply we adults can actually make
some effort, once we pass 13 years old, to wonder.

Practicing wonder as writers does more than open us up to a day's quirks. It is to understand as writers that our imaginations, our physical existence, and our most mundane moments give us infinite possibilities to create for our readers fresh worlds made of words. Wonder proffers us novel topics, uncommon angles, and untrodden insights on familiar subjects without our having, necessarily, to trek to Kilimanjaro. For such is the stuff linguistic dreams are made on.

Authentic freshness lacks gimmicks or cheap trick endings or gratuitous experimentation, showing its cleverness for cleverness's sake. Its novelty instead might provoke readers to view their own world and reality anew, to consider being human in a new light, or to open their hearts and imaginations to someone else's perspective. With regular practice, your imagination may find new stepping-stones for your characters to hop across. Your fictional plots, your nonfiction narratives, and your poetic situations may stay alive because you let your imagination wander into the land of "What if?" and, to borrow Borges's title, into the garden of forking paths of possibilities.

"Life is a spell so exquisite," Emily Dickinson wrote, "that everything conspires to break it." Wonder holds us spellbound. It does so in part by calling everything we think we know into question. For a moment, we cease to know. What we deem real is a dream. What we dream is real. And what better way to understand this incomparable spell we writers weave than to explore that peculiar space where wake and dream converge.

This way of experiencing wonder on consciousness's borderlands—much more than mere curiosity—is more Eastern than Western. The *Shiva-Sutra*[2] is one of the few Yoga texts to reference wonder. It describes "joy-filled amazement," the state of being "wonderstruck" with life, awareness, and reality. Called *vismayo* in Sanskrit, it's an essential though rarely discussed quality for yogis and writers. When a person experiences wake, dream, sleep, and the reality of realities as one, the text says, that person embodies *vismayo*. This description may seem a little heady, but bear with me.

In what in Yoga is waking reality (*jagrat*), we're aware especially of the outside world of things—apple trees and traffic jams—when awake. Keen presence to this world helps us later retrieve details from our reservoir to create the basis of, say, Yoknapatawpha County. But the details that—whether in fiction, nonfiction, or poetry—help writers create compelling "alternative realities" don't come solely from memories of the waking world. And this reality alone of data, facts, and what we call memories are not all there is.

What we see is not what we get. In Yoga's dream reality, *svapna* in Sanskrit, we connect with the image-laden world of our unconscious—a veritable treasure trove for imaginative writing. "Imagination is reality," wrote Wallace Stevens—a three-piece suited poet-yogi if there ever was one. And writers of non-fiction and memoir from Annie Dillard to Toni Morrison attest that imagination, not fact-checking, writes the truth. Imagination and dream are not illusion. Memory needs imagination.

Just imagine Nicholson Baker's narrator, or Baker himself, drifting through the dark kitchen spellbound in that space where the cold feel of kitchen tile laps over images of tiles from dreams and memories. Where waking consciousness, dream, and memory mix it up, and you cannot tell the dancer from the dance, the writer from the words, wonder happens. This way of wonder strikes us at the marrow. For a moment, our skin unravels, and our sense of reality turns upside-down and inside-out.

And Yoga like much good writing essentially loosens our tight grip on reality. Regularly practicing Yoga's physical, breathing, and meditation tools can quiet our brain's "control center," that part of the brain stimulated by analytical activities and ego-defending activities we might associate with waking reality. Analysis alone does not a good novel make. Regular Yoga practice arouses other parts of the brain and of consciousness we might call imagination and intuition, the deep unconscious that influences so much conscious thought. Yoga actually brings some of these faculties' nebulous murk to conscious light.[3] We dream with our eyes open, so to speak. Call it lucid waking. Call it lucid writing.

Brain activity in the frontal cortex, the control center, mirrors some of what we're calling waking and dream state. Earlier in this book's reflections on concentration, I mentioned that when our minds kick into high multi-task, analytical, or anxious gear, our brain waves vibrate like fleas in a dirty dog's bed. These fleas are called Beta waves. Slow down your breath, center your thoughts, and move in tandem with breath and thoughts, and your brain waves slow down by half as if the fleas became caterpillars of concentration. These caterpillars are called Alpha waves. Sustained Yoga practice followed by deep relaxed alertness shifts your brain's waves to an even slower pace we might describe as caterpillars with wings. These winged caterpillars are called Alpha-Theta waves (theta brain waves being characteristic of what we traditionally call "dream state").

Apparently, for us to recall unconscious imagery or memories, our brains must contain some alpha brain waves mixed with theta. When advanced yogis, inventors, writers, artists, scientists, and others report thinking lucidly in images, their brains also likely shift between low alpha waves and high theta waves[4], so no wonder author Joel Agee, highly attuned to his faculties' functioning, seemed confused about what was real, what was remembered, what was invented when he wrote his last "memoir." Neuropsychologist Erik Hoffman, who led a study on eleven experienced yoga teachers in Scandinavia, used an EEG and follow-up psychological measurements to measure the yogis' brain-wave activity after two hours of a form of Yoga called Kriya Yoga. The study revealed significant theta-wave activity in both hemispheres, especially in the less dominant right hemisphere, often, but not always, associated with more intuitive functions. Some neuroscientists claim that practices that induce an alert theta-wave state help people access their unconscious feelings, images, and memories. Neuroscientists call this experience a hypnagogic state. Call it "writer's flow."

In a state of "writer's flow," we experience easier access to thinking in images—the heart of creative language. One study suggested that 70–77 percent of people experience this hypnagogic state but aren't aware of it, yet through some simple Yoga tools writers can become aware of their interior reservoir.

To invite a wondrous state of consciousness, I have experimented with some simple breathing tools. MOON BREATHING (*candra bhedana pranayama*), for instance, involves breathing in through the left nostril and out through the right nostril. Breathing through the left nostril has been shown to stimulate the brain's right hemisphere. The left nostril, often associated with the cool moon, also stimulates a channel of energy called the "comfort channel" *(ida-nādī)* that correlates to the parasympathetic nervous system, which in turn cools down a person's energy.

Writing with wonder happens when we navigate the dream reality in our waking world. Imagine your eyes are centered upon the oak chair before you as your imagination concocts images of termites burrowing holes and corridors inside it, and while you stare at an ivy plant, your dreamlike imagination might imagine the vines reaching out like arms as you invent a gothic story of a "still life" living room grown wild. When you're consciously entertaining random imagery while awake, you're not daydreaming (or hallucinating, you hope) as much as you're living in the reverie of being a writer. Your imagination animates this physical world. Joy-filled amazement (*vismayo*) and being given to play (*kaimura*) are tell-tale traits both of the yogi who experiences these simultaneous and overlapping realities and of the writer given to delightfully questioning reality.

Essayists such as G. K. Chesterton (1874–1936) have a ready wonder with the real. In the essay "A Piece of Chalk," the British writer describes himself in despair because he came to a hill to draw with his colored chalk onto brown paper only to realize that he's forgotten "the most exquisite and essential chalk": the white piece. This leads him to argue—nay, to wonder in such a way that we almost cannot help but agree—that drawing with white chalk on brown paper illustrates that white is a color, a positive presence of color, not an absence of color. This assertion then sends his mind inventing a moral analogy that a virtue is not an absence of vice but a positive action: "Chastity does not mean abstention from sexual wrong; it means something flaming, like Joan of Arc." From personal fact to inventive assertion to risky analogy, this writer kept his boyish imagination alive throughout his writing life.

We can keep our writing fresh, too, by questioning our own constructs of reality. How we view time and space, our notions of "inner" and "outer," the material and immaterial, may be turned inside out and upside down. Jorge Luis Borges, like a curious boy, poses "What if?" questions and then lets his stories work them out to their logical or absurd conclusion. In "The Circular Ruins" the trickster author explores not only "What if a magician could imagine a boy into being?" but also "What if the magician were dreamed into being?" which leads us to wonder, "What if we each are someone else's image?" All characters do, and in some sense each of us does, indeed exist in someone else's imagination. Gabriel García Márquez also blends the fantastic with the ordinary in the oft-anthologized short story "The Very Old Man with Enormous Wings." Set in an impoverished South American village, the story is fueled by the question "What if an angel appeared in our own village?" Most readers may experience complex feelings, including disgust, when a poor couple cages the creature and sells tickets to view him, but we also likely feel strange wonder when the very old man, perhaps content that the couple with a new baby has made a stash of cash, rises from the sand and soars off.

This openness to surprise and wonder begins with presence of the ordinary waking world (*jāgrat*).

Any place, any moment, can suspend us in surprise. I was once standing in the middle of our road and staring at the glowing moon and blowing mist. I hadn't planned to stop there. I had intended to find the owners of a manic barking dog that kept interrupting my dreams, but once I stepped into the road, unable to follow the rude mongrel's path, I looked up and was struck by the hazy moonlight and translucent sheets of mist, by the buzzing power lines and power box in front of our neighbor's house, and by the street's stillness. For a moment everything floated as if the street had become an ocean floor, and I wondered if I were back in bed asleep and finally dreaming. But I was not. I don't think. Maybe the delirium of dreams and dogs' voices filtered my perception, but I savor such small surprises that inform much of how I write.

Try it: Get up in the middle of the night. Walk through your house in the dark. Walk down your street at 3:00 a.m. You might feel as if you're walking through someone else's dream. Write about your house or street's night side.

Or log a day and night. Keep a list of observations from the moment you arise, recalling brief dream images from the night before; then, note incidents from your morning routine, from work, from dinner, and finally from dreams again. Wonder in your writing like Nicholson Baker's Emmett about the miracle of such small stuff. If at day's end you have fewer than twelve entries, don't flagellate yourself for not heeding everything; congratulate yourself for altering your awareness even slightly. Be persistent. Try more the next day. In Gladys Cardiff's poem "Combing," her contemplation upon the simple ritual of caring for her daughter's hair reminds her of her mother and of her grandmother. This ritual, she concludes, is what women do for one another, "plaiting the generations."[5] Tend to the moment's depth. As you write about such a moment in whatever genre you choose, refrain from over-analyzing and straining for an epiphany (unless such tendencies suit your fictional narrator's proclivity). Keep it simple like the act itself you're performing.

When engaged with this waking world, regularly ask yourself, "What is real?" and "What if?" Get in the habit of listing a series of playful questions about reality. What if deer attacked people? (Horror story.) What if the older woman down the street fell in love with your husband? (Fiction, you hope.) What if we ate with our ears? What if mud made us cleaner than water? How do rose petals swim? (Lyrical poetry.) Pablo Neruda filled a volume with such thought problems, titled *The Book of Questions*. Alan Lightman's novella *Einstein's Dreams* is structured as if each chapter were one of the physicist's dreams about time. Each chapter then plays out the dream, fueled by one of Lightman's time questions: "What if time were at the center of town?" "What if in a village time ran backward?" Writers never stop asking questions (which is one reason we're so dangerous to people with unchecked power and so annoying to our friends).

Dreams also can be an immediate resource for questioning what is real and possible. I'm not into mind trips, but dreams still fascinate me, as they do other writers, because they stir up unconscious stuff that writing can play out sometimes without our readers ever knowing we're drawing from our dreams. Twilight time—that state we usually experience either just as we're falling asleep or as we're waking up—is a rich time for me to try to draw dream images for my writing. Where the waking state (*jāgrat*) and dreaming state (*svapna*) overlap, this twilight time also can be induced through meditative yoga movements and breathwork.

But beware when drawing from random images and dreams: Weirdness alone won't sustain a piece's quality or an audience's motivation to keep reading. "So what?" most readers will ask. And the answer usually must be more than simply revealing something quirky about the writer's imagination, personality, or "id." Most of us don't read to psychoanalyze writers, and writers usually don't write as dream therapy. When we ask, "So what?" we're wanting some glimmer, even if it's ambiguous, about being human and what we think is real.

To sleep, perchance to dream; to dream perchance to see what is real anew, that's what some of us write for and it's what your writing might do for your readers. The imagination offers us an entryway into, not an escape hatch from, reality's corridors.

It's not even 5 a.m. Something—an image of a neon book cover that zapped me awake or the cocoa from the fudge torte I relished too late last night—got me out of bed and to the study not one, not two, but three hours ago. I step out back and stand stunned by the full moon's empty stare. The maples that yesterday lit up with proud gold hats this morning look like bags of pale blue bones. Our barn, normally rustic red, residue from the nineteenth century, looks like a blue-faced storage shed. Night and moon make of my world a world of blues.

And then a chilling winnowing waves among the dark blue woods. It is the call of unbidden dreams, the screech owl that rides regret and strips pretense.

I can see nothing but blue. I know so little. I see so little even in my own backyard.

TAKE A BREATH: DREAM A ROUTINE

Intention:

Explore reality to charge your imagination and wonder. This practice might be most effective when just waking up, approaching sleep, or beginning regular routines. You may want to keep wholly open to the experience as it grants you brand new ideas for new material. You may want to resuscitate a near-dead story, essay, or poem that lacks fresh insight or imagination. You may wish to embody a character's point of view.

First, list some daily routines you or a character does around the house that would take no more than ten minutes to complete. Brushing your teeth, checking your e-mail, washing dishes, making oatmeal, hugging someone are some possibilities. Preferably, perform the following practice right before you engage in one of these routines.

Begin in a comfortable **LYING RELEASE / CORPSE POSE** (savāsana) *by resting on your back, knees bent or straight. As your back body melds with the earth, breathe two full inhalations and exhalations. Let this breath clear space for your intention. When ready, ask yourself, "What am I writing for?" After you acknowledge a response, clarify your specific writing intention.*

Then, become aware of how your breath travels through your body. With one hand, close off your right nostril, and breathe in through the left nostril. Then, breathe out only through the right nostril. Repeat this cycle of breath up to ten times while you imagine the breath's path like a colored subway coursing through your nostrils, down your throat, and into your lungs.

As you breathe normally again, imagine yourself or your character dreaming at this very moment. Dream yourself resting on your back here in this room. Don't rush this part. Let your breath be slow, easy, and smooth, even indistinct. Imagine the ground be-

neath you dissolving into ether. Imagine time unbound by clocks and space not driven by dimension.

When ready, actually open your eyes, yet continue to imagine you, your character dreaming. With slow, easy breathing, stand up, notebook in hand, and, in your character's body, walk around your house to begin your routine. You may feel slightly light-headed, but notice how your surroundings look, and notice how parts of your body feel as you walk. As your character turns the bathroom door-knob, for instance, notice how loose the knob is and how its metallic coolness almost stings your fingers. Perhaps the room you've entered sounds louder or quieter than usual. Engage in the routine with as much awareness as possible but with a child's delight.

While in the routine, let your character pose a playful question: "What if hair grew teeth?" "Who is dreaming me here?" "What if I were an eleven-year-old girl? What if I were an eighty-year-old man?" Embody that question.

Once you've finished—the exercise should last no more than ten minutes—begin writing by writing yourself or your character, gifted with this wondrous awareness, into the routine. Don't be shy. Let your readers know rather quickly what you or the character is doing—that is, refrain from making the piece sound like a mysterious dream or riddle. It's your piquant description mixed with authentic playful wonder—not trying to be "mysterious"—that will tantalize your readers. Enjoy the description, the playful speculation, the voice of pensive whimsy.

CHAPTER TEN

RAIN & THE BRAIN:
EMBODIED METAPHORS & SYMBOLS

R AIN, HURRICANE ISABEL'S GIFT blown in from the
Eastern coast, pours on a pond's skin, each drop rippling
shivers through the pond's body. More, more, the pond
utters as it drifts between waking and sleep, lulled by the rain's
caress. With each absorbed drop, the pond expands itself to test
just how much rain it can contain. Slowly, its surface swells over
its edges as its water bleeds into the soil and grass, the roots of
goldenrod and cattails, and, as if relinquishing a part of itself in
near sleep, releases water to the nearby brook. As rain subsides after several hours, the body rests again, content to house the three
box turtles that bark at passersby, the carp that feed off its weeds,
and the few frogs whose bellow brings on dusk. It's a good life this
pond has.

I swim in this pond each week of the warm months, but the
above description didn't come directly from a swim. It came from
this morning's Yoga session. While rain relentlessly fell on the roof
and meadows, I set my twofold intention to focus upon letting my
body grant me some new metaphorical understanding. I flowed
through a series of poses, focused on my breath, and then after
an hour rested in lying release pose (*savāsana*). My body relin-
quished the morning's tension as my thoughts centered at once
on the sound of my breath and that of rain. For a fleeting moment
an image of the pond in my torso surfaced, the rain popping on
my chest and arms, my back melting into muddy waters. Just for
a moment. I didn't force images, and I didn't fight occasional self-

conscious intrusions that analyzed them; instead, I just absorbed what I could. After sitting in meditation for only twenty minutes or so, I went to the desk, turned on the computer, and tried out a few sentences. The experience, primed by my yoga practice, gave me a new view of this pond I hold so dear.

Metaphors, most writers learn, are implied comparisons between two unlike things, as in "The long-necked ballerina glided across the stage" (ballerina to a swan). Similes, another kind of metaphor, make more direct comparisons by using like or as, such as "The unbridled child loped across the room like a wild horse." Symbols, simply put, are tangible things—objects, people, places, animals, events—invested with a meaning larger than what they literally are. Simple words or images or moments become signs to read. An antique writing desk owned by your grandfather means something more to you than treated pieces of wood fashioned into furniture. A friend of mine once said he distrusted poetry with metaphors and symbols. Direct and plain language he equates with honesty; metaphors, with showiness. When not harnessed, metaphors indeed might distort a piece of writing and hide rather than express a writer's authentic voice.

Authentic metaphors and symbols, however, are far more than ornaments to decorate an otherwise dully clothed page. They may be an expression of the body and the brain's innate yearning for meaning as well as for connectedness and interrelatedness among the universe's disparate things. Understood this way, authentic metaphors and symbols may reflect our embodied reality and can give us a powerful way to deepen and to alter our readers' understanding of our subject.

Consider that each of us may be made for metaphor-making. Our brains' synapses seem to delight in our making new connections, in having new thoughts, as some neurological research has shown that a brain's plasticity increases when a person forms new ideas and concepts. The process of making a metaphor stimulates significant regions of both the left and right hemispheres—regions that far surpass the Broca's brain region responsible for the simple utterance of literal words. In turn, when both hemispheres are stimulated, our brains can become primed for such linguistic novelty. In *The Midnight Disease*, neurologist Alice W. Flaherty suggests that metaphors' potency stems in part from the fact that producing and reading metaphors stimulate the brain's more rational cerebral cortex as well as the more affective limbic system. Thought and feeling entwine. Metaphors then can alter not just our minds and physical imaginations; they can alter our brain's shape as they play with our neuronal paths and our cellular dance. As they do for us, so they can do for our readers.

Our bodies shape our metaphors. Exploring the nature of our embodied perception can help us understand why and how we naturally create authentic metaphors. Metaphors are a form of novel categorization and recategorization, and the way our brains operate makes us "categorizing" beings. As George Lakoff and Mark Johnson contend in their book *Philosophy in the Flesh: The Embodied Mind and Its Challenge to Western Thought*, the human eye, for instance, contains a hundred million light-sensing cells but only one million fibers to connect sensations to the brain.[1] Just as a crowd of a thousand people wanting to buy plane tickets may stand efficiently in ten lines according to their last names, so the brain naturally categorizes sensory impulses via certain "fiber lines." The very nature of our bodies, Lakoff and Johnson suggest, make us categorize; it's what we're wired to do. Even how we formulate complex metaphors, they argue, stems from our physical experience. For instance, "Love is a journey" depends largely upon our direct encounters in taking trips, having mishaps, discovering joyful surprises, and questioning whether or not a trip's hardships were worth the trouble. That physical experience gives us the basis for understanding something as abstract as love, also rife with mishaps, surprises, and questions.[2]

Our minds constantly shift from receiving sensory input from the exterior world (what was introduced as the waking state, *jāgrat*, in the previous chapter) to entertaining thoughts and feelings and images in the interior world (the dreaming state, *svapna*). Our imaginations often link an impression from the exterior world to a feeling or thought. A writer's imagination may latch onto the uprooted birch behind his cottage because he's moved recently from his home state of California to Vermont. Much Zen poetry, including haikus, blur these distinctions between inner and outer worlds through subtle metaphor. Ezra Pound's haikulike Imagist poem "In a Station at the Metro" concisely captures this aesthetic: "The apparition of these faces in a crowd;/petals on a wet, black bough." The speaker ostensibly glimpses a faint mass of anonymous faces in Paris's subway station (clue from the title), and imagination's memory and metaphor-making ability links the mass of faces to a branch's petals. Crowd and bough, their sound and concept, bind the two lines and images. Metaphors connect realms of interior and exterior, subjective and objective.

One day within the next week, you might notice how you're feeling or what you're thinking or what you're imagining. Then, while feeling inward, get in the habit of looking outward. One student, for instance, was writing a story about a male character, sixty years old, who was unsure about getting married a second time. As she took a lunch break in Union Square, she noticed she was feeling queasy herself about starting a new job. Then, she looked around her and just noted what she saw: among other things, a man eating a hot dog, a dachshund licking its owner's fingers, and an old oak about to keel over. She penned in her notebook, "Ralph stood in the park, wondering how he could begin this next phase of his life—to remarry. A young man with shaved head sat on the bench next to him. He chuckled as he fed a dachshund bits of a hot dog. Suddenly Ralph felt his limbs about to fall off, his torso hollow and dried out, his whole body leaning, as if about to keel over, uprooted, unable to stand straight and steady. The young guy continued to laugh as the little dog gobbled shreds of processed cow parts." She projected her own queasiness about starting a new job onto her character and used the image of the dachshund munching on a wiener to suggest, comically, that feeling.

Metaphor is no linguistic flourish. Some principles from Yoga philosophy, from Vedanta to Shaivism, can help us understand how metaphors can express the nature of reality. "Yoga," notes the *Yoga-Bija* for instance, "is said to be the unification of the web of dualities."

Practicing Yoga helps us pay attention to how stimuli from the outside world affect and reflect the inside one and vice-versa. We can become attuned to how our mind's habitual thoughts and images shape how we act and what we do in the world, and likewise we might note how the changes in our physical body begin to change the habitual patterns of our emotions, our thoughts, our images—in short, our subtle body. If our bodies influence our perceptions, then when we change our physiology and the ways our brains function, our whole worldview can follow suit.[3]

A friend of mine likes to argue that our bodies' bilateral system accounts for a dualistic reality. "We see with a left and a right eye, we hear with a left and a right ear, we breathe with a left and a right lung; we need dualities." Left-right, left-right, his argument marches along.

Maybe he's correct in some ways, but our body's physiology also complicates matters. Breathing through the right nostril has been shown to stimulate the brain's left hemisphere and vice-versa. And just as the left nostril stimulates a channel of energy that correlates to the parasympathetic nervous system, which cools down a person's energy, the right nostril, which stimulates the brain's left hemisphere, in turn connects to a path of energy associated with the hot sun called the "tawdry channel" (*pingalā-nādi*). Breathing solely through the right nostril has been shown to quicken the sympathetic nervous system and thus heat up the body.[4] These two lines of energy, according to texts such as the *Hatha-Yoga-Pradipika*, spiral up and down on either side of the spine (not unlike, incidentally, a DNA double helix or like the two winding serpents in Hippocrates' caduceus—the ancient emblem of healing and now the symbol for Western medicine).

The practice of Yoga links these seeming left-right dualities of body and energy. In fact, one esoteric translation of *Hatha*, as in "Hatha-Yoga," is "sun-moon" (*ha*=sun; *tha*=moon). Through Yoga, we gradually may be able to experience how what we perceive as light is dark, how we find ourselves in getting lost, for we, too, embody metaphor and paradox. Not coincidentally, a favorite Yoga practice among writers is **ALTERNATE NOSTRIL BREATHING** (*nādī-shodhana prānāyāma)*, a practice that can harmonize the brain's hemispheres and, thus, prime your brain and body for metaphor making. If practiced carefully for long periods of time, not only are both hemispheres communicating but the frontal cortex also corresponds with the emotional limbic system. The brain's boundaries break down.

Some quantum physicists, Western science's yogis, verify the universe's non-duality. The more intricately physicists delve into the universe's laws, the more paradoxical it becomes. Chaos brings order and life, and time may be timeless, as Nobel Prize–winner Ilya Prigogine's research indicates. Nature replicates its patterns, a fact that suggests to several scientists the inherent interrelatedness of all things. A leaf's veins branch out like a tree's limbs. A tree's limbs feather out like a bird's wings or like a brain's neuronal folds. The patterns we find in some snowflakes reflect the patterns that sound vibrations can create in sand. No wonder, then, physicists and science writers recognize that metaphors are not simply flourishes, extraneous to the language of logic, but are expressions of our embodied perception and, perhaps, of nature's nature.

All of this is to say that writers find ways to let language maneuever these realities. We let language flip conceptual categories inside-out because we sense, intuitively or not, that not everything is neatly boxed on clearly labeled shelves.

When divorce or loss leaves you alone, you likely do not feel—if you feel anything—one simple emotion easily tagged as "grief" or "relief." Instead, you likely feel both and more, a complex of emotions, emotions that logically would belong on opposite ends of the emotional body ("Grief on the right; relief on the left," my friend might say.), congealed like a plexus of nerves in your heart. How as a writer do you sort through such a plexus with emotional honesty for a poem's speaker or novel's or memoir's character?

Jane Hirshfield's poem "Standing Deer" meets this challenge. Stanzas mirror one another as she explores a mind's emptying that gets filled, a heart's filling that empties, the dawn's possibilities and the dusk's satisfaction, until barely a line passes that is not a metaphor or paradox collapsing in on the previous one, the poem a universe unto itself. And why not? Among the debris of a crumbled relationship and the reality constructed therein, the poem's speaker rebuilds from the rubble a new set of paradoxical planks on which to stand and move forward. If Blake explores the marriage of heaven and hell, Hirshfield explores the union of emptiness and fulfillment in separation.

Authentic metaphors and symbols hint of such connectivity without forcing mysticism into our writing.

In the essay "Transfiguration," from Annie Dillard's book *Holy the Firm*, the author recounts how she, seeking solitude and rejuvenation as a writer, camped alone for a few days and took with her to reread *The Day on Fire*, a novel about the meteoric poet Arthur Rimbaud, who nearly burned out his creative light by age nineteen. While Dillard read by candlelight, a moth kept flying closer and closer to the flame until at last it found the light literally, its body aflame:

> The wax rose in the moth's body from her soaking abdomen to her thorax to the jagged hole where her head should be, and widened into flame, a *saffron-yellow flame* that *robed* her to the ground like any *immolating monk*.... She burned for two hours ... glowing within, like a building fire glimpsed through silhouetted walls, like a *hollow saint*, like a *flame-faced virgin gone to God*, while I read by her light, kindled, while Rimbaud in Paris burnt out his brains in a thousand poems, while night pooled wetly at my feet.[5]

The religious metaphors (emphasis mine) compare the moth to a saint sacrificing herself to God's light, and—by extension of the author's desire for rejuvenation and her reading of the Rimbaud book—the moth symbolizes the sacrifice sometimes necessary to be a writer, to be transfigured. In the essay's next section, Dillard asks her writing students which of them will sacrifice their lives to become writers. Her metaphors create a bridge within us between our vaporous ideas of "religious sacrifice" and a writer's sacrifice and tangible things like a moth flying into a candle. With these metaphors, familiar distinctions break down. I imagine Dillard opening up a window to see which metaphors fly on the page's white sky.

We do not have to set out to write with metaphors. Just as personal symbols emerge naturally from our own experience and environment, so, too, do some authentic metaphors and symbols in writing emerge from the body of work itself, from the act of writing itself, and from a story's context and language. In Flannery O'Connor's short story "Good Country People," for instance, a girl has a wooden leg. O'Connor said that while writing the story, she didn't know the leg would become symbolic of the girl's vulnerability and limitations. But by the time O'Connor was writing the climactic scene, in which a con man dupes her by posing as a Bible salesman, has sex with her, and then takes her leg and leaves her, O'Connor knew the leg had become symbolic.

Similarly, many of the moth metaphors and symbols from Dillard's experience came only years later when Dillard felt compelled to revisit her journal's notes and begin weaving her memory's images into the essay. Each of those religious metaphors contributes to the others' meaning, and they wouldn't have the same resonance without Dillard's situation of seeking some insight to rekindle her spark to write. An authentic metaphor derives its charged meaning from its relationship to other words within the same piece, just as part of a body functions in accord with the other parts. Otherwise, lavish metaphors and symbols seem forced and disembodied, or removed from the text's body.

Take a walk and try to find at least ten leaves not on or from trees. That is, try to find ten things whose shape and/or function resembles trees' leaves. Or seek out ten things whose shape resembles a hand or a face. Look up, down, upside down. Doing so will remind you of nature's and our bodies' self-replicating patterns. Then, write a prose description of the items, in which you seek to explore their metaphorical reality. As you write, start heeding the words you employ to refer to the things in the world. How does the word *tree* relate to the wooden form with leaves we call tree? How does the word *sidewalk* relate to the squares of cement we call, without thinking, sidewalks? What other concepts nest inside tree or trunk? What's the root of *tree*? Play with the words to see what surprising revelations and connections surface.

Dig around in words' roots. Writers often unearth words' metaphorical origins and discover language's metaphorical nature, a realization that readies writers to derive the most charge from their words. Rummage through a source such as Eric Partridge's *Origins: A Short Etymological Dictionary of Modern English*, and you'll discover that many words, born from our physical and sensory experiences, reveal a metaphorical base. The root of courage, for instance, is the Latin cor, meaning "heart." I imagine some twelve hundred years after the Romans named the physical organ, the Medieval French—based upon their immediate wartime experience of blood rushing through them, chests swelling, and brains reeling—formed a word that may translate to "full of heart," *curage*, which gave the English not only courage but the siblings *encourage* and *discourage*. Similarly, after the Romans named the mouth's slippery but tangible organ *lingua*, the French named the abstract phenomenon of words uttered from the mouth and tongue *langue*, which gave us the English "language." The tongue gives us *language*. Many of us may know our words' roots. My point is, though, that we form words that express abstract concepts quite often from immediate, concrete experience. Our body's myriad nerve endings and our brain's sensory receptors, imagination, and intellect compel us to generate, utter, sputter, and write metaphors.

Language is metaphorical. A story among some Northeastern American Indian tribes tells of a young man asking a wisewoman, "What does the earth rest on?" "A turtle's shell," she said. "And what does that turtle stand on?" "Another turtle," she said. "It's turtles all the way down." A friend of mine once said the same thing about language and its reflection of reality: "It's metaphors all the way down." The authentic metaphors we discover in writing extend language's nature in an artful and pleasurable way that can change how our readers feel and think. Perhaps such metaphors delight us because they can alter our constructs of reality. When boundaries break down, we're one breath away from bliss.

The pond has fractaled into ice patches over night for the first time this season. The thin ice sheet looks like Saran Wrap pulled tight over Big Mama's bowl to be stored in her invisible freezer. The wrap wrinkles in shapes of arrows and heron tracks, though no heron would dare walk this thin ice. The patterns reflect how the pond's liquid body is drawn in, constricted by cold. She's an old one, this pond, by farmer's standards, but each winter she reveals her innate intelligence.

My muscles, too, have tightened in the few weeks leading up to Thanksgiving. Cold air winds up my hamstrings, and my lower trapezious attached to my rib cage aches. But this morning, like every morning, I get on my hands and knees and trust that this one complex shape-shifting metaphor and reservoir of metaphors has tracks to follow.

TAKE A BREATH #1:
MINE THE MOMENT FOR A METAPHOR

Intention:

Engage this practice when you need an original metaphor that comes directly from your environment. You may simply wish to heighten your innate ability to create metaphors. This practice introduces you to **ALTERNATE NOSTRIL BREATHING** *(nādī-shodhana prānāyāma)*, which can harmonize the brain's hemispheres and, thus, prime your brain and body for metaphor-making.

Sit comfortably. **EASY CROSS-LEGGED POSE** (sukhāsana) *or* **ADAMANTINE/KNEELING POSE** (vajrāsana) *or even sitting in a chair will work. Take in at least two full breaths. Then, ask yourself what you are writing for. Once you've absorbed a response, clarify to yourself your specific writing subject. Simplify the subject into a core noun, abstract or concrete, such as* Mother, Gerald, basketball, heavy metal music, grief. *Clarify, too, that you seek metaphorical insight into this subject.*

With eyes still closed, hear with your inner ear the noun for your subject, and notice how the word feels as it courses through your body with your breath. Notice if it sticks anywhere in your body. Let it settle there.

With your subject sufficiently embodied, lengthen your spine, and rest your left hand on your thigh and lift your right hand. Fold the index and middle finger in toward the thumb base, and bring your right hand to your nose. Set your thumb tip on the outside of the right nostril; your ring and little finger along the left. Close your eyes. Close the left nostril, and slowly exhale through the right. Fill your lungs with an inhalation through the right nostril. Close the right nostril, open the left, and exhale all of the way through the left nostril. Inhale fully through the left nostril. Repeat three to five times.

Sit for a few more breaths, and fine-tune your outer senses. Hear what's going on outside of you. Take in the aroma of the air with your next inhalation. Coat your tongue with saliva. Feel your skin. Then focus on the backs of your eyelids.

When you open your eyes, notice what object, sound, smell, taste, or sensation seizes your imagination. A cardinal's chirp near dusk. The slant of smoggy light sneaking through the window slats. Whatever the sensation, absorb it.

When ready, begin writing a piece of prose or poetry that metaphorically links your subject to whatever image seizes you. Refrain from forcing obvious connections. Describe the subject and trust that a link to the external sensation will surface, or describe the sensation and write your way to the subject. Or you can begin with a direct sentence such as "My mother stretches and looms like the hickory in our front yard" or "Grief spreads out and dampens the ground, the aftermath of a good rain that has cooled you down, brought you down to the soil." Then allow connections to surface. Be receptive to the piece of writing's context so that the metaphors spring naturally both from your body and from the body of words.

TAKE A BREATH #2: RE-IMAGINE A BODY

Intention:

Reimagine metaphorically the nature of your body or the nature of a character's body for your writing.

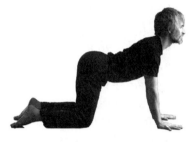

Come onto your hands and knees, aligned beneath your shoulders and hips respectively. Let the tops of your feet rest on your mat or blanket. Eyes closed, take at least two full breaths. Set your intention by asking yourself what you are writing for. Then clarify your more specific writing intention. If you're writing personally, set out to imagine your body metaphorically, or, if you're writing about someone else or a fictional character, ready yourself to project your experiences into his or her perspective. Take another three full breaths as you feel the connection between earth and your hands.

While you center on your breath's movements, sense what it feels like to inhabit this body. Does it move with grace and ease like a river or a greased machine? If it had its choice, what would be its preferred mode of travel? Flying? Crawling? Swimming? Hang gliding?

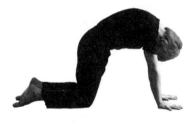

Keeping firm in your hands' mounds and base knuckles, experiment with moving in this pose: Inhale to let your back curve as your heart sinks toward the mat and as your tailbone arches upward; exhale to arch your upper back toward the ceiling and drop your tailbone. Then, look over your left shoulder while you curve the side of your torso to the right and repeat on the other side. You can drop your hips toward the floor on each side to stretch your torso and the hips' external muscles, and you can bring your hips toward your heels to stretch your shoulder girdles. Intuit how this body wants to move the self that inhabits it. If the body wishes to shift the pose in some way, follow it.

As you glide in each position and from one to the next, appreciate the sensations in your body and any images from your physical or subtle imagination that may surface. What is this body? What is this body like that resonates with your self or with the self of your subject? Is it something from the natural world? Could something from the city express its core? For several breaths, just move with this pose, your body, imagination, and the language that surfaces.

The pose you've been playing with is called **CAT POSE** (marjarāsana). *So you might explore whether or not this body metaphorically could curl up on branches or tops of doors and whether or not it could chase after birds and mice. This body may creak a bit like my twelve-year-old gray cat's arthritic body that still musters enough courage, enough heart, to fend off dogs and deer. If so, acknowledge it.*

Then, begin writing a piece that explores one of the metaphorical connections that seemed most authentic. I suggest you place your narrator or character in a situation or place to give the writing context. Describe the subject's body in action and let the metaphorical connections unfold naturally. As you write a piece of prose, fiction, or poetry, be open to how each word's nuance may proffer new insight. Assume whatever tone—serious, humorous, a favorite cat's point of view—that suits your experience and your intention.

CHAPTER ELEVEN

BLISS IN A TOOTHBRUSH: WRITING INTO THINGS

I T'S POSSIBLE, I KNOW IN MY BONES, now. You can become, if only for a fleeting moment, a birch tree standing stalwart on a hill whose limbs the animate air invigorates, a beet in a lover's salad that drips with passion, a humble stone rubbed against another that sparks messages from its inner walls. You can be in bliss. To be in bliss, to be bliss, has been one of Yoga's ancient ends. To be in bliss is not simply to be giddy with delight, nor is it something that need be mystified. Bliss, *samādhi*, is a state of being wholly content while connected with, not transcendent of, this material world of toothbrushes and turnips.[1] We enter bliss when, even if only for a breath or two, the ego self releases its conventional view of reality, we glimpse the essential nature of some object, and our thoughts and sense of self merge with the thing and its referent. Borders between subject and object dissolve. Thus, one of the oldest and most effective ways for being in bliss is to concentrate on an object.

To be in bliss as a writer you need not go into trances or have visions of deities. And I would never promise that you will or even should be in bliss. I'll just posit that it's possible and perhaps desirable as a writer. To write in bliss is a natural way to extend what we've considered in earlier chapters: concentration, voice, presence, wonder, metaphor.

Reality—a word whose root is res, Latin for "thing"—involves our awareness of thoughts and of the material world. This interplay between thought and thing prompts many of us to write, for writing is an open inquiry into the nature of reality, however seriously or comically we wish to approach that inquiry. Our writing, in turn, can become a vehicle that prompts our readers to reflect upon their own reality, the way in which their own thoughts weave through this world of things.

Around a hundred years ago, poet Rainer Maria Rilke, in his early thirties, received some advice from the sculptor Auguste Rodin that changed Rilke's view of reality and writing. Stop thinking in the abstract, the sculptor told the poet, and work with your eyes, learn from your eyes. Rilke took the advice to heart and wrote to a lover-friend, "Somehow I, too, must come to make things; not plastic, but written things—realities that emerge from handwork." And so Rilke did. In the next six years he would write about two hundred such poems, whose subjects range from a panther in a zoo, to a candle, a bed, and a statue of Adonis. The writer's task, Rilke writes in his *Duino Elegies*, is to imagine and to say this world's objects in ways that not even the objects themselves could imagine being. Bridge. Tree. Jug. These become the poet's subjects.

During the twentieth century, a century of mass production, numerous writers heard Rilke's cry to tend to these things. Francis Ponge. Zbigniew Herbert. Wysalla Zymborska. Jane Hirshfield. These poets also let a world of objects float in their hearts.

But before you fiction writers turn the page and think bliss be the fanciful province of poets alone, consider the question, "Can forks talk in fiction?" That's the question, in essence, Charles Baxter explores in an essay titled "Talking Forks: Fiction and the Inner Life of Objects." Baxter reviews John Ruskin's idea from the nineteenth century that writers should avoid projecting their own emotions onto objects—an "error" Ruskin calls "the pathetic fallacy." Objects and place, so the theory goes, are there simply as props for the human agents, the characters, nothing more. Modern fiction and poetry allegedly got a divorce over the issue, leaving objects in the emotional custody of poets. "According to the terms of the divorce," Baxter says, "sentient objects can appear in poetry such as Rilke's, but not in fiction. The blunt materialistic common sense of fiction is supposed to resist this reconciliation [between subject and object]. But it doesn't, anymore, if it ever did."[2]

I would add that fiction writers such as Nabokov, Tom Robbins, Nicholson Baker, and nonfiction writers such as Annie Dillard and Nancy Mairs so illuminate this world of small things that as the writer's eye and tongue and imagination play with and identify with the object, that your sense of self, if only for a moment, can shift, heighten, even dissolve.

Your discovery of bliss in being a writer won't happen necessarily in a meditation hall or even in a yoga class. A meditation cushion and a mat can prime your body, imagination, and spirit for the real deal, which often visits writers in the living room, on a street or basketball court, and at the desk. In Lucille Clifton's poem "Cutting Greens," the speaker, preparing a meal, loses herself for a moment, in love with the blackness of everything around her and on her, including her skin, feeling "the bond of live things everywhere." Bliss flashes in the flesh. Maxine Kumin feels the bond while raking horse dung in "The Excrement Poem." Infinity is in the ordinary—a flower bed, a bowl of oatmeal, your blouse, a letter. The subtle surfaces of the plastic toothbrush you've used to scrub the tub for five years can become a primer for bliss.

Your description of toilet paper or crepe myrtle anchors your readers in a bathroom or in the South. They get their bearings. But an extended description of a thing also can become a form of aesthetic concentration and meditation in which the writer artfully follows the ways thing and thought relate. Take the protagonist in Nicholson Baker's *The Mezzanine*. The entire action of the novella takes place during a young businessman's escalator ride as he returns from his lunch hour. One escalator ride, 130 pages. The first eight pages detail why he asked a clerk for a plastic bag. Another eight pages follow his thoughts on broken shoelaces. Near the novel's middle, he observes his own crisp dry-cleaned shirt, which prompts him to describe for eight pages a memory of putting on one of the five shirts, newly dry cleaned, that he owned when he first got his job. The memory of opening the package leads him to observe, among many other facets of dry-cleaned shirts, that they were "wrinkled with positive kinds of semiintentional knife-edge creases and perpendicular fold-lines that only heightened the impression of ironedness, having come about either as a result of the occasionally indiscriminate force of the pressing and starching machines (such as the crow's-feet on the sleeve near the cuffs) or as a result of the final careful foldup."[3] This guy loves the textures of things.

In this same memory, he recalls how on the subway to work he had had a startling self-realization: He's the sort of person who doesn't think about, say, economics or politics or even his own personal demons, but about buttering raisin toast. As Baker's characters think thoroughly about superficial surfaces—a contemporary Proust with a busier life and less predictable wit—his descriptions and trains of thought keep us suspended in pregnant present moments whose edges round out like bowls around the past and future. As delightfully self-conscious and hyperobservant as Baker's protagonists may seem, they're also quite content, if not blissful. No pages here of psychoanalysis, of anxious fretting about the world's or a marriage's end, of guilt-laden confessions. They—and by extension, we the readers—find bliss in this world of things. We could do worse as writers whose grandest epiphanies have to do with, say, dog smells instead of God's scent. It's easy to bemoan this world of things; more challenging to praise it.

Although gazing on and receiving objects actually is an ancient Yoga practice, if practiced well, it can constitute a new encounter each time. Think about what can happen when you direct your thoughts toward an object. Mind and object engage in a reciprocal communication. We practice one-pointed concentration.

If you focus on the lampshade on your desk, your eyes, fingers, and your brain's nerve receptors take in the thin, smooth, barklike lines of the cloth stretched from end to end. You consider the word *lamp*, and subtle thoughts and images may surface as you explore its relationship to the desk, the electric current buzzing through its body, its willing gift of light. Memory may intervene as you recall your poor grandmother's house full of shadeless lamps, this being one of them, the naked bulbs exposed and proud. Awareness of the future illuminates that in a hundred years this lamp may be disposed of and disassembled into so many glass shards, screws, and wires. Your mind and imagination reveal the thing's nature, and it in turn reveals your nature—ephemeral yet part of the same basic atomic stuff.

This contemplation is the first step of what Patanjali calls in the Yoga-Sutra "bliss with support" (*samprajnāta samādhi*). Possibly, for a moment, these associations, analogies, temporal references, and thoughts such as "I am observing a lamp" vanish while thoughts merge with the thing, and the thing's essential meaning reveals itself. You simply stop thinking if only for a breath. When you approach an object anew, when you forget your preconceptions of a thing—its typical function, its socially constructed significance— you also can awaken a dormant part of your consciousness that offers you insight, however poignant or banal, into the nature of a thing and into material reality. Blake sensed it in a grain of sand, Whitman in a blade of grass, Ginsberg in a building's bricks. Now, what that revelation is—or "epiphany," to evoke Joyce's similar process based on St. Thomas Aquinas's ideas—will be, should be, unique for each of us in each new encounter.

Our brains must love such fresh insight. As mentioned before, several studies performed on advanced meditators indicate that their brain waves slowed down to the alpha state with some traces of theta brain waves (four to eight cycles per second). In this state, a sort of relaxed yet alert state, the embodied unconscious raises random images and impressions to awareness. Such suggestions may be the stuff of what in Yoga we call *dhiti* or revelation. Some recent studies show how, when highly creative people are engaged in creative work, cerebral blood flow increases significantly, the activity stimulates considerably more parts of the brain to cooperate, and nitric oxide releases neurotransmitters that release endorphins, the brain chemicals that induce deep pleasure and contentment. Similar physiological responses have been measured in people in deep relaxation.[4] Another study in Holland illustrates that nitric oxide, abundant in the sinuses, can be stimulated through conscious nasal breathing and humming on the exhalation. No wonder being creative and breathing deeply can be blissful. Bliss has a biological basis. Certain yoga practices that increase cerebral blood flow, stimulate nitric oxide, and slow down our brain's waves can be ideal ways to prime our bodies and imagination for bliss.

Your writing itself can be blissful. Of course, it can be excruciating as well and involves a heck of a lot of clipping, cutting, grimacing, complaining, and tossing. But if we're open to the possibility and prepare our bodies, we also can have at least a few moments of unmediated bliss. Sustained observation causes images to be stored in the physical imagination. In the writing process, as the brain and the body's cells and nerve receptors orchestrate a concert for a piece of writing, these stored images can mix your immediate experience with words on the page, as well as with your subtle imagination's seemingly random associations and imagery. The self gets out of the way, and language and imagination take over. Fresh images, metaphors, and music arise to bring things together, to unify, to make bliss.

We don't need to mystify these "experiences," for they're rare for me and other writers I know, mixed between a lot of patient pushing and waiting, of tinkering with and trashing drafts. Yet, something significant occasionally does stir me in the moment of writing as thought merges with words—the sense, the sounds, the innuendos—and rather than pushing words up a hill like a chugging locomotive, the train of thought and the words and images and their referents themselves carry my self to forgotten villages. And then it's back to the joys of clipping, cutting, pasting.

We can avoid mystifying writing while at the same time celebrating ordinary life's mysteries. That's my main caveat here and elsewhere in this book. To chase after bliss or mystical moments at the expense of this life, this world, this sentence, both misses the point and sets you up for disappointment and frustration. I think of Edward in Eugene O'Neill's *Long Day's Journey Into Night*, who pines to his father about how all he wants is to experience again what he experienced on a boat years before: with the wind howling like a hungry dog, mist flying from the waves that rocked the boat, the sky dark and vast above him, his body meshed with everything. He was everything. He was bliss. As his father sneers that Edward's idealism will doom him, Edward recites Baudelaire's poem "Be Intoxicated." Sure, you can take Baudelaire's advice and get drunk with wine, with poetry, with virtue, or with altered states of consciousness, but a startling sobriety that awakens you to this world of things isn't such a bad path either.

It's a humbling act. Giving your attention for several minutes, hours even, to coffee grains or worn-out socks rather than to "big" ideas like global warming or economics sends your ego and mind a message: "Be small." The ego can quiet down as it stops trying to figure out things and instead appreciates and receives a thing; our sense of separation from the world's things changes and potentially widens our heart's and our readers' heart's field.

TAKE A BREATH: GAZE

Intention:

This practice can increase your cerebral blood flow, slow down your brain waves, and prepare your embodied imagination for a fresh perspective into the nature of an object, of thinking, and of consciousness. Set a specific intention to perceive the animate quality of an object.

Choose an object, or, better, let one choose you. A kitchen utensil, a tool, a pair of socks, something without preconceived sentimental value, works best. Or step into some woods or on a street. Walk with your breath until you happen upon a simple totem—a river stone stranded beneath some leaves, a turtle shell becoming dust, a tossed mailbox half-buried in the soil, a piece of bark shaped like your home state. Sit before it. **ADAMANTINE POSE** (vajrāsana) *or* **ADEPT'S POSE** (siddhāsana) *works best for this practice, but please choose a pose in which you can feel at ease but alert for several minutes. Close your eyes. Grow firm but soft in your seat. Take at least two full breaths and ask yourself, "What am I writing for?" Be patient. Then, clarify that you intend to see some object anew for your writing.*

Open your eyes and practice non-attached looking. For two breaths, move your eyes up between your eyebrows without looking. Then for two breaths, shift your eyes as far to the right as they will go without looking or fixing your eyes and thoughts on anything. Then do the same by moving your eyes down, then to the left.

When ready, close your eyes and perform the same rotation measured by two breaths each.

After five breaths, open your eyes normally, and as you let your thoughts hover upon the object's general outline, acknowledge the common word used to refer to it. Take in its shell in form and name: "tree," "ball," "nail clipper." Close your eyes, and let the image's imprint rest on the insides of your eyelids. From physical imagination's memory, fill out its edges and colors, its textures and surfaces. Then, open your eyes halfway and scan the object from left to right, up and down, noting each nook, crevice, scratch, shift in shade.

While you hold your gaze like a rock in a stream, let your thoughts float by like sticks in a stream. Imagine its history. Its origins. Its multiple functions and roles in the world and its future.

Close your eyes again, and imagine its interior life. Breathe deeply and let roll from your subtle imagination a stream of visual and other metaphors that illuminate the thing's thing-ness.

Then, follow your breath from your belly's base to your third eye as you envision the object as yourself. You may see the object overlapped upon your body's form or vice-versa. You may imagine yourself as having no form, only some essence that enters the object's form. Stay with this image for several breaths and observe what it feels like to be this thing without forcing its qualities into the human realm, without projecting your personality into it. Instead, let it enter you.

*Whenever you're ready, open your eyes and write a prose piece or poem in which you try to capture in imagery and rhythm this thing's nature in relation to "I." Yet, do so with a natural voice, without seeming cryptic or obtuse. A **narrative piece** may recount parts of what your narrator just experienced or may follow the thing's history. A **lyrical piece** may begin praising the thing's qualities. An **exploratory piece** may move back and forth in perspective between your narrator's "self" and the thing. Perhaps there are moments of mergence and of separation. Maybe metaphor links the two. Of course, you can experiment with point of view as well, particularly if you're writing fiction. You might aim to describe the object's es-*

sence. Select concrete, sensuous words, and honor the object's uniqueness by finding the particular details that distinguish it. Try not to follow personal streams of association or sentiment. Instead, be open to the bliss of writing itself. Let one word, one image, one sound, lead you to the next, not knowing exactly to which cobblestone streets or cedar-chipped flower beds that words will lead.

CHAPTER TWELVE

LISTENING TO THE SUNRISE: MUSIC IN POETRY & PROSE

I N THE DARK EARLY MORNING nearly fifteen years ago, a silhouette of a man stood outside my house at the corner sidewalk. For several minutes I watched him from my bedroom window as his form barely moved. An hour later, when I pulled out of my driveway to go teach, he still stood there utterly still. I drove past and waved, but he didn't flinch. It was Edward, a retired fellow who lived five houses down the road. This same thing happened for several weeks. After the fourth time, I stopped waving.

One Saturday as I mowed my lawn, my one physical respite at the time, Edward walked by. I waved. He waved back and smiled. I stopped the mower and walked toward him. His red cardigan, checkered pants, and patent leather loafers assured me I was in Mr. Roger's neighborhood instead of the urban 'hood the area had a reputation for being.

"Can I ask you something?" I said. He nodded. "Each morning I notice you standing at the street corner, and you don't move. Are you concentrating on something?"

"Yes," he said dead-panned. "I'm listening to the sunrise." My eyebrows furrowed. He explained that if you (he, I) stand perfectly still in the right place at the right time you can hear the sunrise. He had tested out several spots along the street, and the corner had the clearest signal.

"Oh," I said. "I was just wondering." I nodded and returned to the vibrations of the lawnmower and my rattling head.

Several years and an unwound body later, I still have never heard the sunrise. Still, I have learned to hear other things.

Rain "thwapping" between evergreens and service berries dots the early autumn forest floor of fallen leaves. Its sound beats irregularly against the steady stream that falls over the small dammed wall a few yards away. My car's transmission could drop to the street, a tree could fall on my roof, but if I can walk into the woods to listen to nature sweet-talk me, then all is right, and I'm in love with the world again.

Most of us, I suspect, are suckers for such sounds. They vibrate us on a frequency we rarely detect in our workaday world. A million people a year visit Niagara Falls, not only because of the spectacle but also, I suspect, because of the audible. Its water drum quivers our body's dancing atoms as if experiencing the universe's creation itself. The Judeo-Christian Yahweh uttered speech to create the world in six days, St. John's famous book suggests "the Word" (the Greek logos) started spinning things into shape, and the Hindu Shiva's rattling drum beat into being the patterned matter of creation. (Imagine how we'd dance together in the streets if Yahweh could sing to Shiva's drum.) Some scientists contend it all started with a loud sound, a bang. Pythagoras, that figure who haunted our geometry classes, intuited this music of the spheres as did the scientist Johannes Kepler. Whether that sound was God's voice, Shiva's drum, or exploding atoms, this planet we inhabit nonetheless circles to a series of musical rhythms latent within its rivers and stones, even within its roads and streets. Our bone marrow may contain the same sonic stuff as the melody of a stream, the cacophony of a street, or the symphony of a star.

No wonder certain words, combined in a sentence or series of sentences, ring true and bring joy. The first sentence of Joyce's Portrait of the *Artist as a Young Man* suggests a primordial relationship between narrative's music and the birth of consciousness: "Once upon a time and a very good time it was there was a moocow coming down along the road and this moocow that was down along the road met a nicens little body name baby tuckoo....."[1] Such was Stephen Daedalus's earliest memory, a story his father invented and near-sang. Several writers sense that combinations and repetitions of sounds in prose or poetry, repeated with the right regularity, bring us delight or delirium.

"I just don't hear the music," a writer once bemoaned. "I guess my ears don't work that way." But I suspect each of us has an inner ear that lets us hear how words work on the inner vestibule. It's a matter of tuning in and of dropping deeply in. When we tune in to poetry's and prose's music, then sense and sound can play off of one another, and we can hear how repetition of sounds can imbue our writing with authentic musicality.

Sound clusters in English, the tongue of engineers, hold incantory power. The poet Gerard Manley Hopkins sensed it so. In his journals, he lists groups of words with similar sound clusters and then beneath or beside such a cluster writes a word that seems to sum up some essential resonance. He writes, "mead/meadow/ meat/maid" and beneath it, "(blooming and bearing fruit")." He writes, "crook/crank/crick/cranky" and beneath it, "(not straight)." What is it in the *cr* and *k* that holds this family of words together? Is it something in the way our mouths move to shape the syllables that vibrates some sense beyond meaning? Hopkins not surprisingly strings his poems with finely tuned combos.

This sound stuff isn't just a poet's province; the best prose writers sense it too. William Gass claims, "No prose can pretend to greatness if its music is not also great; if it does not, indeed, construct a surround of sound to house its meaning the way flesh was once felt to embody the soul."[2]

Some novelists follow words' undulations and not just their definitions, as Faulkner so often did. In the following passage from his short story "The Bear," the boy protagonist stands next to his mentor, Sam Fathers, who has taught him for years how to navigate the woods among men so he might spy the mighty bear that his father and his father's father have hunted for generations. The boy suddenly feels in his body the looming meaning of hunting the bear. It's a terrifying exhilaration of primal wilderness itself, that link between us and the natural world that is raw strength and courage and instinct:

> Then, standing beside Sam in the thick great gloom of ancient woods and the winter's dying afternoon, he looked quietly down at the rotted log scored and gutted with claw-marks and, in the wet earth beside it, the print of the enormous warped two-toed foot. Now he knew what he had heard in the hounds' voices in the woods that morning and what he had smelled when he peered under the kitchen where they huddled. It was in him, too, a little different because they were brute beasts and he was not, but only a little different....[3]

The woods' atmosphere, combined with the sight of the bear's spoors—the gutted log and the footprint—trigger in the boy a visceral sensation that connects him to what the hunting dogs feel and know. In the first sentence, the hard "oo" of gloom and afternoon plus the soft "oo" of woods, looked, and foot hold these words together in their mutual combined effect on the boy. His connection with the hounds' instinct is reinforced subtly in the second sentence through the repeated whispering h's and the thudding d's. Words' sounds as much as sense hold together this passage's effect.

Some sounds can just crack us up. The following not-so-subtle excerpt comes from the closing of humorist Suzanne Britt's essay "That Lean and Hungry Look," in which she reverses stereotypes about fat people versus skinny people:

> Fat people will grab, giggle, guffaw, gallumph, gyrate, and gossip. They are generous, giving, and gallant. They are gluttonous and goodly and great. What you want when you're down is soft and jiggly, not muscled and stable. Fat people know this. Fat people have plenty of room. Fat people will take you in.[4]

The last paragraph's repetition of sounds builds upon the essay's rhythm to a comical climax. The repeated hard g sound almost imitates the gurgling chortle and jiggling gut of the essay's heroic Everyfatperson. Too, we can't help but notice how she reverses the stereotypical virtues of our Protestant work ethic and Catholic cardinal sins when she conjoins "gluttonous and goodly and great," the added ands echoing the King James Bible's incantatory cadences.

In the chapter "The Present" from Annie Dillard's Pulitzer Prize–winning nonfiction *Pilgrim at Tinker Creek*, Dillard stops at a gas station for some coffee after hours of driving along a mind-numbing freeway. There, she steps behind the station, pets someone's puppy, and watches the sun set. Suddenly, the present strikes and absorbs her consciousness. Whereas describing a sunset could be material for clichéd reverie, in Dillard's hands and imagination the description gives readers a dazzling experience of being—and reading—in "the present":

> Shadows lope along the mountain's rumpled flanks; they elongate like root tips, like lobes of spilling water, faster and faster. A warm purple pigment pools in each ruck and tuck of the rock.... As the purple vaults and slides, it tricks out the unleafed forest and rumpled rock in gilt, in shape-shifting patches of glow.... The air cools; the puppy's skin is hot. I am more alive than all the world.[5]

Your mind might draw virtual lines among *shadows, lope, lobes,* and *glow* because of the *l*'s and the long *o*'s. The first sentence actually contains six more l sounds. This moment of shifting light at once envelopes the landscape and Dillard's perception and strings together the landscape's disparate parts—the rock and water and mountain and light. So the *puhs* and the *ucks* and the *ruhs* and *shs* also string together the various words in the reader's inner ear.

I suspect Dillard hears words' internal sounds as she writes. So the sound of *ruck*—which means an indistinguishable jumble and thus makes a perfect word for how, at dusk, forms begin to meld into one another—leads her to *tuck*—which at once suggests a rock's pocket in which light could be tucked, as well as the definition of a drumbeat. "Ruck and tuck of a rock" reverberates with meaning and reflects a focus on the feast of writing itself: Sometimes we worry less about translating an experience into denotative words and center more intuitively upon letting one word's sounds unfold another word. Whether or not Dillard herself could actually *hear* the sunset doesn't matter; she *can* hear the ways words settle in the inner ear.

The body and brain are the inner ear's tuning fork. The inner ear appears to arouse the brain as well. Musical prose and poetry stimulate more parts of the brain than plain, literal language. Writer and former *Kenyon Review* editor Frederick Turner is cofounder of the international poetry movement Natural Classicism, based in part on his extensive research with neurologist Eric Poppol on poetic meter and the brain. Their research suggests the human brain is genetically coded to need measured narrative, for his research reveals that narrative meter with regularly paced lines especially stimulates the forebrain—the brain's bridge between left and right hemispheric functions.

Yogis have been tuning in to this deep source of language for over two thousand years. Similar to Pythagoras's view of the music of the spheres, the ancient Indian text *The Upanishads* claims that patterns of sound lie latent in the universe's rhythms (I hear the first über-note of Strauss's tone-poem *Also Sprach Zarathustra*). The Vedic bards, called rishis, tuned their ears to hear these pulses that they, then, translated into mantras. Mantra is an instrumental sound wedded to thought and intention (man meaning "to think"); it is a charged combination of sacred sounds and syllables that shape energy. Perhaps my neighbor, Edward, was onto something.

The Sanskrit language unfolds, then, more from mantra than semantics.

Take this family of words, for instance: strong/steady/stalwart/steel/stance. The mother word for this family seems to be the Sanskrit *sthira*. What Hopkins sensed about English clusters stems, in some cases, from such Sanskrit roots. *Sthira* embodies the qualities of strength and stalwartness, a confident stance you can learn to feel in your marrow. Such a quality is not an intellectual abstraction. It is a way of embodiment. *Sthira* is one of two qualities that the author of the two-thousand-year-old *Yoga-Sutra* says defines a Yoga posture.

Mantra is one way to help writers tune in. Through mantra practice, we learn to speak a mantra out loud (*ucca*), whisper it (*upamshu*), and then speak it within (*manasa*). Repeating it and keeping its sounds vibrating within your inner vestibule at once can heighten the word's energy and adjust your inner ear. Although Mantra Yoga can entail taking elaborate steps (sixteen according to one yoga text) for mantras to manifest their sacred power, I'm more interested in mantra as a way to help us hear how words, even seemingly ordinary words, can carry charged sound when bounced with other words' sounds.

Chanting freaks out some writers. If chanting evokes, as it once did for me, images of beatific middle-class Hare Krishnas who had tuned in and dropped out in the 1970s, think Dada instead of Krishna. Hugo Ball, who founded and hosted the Dada Cabaret in Berlin in 1912 would come dressed in a metallic suit and cylindrical helmet; he looked like the Tin Man from Mars. He invented what he called "sound poems," poems composed of syllables without reference, sound clusters that when combined and chanted evoked emotional clusters. *Gadji beri bimba sa la la / rim rim rim.* Something like that. Most of the crowds hated them and threw more than invectives his way.

But Hugo Ball, though quite the provocateur, wasn't simply provoking for provocation's sake. He wrote and spoke extensively that if language (often abused on behalf of reason to justify, say, a world war) were to be revolutionized, we must access language's core, pure sound. His sound poems, he hoped, would open people's ears to language's heart.

They did mine. When 22 years old, fresh out of grad school and living in Edward's neighborhood, I latched onto Ball's sound poems as if they were some secret text that uncoded poetry's mysteries. I was teaching American literature at a blue-collar suburban school attended by mostly well-mannered kids in a largely Christian community. To introduce early twentieth-century Modernist literature—not the easiest literary era for teenagers to embrace—I surprised the students one morning. The desks re-arranged in odd shapes, some stacked like Duchamp-esque found objects, I entered the room dressed in a costume concocted mostly of poster boards spray painted silver and wrapped around my limbs and strapped on my head with shoelaces. Hugo Ball visits the suburbs. I assumed some unidentifiable accent and ran the class as a Dada Cabaret complete with numerous incantations of Ball's sound poems that I had reprinted on the chalk board. The students lit up. Some of them probably wished Hugo had remained their teacher the rest of the semester.

After that day I likely was on parents' "suspicious activities" list. But for an hour, some of those polite yet anxious teenagers traveled to another world, one of spontaneity in which the delights of language so common to children came rushing back to them. When was the last time they were encouraged to play with language's sounds?

In mantra practice, I have discovered ways to help tin-eared writers enter the tin house where that "surround of sound" in prose and poetry dwells.

We often begin with four mantra seed syllables. Seed syllables are clusters of sounds believed to resonate energetically within parts of the body. Playing with them helps some writers embody sounds and feel how words both originate from the body and vibrate parts of the body. Most of us are familiar with the seed syllable with which we begin, *om*. After writers get in a comfortable seat and follow their breath for a few minutes, we focus on the third eye region between our eyebrows and utter *om*. The m sound vibrates from our mouth's roof to the pineal gland located near the third eye. We then work with other seeds syllables, *ham, yam, ram* (pronounced "haum," "yaum," and "raum"). Then, we try to vibrate these places by repeating each syllable to ourselves.

We also follow Hopkins' lead. We'll choose a simple word to sound out and write into such as "butter" or "listen." We each utter our respective word aloud a few times, listening especially to the consonant clusters and separate syllables. Then, we list other words whose sound combinations seem related. For "listen," I might list list/lost/lessen/loose/lasso. From that list, we write into a word to evoke some essence not often heard when the word is over-used in rational discourse. We retrieve something of this ordinary English word's sacredness.

Hugo Ball still works through me. I often have writers stand, voice out their words like rhytmic incantations, and move rhythmically in tandem with the word. We create something like a mantra Dada Cabaret. Once, after I led a group of writers through these practices, the same writer who had told me she couldn't hear the music approached me. She said that although she had been writing nonfiction for eleven years, she'd never noticed how physical language can be. She later wrote me to say that not only does she take more pleasure, if not measure, in speaking, but her writing experience, now, seems more visceral as she can hear how words hum from her body to the page.

Start with something simple. Take at least two full breaths just to quiet your inner noise and to make space for music. Aim quietly to voice a word's wondrous sounds, to let them vibrate in ways you've never felt before. Take the word *reuniting* if you cannot hear your own. Forget for now its meaning and just enjoy its sound as if you spoke it for the first time. Speak it out loud five times. Let your mouth, your word-organ, play the invisible word's notes one rebounding syllable at a time as your tongue and breath, your throat and lungs and heart and belly, all work together. Now, without moving your mouth or making an audible sound, hear the word being uttered within over and over. If doing so triggers an image or another word, heed it. You might write a brief sketch devoted to exploring this word's unique power or that of any word you choose.

Read a passage by a prose writer who listens to words' music. Something by Gass, Constance Hale (editor of *Wired* magazine), G. K. Chesterton, Arundhati Roy, Rick Moody, or Toni Morrison should suffice. First, put the passage's sense in the background, and its sound in the foreground. Read it aloud with the same savor you did with the word *reuniting* and notice what parts of your body seem especially tweaked. Then reread it to yourself to hear and feel how sense and sound in the passage may work together.

Listen to and utter words whose meanings you don't know. At the Zen Mountain Monastery, we chanted *dhvanis* ("sound" in Sanskrit), chants whose words mean nothing other than their sounds. I relished just letting my tongue roll with my eased mind and breath. So, read a story or poem in a tongue you don't know. Read some of it out loud. Then let its sounds sink into your skin.

There's something to be said, too, for stepping outdoors to listen. Sometimes, numbed by the computer buzzing and my head humming, I have to walk out to the wood stream near our farmhouse and sit. And listen. If I wish to recall the baseball bat's sonic pock that smacked the ball the one time I got a triple as a Little Leaguer, then I must listen. So, practice listening outdoors. Then, move inward.

It's not yet 7 a.m. and still mostly dark, the sun more reluctant to leave the covers these chilly November mornings. Brown leaves crush beneath my boots as I saunter toward an old log in a meadow that faces east. I step across the old stone wall and sit on the log. I have sat here a number of times to think and to cry and to be still. Layers of stuff have fallen away these past several years, layers that once stuffed my skull and blocked my ears like boxes packed with photographs stacked in front of an attic's window. I am still waiting to hear the sunrise. I am still, waiting. I am still.

TAKE A BREATH:
SOUND OUT YOUR EMBODIED WRITING

Intention:

Find a piece of your writing whose thudding sounds you'd like to tune up. Maybe the piece needs fine tuning for tone or mood, and changing its sound quality may just do the trick. Or you might simply want to sound out a new piece.

For this practice, you may either sit in a comfortable position and let your spine lengthen up and down, or you may recline in LYING **RELEASE POSE** *(savāsana). Feel your breath draw in and out as your belly expands and contracts. After at least two full breaths, ask yourself, "What am I writing for?" Tune your ear to whatever inner sounds or sights emerge. Then, clarify your specific writing* *intention for this session. You might acknowledge that you wish to hear the innate sounds of words for a specific subject or scene—either one you've been writing about or a new one.*

When ready, take a deep inhalation, and as you exhale, hum with lips and eyes closed for as long as you can. As you do so four more times, play with the pitches and tones your throat, mouth, and breath can create. Focus on the third eye region between your eyebrows, and voice om *("aum"). Notice where in your skull the vowels and humming consonant vibrate. Then focus on the throat and hum* ham, *"haum." Notice how the* h *sound tweaks your throat. Then in your heart you can feel the shake of the syllable* yam, *pronounced "yaum." And, finally, the fiery seed syllable* ram *("raum") pulls your abdomen back and so arouses your solar plexus, your inner sun. After you've played with and felt the sounds for a few minutes, breathe and quietly try to re-create some of the sounds internally.*

Then, with your inner vestibule tuned up, heed and hear a core word or two that pertain to your writing subject or scene. What core words and syllables seem to be essential to your writing piece? Maybe mother *and* cutlery *or* angel *and* desperate *suddenly surface. Sound out each one in your mouth. For the sake of experimentation, notice how their different sounds might vibrate different parts of your body. Then, as you breathe fully, hear a new line or a sentence for your subject or scene that surfaces naturally. For now heed sound more than sense.*

With eyes open, slowly write down that line or sentence. As you do so, hear each word's sounds that may trigger another word whose sounds may rebound off of yet another. The sound of mother *may trigger* mutter, *and* angel *may lead you to* bagel. *Continue to write this way, following each syllable like a foot's beat, tending for several minutes or longer. When finished, read the piece aloud and hear how parts of it sing and vibrate. Double-check your words' meanings to see if their sense and sound wed. If some parts seem forced, a tank of tintinnabulation roaring through your ear like lines from a Poe poem, rewrite it for subtlety.*

CHAPTER THIRTEEN

THE KISS OF SYNTAX, RHYTHM, & KIRTAN

"**W**HOEVER PAYS ATTENTION to the syntax of things / will never wholly kiss you," e.e. cummings writes. With all due respect to the master of grammatical lyricism and whim, I disagree.

Syntactical patterns haunt and shape our thinking. Sentence rhythms that we hear and read can recall, in our brain's neuronal wiring, the ebb and flow in which predecessors uttered first syllables and words. Over years of thinking, of breathing, of listening and of reading, in certain patterns, we're drawn back along ancestral waves to interior caves where we write in patterns that we've unconsciously inherited.

Irish writer Seamus Heaney knows it's so. The Nobel Prize-winner says that as he struggled with the translation of *Beowulf*, he intuited a deep need to sustain the project as he realized that the project involved his "own linguistic and literary origins": "I had noticed, for example, that without any conscious intent on my part certain lines in the first poem in my first book conformed to the requirements of Anglo-Saxon metrics."[1] In other words, decades before Heaney started the translation project of the classic Anglo-Saxon poem, the Anglo-Saxon syntax—rooted as much in the Irish soil, in the Ulster taverns and farms, as in any book's pages—had shaped how Heaney heard words and rhythm bead together in his earliest poems. We inherit syntax.

Syntax, simply defined, is the patterned structure of words in a sentence. Over centuries, each language's speakers develop, consciously or not, what they consider predictable and unpredictable patterns, what they regard as regular and irregular, pleasurable and annoying. Syntax is not an arbitrary term devised by rhetoricians; it is a natural expression and translation of our body's (especially our central nervous system's) rhythms. Our body's natural rhythms suggest that we're formed as much for sentence shaping as for lovemaking. And Yoga helps us heed those rhythms.

Although thinking about sentence structures while enjoying writing might seem like being on vacation with an uptight lover obsessed with rigid rules, tending to the syntax of things actually may liberate us from unconscious patterns of thinking and writing. Words and sentences are writers' raw material, and if a writer has no love of them, then her writing likely may never move beyond the transliteral or the purplish. Our sentences may pucker up and peck or be way too much tongue and saliva, but a writer tuned into syntax's rhythms may be able to wield sentences and lines that will kiss a reader from cell to sole.

Each of us likely begins to write a sentence, any sentence, somewhere safe, a sort of toe-dipping by word and then phrase. Until we can glide across the page in a breast stroke and dolphin kick, we may be unwittingly content to dog-paddle in the shallow end of simplistic sentence structures. Tending to and shifting undesired unconscious patterns is the heart of my Yoga practice. If we return, for a moment to the recognition that ninety-five percent of our thoughts are unconscious, then we also might understand how unconscious are our syntactical patterns. These unconscious thoughts shape the sentences that our conscious thoughts, imaginings, and feelings assume when they dive on the page. These unconscious impressions that shape our actions—"subliminal impressions," as B.K.S. Iyengar describes them—are called *samskāra*. Part of my Yoga practice aims to do three basic things with *samskāra*: help detect these impressions' patterns, learn how to use them, and learn how to alter them. Learning the ins and outs of syntax can follow a similar process.

First, we recognize an obvious grammatical pattern engrained, consciously or unconsciously, in our minds if not in our brains.

The English language's most fundamental sentence pattern is the S-V-O, or Subject-Verb-Object. Here are some simple examples:

The singer (subject) belts (verb) her tune (object).

Jonathan (subject) broke (verb) his leg (object).

This dog-paddle pattern locks in many writers' thinking. Their thinking plods in the same rhythms. Their sentences follow the same beat. Fine, if you intend to do so to make a point or to arouse monotony in your reader. But once aware of this basic pattern, you can create limitless variations of it to bring forth not just what your authentic voice needs to say but also how it needs to say it.

If we can hear syntax's rhythms, we can learn how to use or vary them according to our intent. A sentence often spirals or shrivels depending upon its rhythm—a sentence's basic unit that gives it musicality. Rhythm is patterned repetition. A sentence can repeat words, phrases, or clauses for a consistent musical rhythm and for emphasis of ideas or feelings; a sentence can repeat grammatical structures and parts of speech, too, to play upon readers' conscious or unconscious expectations of what idea or impression will come next.

So, there's merit in some repetition. Sometimes our writer's body and authentic voice need us to repeat this subject-verb grammatical structure to emphasize an idea or to evoke a feeling. The opening of Don DeLillo's *The Body Artist* describes the morning routine of a couple who has been married only for a few years: "She poured milk into the bowl. He sat down and got up. He went to the fridge and got the orange juice and stood in the middle of the room shaking the carton to float the pulp and make the juice thicker. He never remembered the juice until the toast was done."[3] These sentences' repeated subject-verb structure hammers the drudgery of the husband and wife's physically monotonous and parallel lives that only occasionally, if not accidentally, collide. She pours. He moves. She shakes. He pours. She nor he pays much attention to the syntax (or samskāra) of things, and neither (we can infer) has wholly kissed the other in quite some time.

Some writers' sentences, though, do kiss. In *A Natural History of the Senses*, Dianne Ackerman recounts how in the early sixties many girls made kissing an art form:

[W]e kissed inventively, clutching our boyfriends from behind as we straddled motorcycles, whose vibrations turned our hips to jelly; we kissed extravagantly beside a turtlearium in the park, or at the local rose garden or zoo; we kissed delicately, in waves of sipping and puckering; we kissed torridly, with tongues like hot pokers....[4]

Ackerman knows how to kiss with her lips and with her tongue (her language, that is). The repeated subject-verb-adverb pattern torques her idea and reinforces how inventive the teenagers were with their kisses just as the writer is with her sentences. The opening of Rick Moody's *Purple America* uses a similar pattern for a different effect: The repetition of the arcane "whosoever" elevates the protagonist's personal sacrifice to something religious and reinforces the overwhelming nature of being a middle-aged son who must care for, in every way, his debilitated mother:

Whosoever knows the folds and complexities of his own mother's body, he shall never die. Whosoever knows the latitudes of his mother's body, whosoever has taken her into his arms and immersed her baptismally in the first-floor tub, lifting one of her alabaster legs and then the other over its lip, whosoever bathes her with Woolworth's soaps in sample sizes ... he shall never die.[5]

That last sentence runs for four pages, its momentum overwhelming the reader. Nonetheless, this sentence's kiss is so tender, so complex, so angry and confused and loving.

Bhakti Yoga offers ways to explore the syntax that rings right with a writer's body. Bhakti is an ancient form of Yoga devoted to praising the self's qualities by chanting. Quite often, Bhakti yogis chant in what is called a kirtan style—one person (often a teacher) calls out a chant to a certain rhythm and pitch, and the group (usually the students) responds by repeating the chant in the same rhythm and pitch. The predictable patterns give each voice a form in which to soar, and you learn that a chant's basic structure can have limitless variations.

A word of caution: Bhakti Yoga unravels armored hearts. A few years ago, I returned home one spring after spending several months in India with my first wife; she had chosen to stay there. I knew in my hard heart we were all but through. My 21-year-old cat had died while we traveled. Snow remained on the ground. The house was quiet.

Within a week and with the help of some friends, I started hosting a small kirtan event at a local bookstore in Woodstock. Members of the greater community, most of whom had never chanted anything, and some accomplished musicians packed into a small room. This skeptical writer, soon to be single, let down his guard and let a room of people, from their 20s to their 60s—former hippies, current preachers, therapists, carpenters, and professors—enter. After a few months of my hosting this kirtan, the kirtan teacher to and friend of Ram Das said to me, "You look softer. Your edges aren't so distinct." I didn't know what he meant; I felt it, though.

I was working on a collection of poems, many of which were told from a female speaker's points of view. My writing assumed a different texture as if the words stemmed fom a source a little lower than my skull. Something more than that 5% of quotidian conscious thought came to the surface. What the Yoga poses and the breath work could not penetrate at the time, Bhakti did. *Bhakti* means love.

So, I often encourage writers to explore syntax kirtan-style. I "call out" a syntactical pattern, and they repeat it in their writing. They become aware again of the basic subject-verb pattern and then feel in their writing how repetition with this structure gives our writing bodies some new strokes. Then, once their body and brain assimilate the patterns, they can learn to vary according to how their voice most needs to express an idea or feeling.

We start with parallelism. Possibly the foundational riff for writing musical prose, parallelism is the similarity of structure in a pair or series of related words, phrases, or clauses. In parallelism, we usually express a balance of ideas and images. In both of the following examples, notice the similar length of each unit, a quality that adds to each sentence's harmony. This simple student example repeats verbs to emphasize the bird's grace as it hunts: "The <u>eagle</u> glides, <u>swoops</u>, and <u>grabs</u> its meal." I encourage students to take their own subject ("my husband," "the waitress," "my body") and write a similar sentence: <u>X</u> <u>verb 1</u>, <u>verb 2</u>, and <u>verb 3</u>. An object can follow or not depending upon the verbs. We then take the pattern a step further and construct parallel phrases that begin with verbs (verb phrases). Read the following example and let your own subject soar:

The <u>sparrow</u> <u>sings</u>   <u>its song</u>,   <u>flings</u> <u>its feed</u>, and <u>flicks</u> <u>its wings</u>.
  X   verb   phrase 1,   verb   phrase 2,   verb   phrase 3.

For a dissonant effect or for surprise, make the third one stand out in length, meaning, or sound, such as this student sample: "The chef sliced the rutabagas, stirred the broth, and concocted new recipes to leave her lover." These rhythms can lull our readers asleep or rock them awake depending upon our intention. They surface naturally in our writing when our whole body seems to beat to the suite of our sentences in a desire for balance.

We can find balance, though, not just in harmony but also in contrast. Thus, writers also find antithesis useful. A type of parallel sentence in which two parallel elements contrast one another, antithesis can register in us a subtle pleasure when we define something by what it's not: "My mother taught me that my color was not a mask but a shield," writes Alice Walker, and in Clinton's early days of optimism he said, "We must be the architects of our children's future, not the demolitionists of their dreams." More than one scholar recently has pointed out that in Lincoln's Second Inaugural Speech, his voice latched on to antithesis as an artful rhetorical tool to try to bridge divisive factions during the Civil War. To try out antithesis, write your subject in the first blank of the following line. Think of two contrasting metaphors or images to describe your subject:

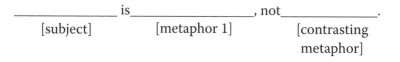

_____ is_____, not_____.
    [subject]   [metaphor 1]   [contrasting
                                                     metaphor]

It's as if the subject's pull and push, in and out, work together.

Emotion has its own rhythm and syntax. Sometimes, we write with such fury or reverie, disgust or jubilation, that our voice beckons us to repeat phrases and clauses. In such writing, our writing bodies and voice may need the shapes of anaphora or epistrophe. Ackerman's kissing sentences and Moody's caretaking sentences excerpted earlier in this chapter employed anaphora, the repetition of the same word or group of words at the beginnings of successive clauses or sentences. One student wrote the following sentence, not to evoke emotion but to describe a character's obsession: "She writes at dawn; she writes at noon; she writes at dusk." Epistrophe is the repetition of the same word or group of words at the ends of successive clauses or sentences, as in Franklin D. Roosevelt's example that aroused Americans' feelings of unfairness: "In 1931, ten years ago, Japan invaded Manchukuo—without warning. In 1935, Italy invaded Ethiopia—without warning. In 1938, Hitler occupied Austria—without warning. In 1939, Hitler invaded Czechoslovakia—without warning. Later in 1939, Hitler invaded Poland—without warning. And now Japan has attacked Malaya and Thailand—and the United States—without warning." A student wrote the following sentence in a creative essay about the virtues of living in uncertainty and dealing with ambiguity: "Gravediggers work in the dark; politicians speak in the dark; poets live in the dark." Learning this structure is easy. Take your subject, feel a phrase that will resonate each time it's repeated like a song's refrain, and follow a form similar to this one: X verb 1 phrase 1; subject 2 verb 2 phrase 1; subject 3 verb 3 phrase 1.

But to write from our syntactical core, so to speak, requires more than learning twisty, tricky patterns just as practicing Yoga requires more than learning twisty, tricky poses or chants.

At this moment, your body breathes. We each breathe about 23,040 times a day. The palpable fact of breath's undulations reminds us of our body's rhythms. An inhalation brings oxygen to our cells; our cells release carbon dioxide to our blood capillaries; our blood capillaries send carbon dioxide to our heart; our filtering heart, drumming our destiny's beat, gives oxygen back to the blood; our veins channel oxygen throughout our bodies' cellular makeup. Our whole body breathes; our whole body beats. Its tempo, subtle and individual. My mother's body steps to the beat of a different drummer than mine, than yours, than your daughter's, than Thoreau's.

You played with your breath when a boy or girl. You'd hold your breath underwater or challenge your friends to breath-holding contests. You'd hold your breath so long you made yourself dizzy, and the world's form for a moment jiggled like Jell-O—your first taste of altering your own state of body-mind-imagination.

Prāṇāyāma is the yogic art of becoming aware of, using, and altering breath to vitalize the body, to alter space within the body, and to extend the life force. Once we learn our breath's basic structure, then we can begin to work and play with it, not so much for child's play but for writer's playful work. To explore how our bodies' authentic rhythms may influence our writing's rhythms, we work with breath.

Just as a sentence has a structure, so, too, does our breathing have a basic three-unit structure: inhalation, exhalation, retention. Simple, it would seem. But as you read this paragraph, notice from where your inhalation begins. Are you still breathing primarily in your chest? Can you drop your breath's point of origin below your rib cage? Three fingertips below your navel? Place one or both hands below your navel, and on the inhalation let your belly expand and blossom. As you exhale, keep your fingers on your belly and lightly draw in your navel toward your spine. Keep your awareness on this movement for five breaths. Appreciate any differences you feel when breathing from this place versus from your throat or chest.

Retaining your breath on the exhalation (*bahya kumbhaka*) is the next step in harnessing breath. We taste stillness for a moment as our lungs rest and as our inner ears grow quiet. When we suspend our breath for a few seconds, we train our minds to heed our thoughts as well. By suspending our breath, we can almost suspend our thoughts like a diver caught in midair. An advanced Yoga practice is to catch a thought in midair and reverse it like a film image of a diver who almost reaches the pool lip before the film projector halts the image and then lifts the diver right back up to the diving board. For those of us whose thoughts constantly plunge into the deep end and who find ourselves almost drowning from exhaustion, this practice can help us harness thoughts into the shaped sentences our authentic body and voice need.

Be cautious, though: It's best to practice *prāṇāyāma* on an empty stomach so the body and mind's focus is not divided. Begin *prāṇāyāma* cautiously, noting your limits as you proceed. Refrain from retaining your breath until you've worked for a few weeks with elongating your inhalation and exhalation. Also, refrain from retaining your breath after the inhalation (*antarā kumbhaka*) until you're comfortable with doing so after the inhalation; otherwise, you may disrupt your nervous system. If you have high blood pressure or heart ailments, forgo retaining your breath at all. You can retrain your breath without retaining it.

As you read the following lines from Maxine Kumin's "Morning Swim," try to read as you heed the rhythms of your breath. That is, inhale as you read the first line, exhale as you read the second, and so forth:

> and in the rhythm of the swim
> I hummed a two-four-time slow hymn.
>
> I hummed "Abide with Me." The beat
> rose in the fine thrash of my feet.
>
> rose in the bubbles I put out
> slantwise, trailing through my mouth.[6]

The line's steady length and rhythm reinforce the speaker's bodily rhythms and the song's rhythms. Each line's pace follows your breath's pace, each inhalation and exhalation's length approximately a four-count. Most of this poem is written in what is called iambic tetrameter. An iamb is a measured unit of language made up of two syllables—an unstressed syllable followed by a stressed syllable. A line of poetry composed of four iambs is tagged iambic tetrameter. *Tetra* is Latin for "four," and meter simply means "measure," so iambic tetrameter translates to "A line of poetry measured with four iambs." Before you break out into a cold fever as you fret over marking a poem's rhythms, simply notice and hear the iambs in the poem's first line (with the stressed syllables italicized): and *in*/the rhy-/*thm* of/the *swim*. That English-writing poets for centuries have written verse so often in these four-beat and five-beat (pentameter) lines should be no surprise: They wrote with what came natural to their breath and with what brought the most embodied pleasure to their audiences.

Most prose writers also know the value of writing with measured rhythm. "The mass of men lead lives of quiet desperation," Thoreau wrote, wittingly or not, in a mostly iambic beat. And whereas the following sentence from Annie Dillard's *Pilgrim at Tinker Creek* follows a more complex measure (mostly iambs and what are called anapests), it does have a steady beat: "The sign on my body could have been an emblem or a stain, the keys to the kingdom or the mark of Cain."[7] The prose sentence's rhyme of stain and Cain is a bonus for the inner ear, the rhyme words' meanings reinforcing one another as much as their sounds.

Once we sense how a basic sentence's fundamental rhythms work, we can play with our sentences' breath, so to speak, by repetition and length. When we deliberately alter such patterns, we move to the third step of working with *samskāra*, those subtle impressions. This step involves consciously altering thought patterns. As with our breath, so, too, our syntax. It can expand or contract depending upon how we work and play with its rhythms. Each sentence breathes. Some stutter. Raspy heaves. Hacks. Other sentences blow on, their momentum carried by a phrase's or a clause's wind, sometimes their subject, hidden behind a flock of geese or an amateur glider, separated from its action. Take this student example of three sentences: "The clients, the meetings, the conference calls, the e-mails—everything about her job seemed to add weight to an imaginary board on her chest. She needed a break. A wake." These three sentences' pace follows roughly a 10-3-1 count to reflect the character's near breathless exhaustion.

Once writers set up patterns—as we've explored—they break them. Vary them. Twist them. Writers do riffs on the basic

Subject-Verb-Object structure like a guitarist who can play variations of C for five minutes or longer. Sometimes the order of the subject, verb, and object writers invert—as in this sentence (O-S-V). Sometimes a subject, modified by a flighty image or breezy phrase, gets separated from the verb—as in this one. A writer or narrator's worldview, aesthetic tastes, and philosophical disposition can each influence sentence lengths and structures.

The first paragraph of Hemingway's short story "In Another Country," for instance, contains all compound sentences. The narrator is wounded, physically and emotionally. He makes observations that are equally conjoined, and no thought ventures a complex cause-effect relationship. The past was then, and now is the present. Things just seem to happen, and the narrator just seems to blow in the wind. Faulkner, on the other hand, with the weight of the past and the weight of place always bearing on his protagonists' shoulders, exhales sentences that go on for two pages or more. In some writing, shorter sentences constrict. We feel tense. Or we feel relief. A character's fragmented thoughts might follow short patterns, whereas the thoughts of an effusive narrator, excited or outraged and openly expressive like a wild mare loping across a page's prairie, can only be reflected accurately in longer, rambling sentences.

With practice, we get the hang of some basic patterns, and then we alter them. As we learn to respond to how our body, breath, and imagination need a thought and image to unfold, writing memorable sentences that swim into our reader's unconscious, while still a miracle, may no longer be such a mystery.

The spring I returned from India, I kept writing alone and attending kirtan. Someone from the kirtan group introduced me to the fourteenth-century Sufi poet Hafiz. He's like Rumi with a sense of humor. In one poem, he writes, "When I want to kiss God / I just lift my own hand to my mouth." Yes, I thought, a writer could do worse than lift a hand to the page and lay out a line of kisses.

TAKE A BREATH 1:
FINDING A STEADY RHYTHM

Intention:
Try this practice if you have difficulty hearing your prose's space and your sentences' cadences. Try it also when you're writing about something whose steady rhythm you wish to capture in steady syntax. A character walking to the store, a conversation, people in a subway station, a character's morning routine.

This practice asks you to practice **EQUAL MOVEMENT BREATHING PRACTICE** (sama vrtti prānāyāma), *which helps you balance your inhalation and exhalation. Practice it to sense how the length of your sentences' units—the phrases and clauses— can create a steady rhythm. Once you hear the steadiness, you can vary the patterns.*

Come into a comfortable seated position, spine extended. Breathe completely at least twice, noting where in your body your inhalation originates. When your thoughts quiet, ask yourself, "What am I writing for?" Let your whole body take in that question and the ensuing reply, whether in image or word(s). Then clarify that you intend to write intuitively according to the rhythms of your specific subject as your sentences flow with your breath's rhythms.

Balance the lengths of your inhalations and exhalations. Beginning the inhalation from your diaphragm, breathe in to a count of four. Then, drawing in the navel, breathe out to a count of four. In four counts, out four counts. Try this practice for five cycles, then seven, then ten. You're beginning to harness your breath's basic dual structure, the in and the out.

With your writing subject surfing your breath's wave, take in another full inhalation, and hear a short sentence related to your subject that you can complete within an inhalation, followed by a sentence you can complete within an exhalation. You might begin with the basic Subject-Verb structure. Don't sweat the meter. Just hear the general length. Call the first sentence the in-sentence; call the second the out-sentence:

(In) The daffodils have bloomed. (Out) The peepers smell them.

Nothing fancy for now. Then, you can add an and, but, or or to link the in-sentence with the out, the inhalation with the exhalation:

(In) The daffodils have bloomed, (Out) and the peepers smell them.

Again, refrain from striving for linguistic acrobatics. Aim isntead for comfort with the syntax of things. Try to write at least ten same-breath sentences. Then, try to expand your breath's length and your sentence's length to a count of five, maybe six, or seven. Here's a student's example of a slow count to six:

(In) An afternoon in Abigail's alley gave me all I need to know about beauty.

(Out) Truth or not, in that shadowed beauty was where I yearned to live.

Although writers like Emily Dickinson and Robert Creeley seem content with tight breaths, some writers—like Walt Whitman, Faulkner, and Norman Mailer—seem to inhale to a count of ninety (I think Mailer inhales once a page and Faulkner once every two pages). Once you have a paragraph of same-length sentences and one or more longer ones, you have material to manipulate. Break it up if need be. Try the next practice to become even more adept at altering the rhythm.

TAKE A BREATH #2:
RETAIN YOUR BREATH AND MIX IT UP

Intention:

This practice builds upon the first one and helps you alter established syntactical patterns. Use the draft you started in the previous practice, or take another draft whose syntax flops like a swimming dog paddling for air.

The first breath practice **EXHALATION RETENTION** (bahya kumbhuka sama vrtti) *reduces central nervous activity and can alleviate some writers' anxiety attacks, mute writer's chatter, and send them to sleep. For the dormant-minded or sluggish among us, the second breath practice* **INHALATION RETENTION** (antarā kumbhaka sama vrtti) *incidentally increases synaptic activity and arouses the sympathetic nervous system. A useful alternative to caffeine, it also helps writers whose blues or depression make them stuporous.*

With the above cautions observed, come into a comfortable seated position, take two full breaths, and remind yourself, "What am I writing for?" After you feel the reply sufficiently in your body, clarify that you intend to hear how the rhythms of your writing subject need to be varied. When ready, breathe in to a count of four, breathe out to a count of four, and retain your breath to a count of four: In-4, Out-4, Hold-4 (five to ten times). Take pleasure in this breath.

Repeat the above pattern, except this time breathe in to four, hold for four more after the exhalation, and breathe out to four: In-4, Hold-4, Out-4. Be cautious if you attempt it. Notice the palpable sensations in your skull, your neck, elsewhere in your body.

Now, the variations. Not unlike riffs on a 4/4 melody, inhale to a count of six or eight and extend your out-breath to a count of four: In-6, Out-4. Or try extending how long you hold your breath to the following count: In-4, Hold-6, Out-4. The idea is to become versatile in your breath control and awareness so you can note what alterations best serve your mind and imagination.

Then, once you feel fairly adept at playing with your breath's structure, take a section of an existing draft and try to breathe to your sentences' lengths—just as you did with Kumin's poem. Doing so will help you hear whether or not your sentences together drip like water from a leaky faucet or whether they flow like water down a mountain stream. You may want the leaky faucet effect. It depends on what you want your sentences to do. For a section full of monotonous sentence lengths, you might mix it up. Follow three long sentences with a pithy one. Or begin with pith. Then follow brevity with sentences whose phrases and clauses, their grammatical compliance notwithstanding, rollick and ramble down hills of your own devising. Play. Note which rhythm feels right in your body, for your subject, and for emphasis. When you've rewritten the passage, let a friend read it and breathe to see if she has the response you intended.

Once you feel comfortable mixing it up with an existing draft, you may grow more at ease mixing it up while you write. See if as you write you can deliberately stretch your sentences' lengths, intuitively adding and elaborating where you sense such tricks fit. Really roll with the way words unfold one by one or three by three or four by four like planks of wood cut just right for certain purposes and effects. Then cut it short. Enjoy building. Relish the feel of a hammer or an ax fitted in your palm. Love the craft.

CHAPTER FOURTEEN

NON-VIOLENCE & THE ART OF DIALOGUE AS REVELATION

REPORTER AND RADIO ESSAYIST JACK HITT interviewed inmates and explored the stories behind a professional production of *Hamlet* performed by hardened criminals at a high security prison near St. Louis. When Danny, a forty-four-year-old criminal, had the chance to perform, he chose the part of Hamlet's father—the ghost. He said he had never been so moved as when he read such lines as

> *I am thy father's spirit,*
> *Doomed for a certain term to walk the night*
> *And for the day confined to fast in fires,*
> *Till the foul crimes done in my days of nature*
> *Are burnt and purged away. But that I am forbid*
> *To tell the secrets of my prison house,*
> *I could a tale unfold whose lightest word*
> *Would harrow up thy soul, freeze thy young blood.*
> (Act I, sc. v, 9–16)

Hitt asked Danny, "Who's speaking those words when you're on-stage?" Danny paused, then said "I'm the body up there, but the words are coming from mostly, uh, uh, William Pride, the man that I, uh, killed. He, uh, he's mostly the one talking."[1] This prisoner's fragmented words are almost as compelling as Shakespeare's ghost's eloquent speech.

With the radio's advantage, Hitt let this prisoner and others speak "in their own words." How did Hitt get these criminals to unveil their own stories and their own ghosts as they worked on

Hamlet? He inadvertently gave away his secret to good dialogue early in the piece. He said he had wondered—after having studied *Hamlet* and having seen a dozen professional and famous productions—what else he could learn about the play. Then he realized that this play about murder and its consequences was going to be performed by criminals who know firsthand about violence and who are living out those consequences. "After hanging out with this group of convicted criminals for six months, I did discover something," Hitt admitted. "I didn't know anything about *Hamlet*."[2] Such humility and a willing suspension of judgment made Hitt a nonhostile source for these prisoners to speak openly.

Like Hitt, many writers recognize dialogue's broad potential to reveal wisdom. Anyone's talk can be illuminating. Shakespeare's clowns, fools, and gravediggers sometimes speak, after all, with more wisdom than a king and his attendants. Similarly, yogis in several nondualistic schools of Yoga, such as *Vajrayana Tantra*, recognize that any act of speech from any source can be a spiritual tool. I'm not interested, for instance, in branding "vulgarity" as somehow less truthful than a sermon, or in tagging a guru's words as "higher" revelations than those of the woman who operates the Library Laundromat down the road. This yogic openness to wisdom's varied voices, coupled with a good ear and a keen understanding of why we humans talk in the first place, can help us craft artful dialogue.

Crafting believeable dialogue comes back to what almost every chapter in this section has emphasized: Listen. And listen without defense, without judgement. Be like Jack Hitt among murderers. "When a person is rooted in nonviolent speech, thought, and action," Patanjali's *Yoga-Sutra* states, "others relinquish their hostility and defensiveness" (II.35). *Ahimsā*, nonviolence, is a fundamental tenet of Yoga that encompasses everything from diet to thought to speech to action. I don't intend to simplify this practice; rather, as writers we can begin our practice of non-violence as we talk to other people—a practice that can allow you to be attuned to how all of our prisoners' stories are revealed.

Why do we talk? We ask questions. We share stories. We share facts. We warn. We want. We compete. We control. Most of these reasons we talk can be pared down to one: to learn. In talking, you learn what's happening in Liberia or in your ex-lover's heart. In all of this talk, intentionally or not, you learn about yourself—how your childhood experiences compare to your new friend's, how your opinions on hybrid cars compare to the deli owner's.

When characters talk, we also listen to learn. Dialogue informs us about the speaker, the plot, the subject, other characters. Without being didactic, their dialogue teaches us, too, how people talk about themselves, others, and their notions of reality and truth. When we see on the page those floating eyelashes " " framed around someone's words, our inner ear perks as we sense an immediate and accurate source speaks. Even in fiction, dialogue somehow sucks us into thinking we're hearing it directly from the character's mouth, the illusion of speech unmediated by a biased narrator. Those curly punctuation marks grant a story credibility, which is why journalists scramble for the right quotation. If we can keep in mind these basic reasons why we talk and why we read dialogue, we can be more artful with our characters' conversations.

Dialogue reveals. Dialogue can reveal plot information and geographical locale. It also tells us a character's thoughts, tone, age, the discrepancy between a character's thoughts and speech, conflict between characters, and a character's values.

Understanding dialogue's basic function to reveal, we can intuit how not to write dialogue: Refrain from babbling. To prattle is to speak indiscriminately and without intention. Some schools of Yoga contend that in a yogi's path, prattling (prajalpa) impedes a yogi's progress because it wastes a yogi's time and dissipates mental energy. Consider the following example:

> "Hey! How's it going?" Michelle said to Wendy.
> "Hi!" Wendy said. "Fine, although I've been running a lot of errands, and I'm exhausted. How are you?"
> "Good, I guess. A bit bushed and busy myself."

The dialogue reveals almost nothing and neither advances the story nor teases us enough to keep us guessing. Contrast that exchange with the following dialogue from the opening of Charles Baxter's clever fablelike story "The Cliff":

"I used to smoke Camels unfiltered," [the old man] told the boy.... "But I switched brands. Camels interfered with my eating. I couldn't taste what the Duchess cooked up. Meat, salad, Jell-O: it all tasted the same. So I went to low tar. You don't smoke, do you, boy?"
The boy stared at the road and shook his head.
"Not after what I've taught you, I hope not. You got to keep the body pure for the stuff we're doing."
"You don't keep it pure," the boy said.
"I don't have to. It's been pure. And, like I say, nobody is ever pure twice."[3]

In that short exchange, one character's voice conjures an image of a gruff man full of contradictions. The dialogue also veils enough to goad our questions. Who is this old man in relation to the boy? A teacher of some sort, we can infer. We also can guess that the boy is not enamored of his teacher, since he doesn't make eye contact with him and he challenges the old man on principle. The slight revelation contained in his reference to "the stuff we're doing" also teases us. What stuff? What's this talk of purity? Plot, conflict between the two characters, and theme are mixing it up in the dialogue.

A character's speech often betrays more about himself than he intends. In John Cheever's short story "Reunion," a boy sees his father for the first—and, we find out, the last—time since his parents divorced. His father, a busy businessman, wants to take his son to a fancy restaurant in New York City to make a good impression. The father does just the opposite, primarily through his speech. Throughout the story, the boy is quoted maybe twice, whereas the father is quoted constantly—a revealing detail itself. As the father grows impatient with one waiter after another, the story's simple structure follows the two characters from restaurant to restaurant. Here's a typical exchange at a restaurant where, the boy tells us, the waiters wear "pink jackets like hunting coats, and there was a lot of horse tack on the walls":

"Master of the hounds! Tallyhoo and all that sort of thing. We'd like a little something in the way of a stirrup cup. Namely, two Bibson Geefeaters."

"Two Bibson Geefeaters?" the waiter asked, smiling.

"You know damned well what I want," my father said angrily. "I want two Beefeater Gibsons, and make it snappy. Things have changed in jolly old England. So my friend the duke tells me. Let's see what England can produce in the way of a cocktail."

"This isn't England," the waiter said.

"Don't argue with me," my father said. "Just do as you're told."[4]

These one-sided dialogues escalate the story's tension with each new restaurant. Although we hear the father's bullying, Cheever's masterful touch is not to let the boy, the story's narrator, comment on his father's behavior. The boy, like the reader, is an observer—privately mortified if not repulsed—as the father, allowed to talk all he wants, implicates himself.

Simple "small talk" exchanges in a story can become charged with undertones of emotion and meaning. "Where are you coming from?" "Where are you going?" Those two questions are loaded, given certain contexts. They are the two questions Simon Ortiz once told me that he uses to begin a conversation with someone he meets at a bar and for how he begins a story. Imagine: A man and woman stand in a kitchen. The woman, exasperated, grabs the car keys. "Where are you going?" he asks. "Home!" she yells, and slams the kitchen door. A middle-aged woman driving down the highway stops to pick up a hitchhiker, a young man, haggard but handsome. He leans in the window and asks with an Italian accent, "Where are you going?" "Home," she smiles, and opens the car door. A middle-aged woman crawls out of a motel bed, where a young man still sleeps. After she dresses, she takes her purse, leaves money on the nightstand, and, once she's opened the door, turns toward the bed. She extends a lonely grin and faint wave. The young man, groggy-eyed, asks with an Italian accent, "Where are you going?" "Home," she says, and shuts the motel door.

If you stay hobbled in your writing hole as if it were a Himalayan cave and hear how people talk only through television and books, then you may never capture the wonderful and real ways speech unfolds. Consider a passage from Nathaniel Hawthorne's *The*

Scarlet Letter. As Hester Prynne walks through the Puritan village with her scarlet-dressed daughter Pearl, a Puritan child spies the pair, and says to the brood of other children: "Behold, verily, there is the woman of the scarlet letter; and, of a truth, moreover, there is the likeness of the scarlet letter running along by her side! Come, therefore, and let us fling mud at them!"[5] Oh, my. Verily, indeed. For all of his elegant phrasing and insight into the human heart that makes this novel a richly textured tale, Hawthorne needed to get out more often and talk among the villagers. I could identify any number of contemporary romantic novels as having similarly overwrought dialogue.

The voice of daily talk, the chitter-chatter, is called *vaikhari*, according to the ancient text the *Ganapati Atharva Shirsha Upanishad.* The text warns against speaking only from *vaikhari*, the coarsest and most audible of four levels of sound, without other forms of truthful sound frequently mediating. Given to *vaikhari's* own prattle, our speech gets distorted. Hear what's going down only from television, radio, popular music, escape literature, your friends, and you may write with a pastiche of catchphrases, clichés, colloquialisms, and the news's half-truths.

Still, with discipline, we'd be wise to listen to the world's chatter and to popular culture's babel. Writers often catch phrases and rhythms from the Zeitgeist *Vaikhari* and spin them from the air to the page in such a way that we can hear more clearly how daily talk betrays people's concerns and feelings. Like conceptual artist Barbara Kruger, writers listen to the muses of Madison Avenue as they sample commercialese and billboard-speak, radio talk and everyday chatter. Tom Wolfe has made a career of eavesdropping, cataloging, and imitating dialogues in subways, honkey tonks, art galleries, and penthouse parties. He can imitate the voices and syntax of a museum curator as accurately as a stock car race driver. With equal facility, young Scottish novelist Duncan McLean can capture the rhythms of a butcher's voice in Edinburgh or the waves of a waitress's voice in Buda, Texas. He told a group of students a few years ago, "You have to get inside your own head, but you also have to get out of your head and listen to all the voices around you—down your streets, in clubs and restaurants, at gas stations. Just listen."

You never know where a rich piece of dialogue will be given to you. While driving through Arkansas a couple of years ago, I stopped for dinner at a cheap chain cantina next to a Days Inn. The fluorescent lights brightened the queso-colored walls and the plastic daisies bunched in a plastic vase on each table. In a booth across the white-tiled aisle, a girl-woman around twenty or twenty-one and two boy-men, all three white and restless and trying to impress each other, chatted about reading and religion.

"I don't think Jesus was black," the girl announced. "I think he was extremely tanned." The boy-men looked dazed, their chips deposited like coins in a parking meter, their eyes glancing about the restaurant for different company, maybe wondering if she was really religious or just used it as a distraction from what the boys were really interested in.

"J'you see the game last night?" one guy said to the other.

"Nope. Wanted to, but had to work."

Despite the boys' half-interest, or perhaps because of it, the girl's voice pushed its way to be heard, often forced to repeat itself as if the repetition would at last get through. She must have looked over at me, as she seemed to have changed subjects. "I never go to a restaurant alone. I never eat alone. Even at the Wal-Mart—even at the Wal-Mart—even at the Wal-Mart I don't eat alone. If I have to, I have something to read like The Good News. It helps me understand the Bible because people don't talk the same as they did when they wrote the King James Version. J'you ever read it?" She seemed pleased she'd got the subject back to the Lord, so she could perhaps get through to these guys a message or two about the Word.

"Nope. Wanted to, but never got around to it," one of them said. The other one shook his head.

"With The Good News I can understand the Bible, all the stories I remember, even with all the thees and thous and stuff. It's in my car. It's in my car right now."

"J'you see American Pie? Oh, God, that was funny," one guy asked the other.

"Nope. Wanted to."

"It's in my car. Listen. The Good News's in the backseat of my car. Listen to me." Her moment of witnessing seemed to be slipping as the two boy-men washed the chips down with Coke and kept shifting the subject to watching football and to sex scenes in a movie they'd seen.

Her voice and this scene became the basis of a short story titled "Good News" about a girl and two guys traveling across the South. She's seeking love and Jesus; they're seeking sex. Just listening without judgment let me capture the urgency in her manic repetition and in her pleas to be heard, to be listened to. The guys' voices, laconic and lackluster, seemed the comic foil. "Listen to me" becomes the story's refrain of desperation.

So, eavesdrop. You may think this practice unethical, but if you want to hear how people speak without self-consciousness, then listen to a dialogue in a public place—a grocery store, a restaurant, a gas station, a town board meeting (my favorite place to record speech patterns). Note the speech's cadence and texture, half-starts and repetitions. If you make this practice a habit, you may hear how people in ordinary circumstances struggle to communicate ideas and feelings. When you write dialogue for a story or nonfiction piece, try to create dialogue whose rhythms and content may reveal more about the person than the person realizes.

In workshops and classes, I often break up writers into groups of three. I'll give two of the people a topic to discuss while the third person listens in the background and takes notes. The recorder then shares with them bits of noted dialogue and speech traits—accents, dialects, fillers ("uh" "hmm"), broken syntax, repeated words or phrases. The objective is to honor each person's unique speaking voice without judgment.

You also can listen to the electronic *vaikhari*. For at least a day, record the catchphrases, clichés, and telling homilies you hear from electronic sources—radio, television, and automated answering services. By day's or week's end, you may recognize patterns of our culture's flotsam that may give you fodder for creating a fiction or nonfiction scene. Weaving in and twisting these speech bits also can give a poem texture as it comments on the nature of our daily language. One student wrote a short story in which one of the characters spoke almost entirely in commercial jingles and sound bites.

Try combining dialogues with voices of popular culture for irony. Irony is a way of looking at life and saying, "There's much more to truth than we say, think we know, or expect." The main action that readers are noting is the foreground. Something else, though, can happen in the background that subtly "comments" on, highlights, reflects, or counters the foreground activity. In *The Great Gatsby* Fitzgerald weaves in numerous song lyrics and references to popular culture that comment on the characters' situations. In the novel's most heated scene, which happens in New York's Plaza Hotel, the cuckolded husband Tom strips Gatsby of all his glamour in front of his wife Daisy's eyes. From the hotel's lobby, "Mendelssohn's Wedding March" is playing from a wedding party.

In Elizabeth Tallent's short story "No One's a Mystery," popular culture's background meets dead-on with the story's foreground, even providing its title. The short short story revolves around a girl who's just turned eighteen and Jack, a middle-aged man with whom she's having an affair and who has just given her a diary for her birthday. The whole story, mostly dialogue, happens over an hour or so as they drive in his pickup. As the man's wife drives by, the girl ducks and looks at the pickup floor. As she's studying his beat-up boots and the floor crowded with pop tops, Rosanne Cash sings on the tape deck, "Nobody's into me, no one's a mystery." The song doesn't get much direct attention in the dialogue, yet it reflects the story's theme and the predictable outcome, given the almost clichéd nature of their relationship. So, as you create a scene for fiction or nonfiction, notice how the voices of popular culture in a scene's background can play upon your characters' dialogue and situation.

When I was in my twenties I spent a few days in the East Texas Big Thicket that borders backwoods Louisiana. I found a room at the Big Thicket Courts. Near dusk my first evening there, two men sat out on the picnic table outside my room chatting and sharing a bottle of whiskey. One of them, in his forties, I guessed, had a shut right eye and a thick scar above his brow. The long arms of the other man, older, extended out of his flannel shirt. I said hello. They asked if I wanted to join them. I did.

"Where you from?" the older one asked as he handed me the bottle.

"Ft. Worth-Dallas area. I teach in Dallas. Just here for a few days to relax."

They nodded.

"Y'ever do any time?" the younger one asked. "We was just trading stories, how we both done time."

"Not really," I said and swigged. "What were you in for?" I asked non-chalantly as if this conversation came up regularly among my colleagues.

"Used to traffic in black market cigarettes and liquor," the older one said. "Steal 'em from train cars and sell 'em in the next town over. Big bucks for a while." He went on to detail the network between Texas and Tennessee he and five other men had formed, a network of railroad routes, cardboard boxes, and loot.

The younger one said he just flat out robbed liquor stores. "Did it to keep my woman. Then she done run off. I coulda killed her, but I didn't."

Light faded. The younger one said to me, "You know, twenty years ago you'd be run outta this town for sitting here talking to us." The other man nodded. "Yup."

I adjusted my glasses and asked why.

The younger one sat straight and proffered his bare arms on the picnic table. "We're black. You ain't."

I had lived in Texas all my life and had never run up against anything like what they were talking about.

"Wa'n't until I joined the army and got outta here I learned that not all white people are the devil," he said.

"Yep," I chuckled, "not all of us."

The next couple of hours passed this way, mostly the two of them trading stories and me listening and piping in when I could. Gradually, the night darkened all our faces.

That was years ago, before I had even heard the word *ahimsa*.

III.

NAVIGATING EMOTIONAL
CRAGS FOR COMPLEXITY

CHAPTER FIFTEEN

WHEN THE INNER HECKLER CALLS

A ROUND 10 A.M. ON SOME MORNINGS, I receive calls almost on schedule. It's Karen who wants to know why I haven't called her back about the new mortgage rate she can offer. Her recorded voice sounds urgent. Or it's Rob who's still excited to tell me how to bring down my debt. His recorded voice sounds earnest. Or it's that other schlock who says something like, *Still writing, are you? Don't you think you'd be better off selling real estate? or Do you really call this writing? Go back to school, pal, and get an--.* His recorded voice sounds insidious. I usually hang up mid-sentence. Some calls simply don't merit my kindness and courtesy. Although I'm not on the Inner Heckler's No-Call List yet, I do know now how to handle him on most days.

Fear, doubt, and self-consciousness call every writer at random like a desperate, relentless telemarketer.

THE RELUCTANT WARRIOR

Abby, a writer in Woodstock who attends my workshops, had a feature article about Alzheimer's due to a major health magazine in less than two days. A freelance writer for eight years, she felt good about her interviews with specialists and people with the disease; the article, her third feature for this magazine, had the right angle to boost her reputation; and her relationship with the magazine's editor had solidified enough that Abby thought this article could lead to a permanent position on the staff. But then her Heckler showed up. *Do you really think you have a unique angle? Hasn't this topic been overdone?* The questions became relentless.

Aren't you really hacking your way through this "career"? Suddenly, the interviews seemed superficial. The article's tone sounded all wrong. *That personal aside about your own memory loss makes you look self-indulgent, which you are, you know?* The voice undid her confidence, she later told me, and for much of the next day, her neck, shoulders, and right hand ached with doubt and fear that she wouldn't complete the assignment.

Then Abby remembered some ideas we had discussed in a workshop about these very topics. She pulled out some of Patanjali's sutras I had copied for the group: "Fear, subtle and arising from its own origin, visits even the wisest among us" (II.9) and "When doubt disturbs your thoughts, counter it with the opposite frame of mind" (II.33). She later told me that just rereading those sayings, written some eighteen hundred years ago and derived from at least another thousand years of previous yogic wisdom, started to ease her body and to quell her Heckler. She practiced a couple of strategies we had practiced and caught the Heckler off guard by laughing back at it and saying, "Yeah, so what if you're right? What's the worst that could happen?" When she reread her article, she realized that in a few places the tone was indeed off, but overall the piece felt right. She knew it. Where then, she wondered, did this voice come from? Maybe she had let too much ride on the article—her reputation, the prospect of a permanent position. Instead of just focusing on the subject and writing, she was giving way too much attention to the piece's possible success or failure.

With a few harnessed breaths coupled with a concentration practice, Abby soon heard another voice. With no false hope, the voice simply said, "Trust yourself. Keep writing. The ground's not going to fall out because of this article." Within a day, she finished and submitted the article, one that received numerous favorable reader replies. Although she doesn't yet have a permanent position with the magazine, she says the experience of handling this sudden attack of doubt gave her more confidence, and she's negotiating with another magazine editor for a position.

Doubt wracks the best of writers. So does its twin, fear. Whether you've succeeded or failed as a writer, the Inner Heckler's dual voices will call. Yet, I do think it's possible to understand the Inner

Heckler's nature, and in doing so, we can prepare and learn how to deal with it.

One of the Inner Heckler's voices is fear. It usually stems from protecting the ego self, the "I." If you understand fear in this sense, you realize that—unlike most telemarketers—it does have your best interest at heart. Sometimes it's like the overworried parent who wants no harm to come your way. It's like the friend, always aware of death, who suggests you stock up on life insurance for your kids. It's the tendency to avoid pain at all costs. We cling to what comforts the ego self and avoid what threatens and potentially could "kill" our sense of self.

Fears related to writing often stem from fears of death. Fear of criticism—be it from that jerk of an acquaintance who published her memoir before you did or an invective from *Atlantic Monthly's* B. R. Myers—paralyzes some of us. "Her criticism pierced me." "His criticism slaughtered me." "It killed me when my book was dropped." "When they laughed at my poem, I could've died." Our Inner Heckler speaks directly to our ego's desire for self-preservation. This desire, this clinging to the safe and familiar, translates in Sanskrit to abhinivesha, and it ironically is not life-affirming. It feeds the ego and starves our authentic self. The authentic self conversely feeds on exactly what starves the ego: risk, challenge, uncertainty.

I have dual impulses as a writer. Actually, I have a veritable pantheon of impulses as a writer, but two stand out: Apollo and Daphne.[1] The Greek god Apollo tried to woo the nymph Daphne out of the woods with his achievements. Inventor of music, god of healing, voice of reasoning, source of light and harmony, the brilliant god with a luminary's vita tried everything to win her heart. But she fled. The introverted nymph didn't desire the illustrious world of laurels; instead, she sought the mysterious, dark realms of the woods where she (she thought) could be forever free and unattached. With the sun god fast on her heels, Daphne called for help to her river god father, who changed her form into that of a laurel tree. Although Apollo never caught Daphne's bodily figure, now he actually could stroke her grainy-barked torso, hang from her limbs, and lounge beneath her shade. With a telling gesture, his artful, love-hungry hands clipped her branches and wove them into a crown—the symbol of victory. Ironically, although Daphne fled from worldly recognition, a part of her transubstantiated body—the laurel leaves artfully woven into a crown—comes to represent artistic and civic accomplishment.

Part of us like Apollo seeks outward accomplishment. To create beautiful writing that others may enjoy, to get our art in public venues, praise, that laurel crown of publication—yes, that six-figure advance!—these are Apollo yearnings. Yet, another part of us shuns the public hoopla. True, we might naturally incline toward being alone, unbothered by the demands that readers and the publishing world make on us. But fear and doubt also lead us to retreat like Daphne. We might try to deny these feelings and claim we like to write in our own dark woods, not showing our work to anyone else and shying away from Apollo's lures of exposure and prominence. "I'm above all that," one writer told me. I know what she meant, and I applaud her authenticity of not getting obsessed with seeing her name in print as some writers do. Still, many writers fear exposing their writing to the light and risking failure or—as one writer pointed out to me—risking success. For failure and success alike can change a person's life, fatally disrupting some of the ego's former patterns. Whether fear's origin be of failure, criticism, or success's laurels, the effect often is the same: We hide. And we don't change.

The Heckler's other voice is doubt. Doubt's nature in Yoga is expressed as that state of mind in which we have conflicting thoughts (*samshaya*). Perhaps no story from Yoga better illustrates a writer's doubt than that of Arjuna in the *Bhagavad-Gita*. This beautiful poem, composed probably in the third or fourth century BCE, occurs at the onset of a war between two clans of the same royal family. Arjuna, a member of the "virtuous" clan, has for his charioteer none other than Krishna, the god of love. (Who wouldn't want to be driven by the god of love?) Just as the war is about to begin, Arjuna asks Krishna to lead him to the battlefield's center so he can see the faces of the cousins, uncles, and brothers who are about to kill one another. Overwhelmed with grief and compassion, Arjuna collapses, weeps, and wails, for, full of doubt, he's torn between his love for his whole family and his duty to his clan. Time stops. Soldiers freeze. Arjuna, though animate, remains paralyzed with inaction. Does he do battle or retreat?

It's sort of like opening your eyes for the first time at your big family's Thanksgiving dinner table. Your relatives argue all of the time, and none of them "get" why you write. But for the first time, you see their faces for what they are: reflections of the civil war happening in your embattled mind and heart. Do you do resolve the battle or forget about your memoir?

Arjuna is, I think, the first writer wrought with writer's block in all of literature. Wouldn't life be easier if he would just go home, hang on his porch a cobbler's sign, and make a living repairing soles? His indecisiveness reflects our own inaction as writers when doubt sets in. While your partner and the rest of the world work their tails off, you're floating in a world of words and imagination. Shouldn't you be spending your time on something that will pay for your kid's tuition? Shouldn't you be spending your time on something more practical? Fixing the fence? Going on a peace march? Humph. At least clean the bathroom. Doubt divides us. We're torn between doing what our authentic self needs us to do (write!) and doing what we think we should do (be practical and profitable). So as soon as we make time to get to the desk, the Heckler shows up, and we find ourselves sprawled on the battlefield, unable to do the authentic work we know we were born to do.

Reluctant warriors of words, all of us.

THE HOUSE OF FEAR & DOUBT

Fear and doubt can take over our bodies like obnoxious houseguests whom, after a few years, we've unintentionally allowed to move in for the long haul. Pretty soon, they invite friends and relatives. In Yoga-Sutra I.30, Patanjali lists these relatives' names as the most common impediments to a yogi's path. What's related to doubt? Lack of progress on a spiritual path and delusion, for starters. Sluggishness and excitability, sloth, and illness come next. You know these relatives. They're the brother-in-laws who stay for ten days and never get off the couch. And as Sutra I.31 reminds us, such an open house invites other unwanted relatives: disturbed breathing, physical agitation and trembling, depression, and general suffering (*dukha*). Before we know it, a veritable clan of cousins whose names we barely know has taken over our home.

I don't mean to make light of this state. It can be a devastating place to live in. I remember the old house of disrepair where I lived while in my twenties. I drew the blinds and rarely let anyone in. At the time, I could see no way out even though I sensed there was one. I know writers who somehow still write in such a home. Like a kid with six siblings, they learn to tune out the noise and ignore the house's state of increasing disrepair. One of my friends, who writes features for a major newspaper and who has published six novels, says (despite his frequent influenza and colds) he likes his body-mind the way it is: crowded, loud, and broken down. But he's also told me frequently that he often thinks he'd rather write a different kind of novel than the modern Western mysteries for which he has become known. Yet, whenever he starts one of his fantasy short stories, what does he hear? *If you're going to write fantasy, you'd better change your name, or else your fans and friends are going to laugh at you. Don't you think you should focus more on your feature or your novel that's a sure sell?* Success as a writer won't necessarily clean your house of the Heckler and its clan. In fact, success can breed more attachment to the fruits of our writing—the praise, the money, the recognition. Such attachment can become another room for the Heckler.

If we try to ignore doubt and fear over several years, we can unconsciously live in a fight-or-flight response. When fear and doubt heighten, our brain may sense danger, which triggers our heart rate to rise, and the endocrine system starts releasing excess amounts of adrenaline (the adrenaline rush) and cortisol. Although healthy in moderate amounts, too much cortisol can debilitate the immune system and exacerbate a cycle of stress. Our breath quickens, and our digestive system virtually stops functioning. If our fears escalate to anxiety or panic, our abdomen can become distressed. Troubled breathing and shallow breathing, not surprisingly, have been correlated with coronary complications.

Few of us may have panic attacks when we write, but the point is that these strong emotions can override our writing spirit and wreak havoc on our bodies. We don't have to write this way. Yoga can help us shape our fear and doubt. Not just face them and definitely not suppress them. But transform them. Fear is not something to be "overcome," nor is fear a "moral blemish" as some classical Yoga texts suggest. When we write from a yogic place in our body and approach these feelings as something to be acknowledged, expressed, and tempered, we often can channel doubt and fear's fire one line at a time, one sentence at a time.

Given the above explanation of the fight-or-flight response, it should be no surprise that Patanjali recommends in sutra I.34 we take a deep breath and retain our breath after the exhalation (*bahya kumbhaka*). You might think this sounds cliched, but doing so calms the sympathetic nervous system and thus quiets brain activity. Even just lengthening the exhalation to be twice as long as your inhalation without retaining your breath can quiet the Heckler. Just imagine the out-breath as blowing out those annoying cousins. It works. I don't know how else to say it, but harnessing the out-breath with care and over extended periods of time can change the composition of your house.

Yoga can reduce the body's chemistry of fear. One yoga class significantly dropped levels of cortisol in students with mixed backgrounds in practicing Yoga, according to one recent study.[2] Yoga also can reduce fear's effects by its loosening of the "psoas constrictor." A sixteen-inch serpent called the psoas muscle potentially constricts our courage and contains much of our body's and imagination's fear. Imagine a long, snakelike muscle attached near the middle of your spine (at the thoracic vertebra T12, to be exact) that connects to each of the five lower lumbar vertebrae (the lower back), through the pelvis, over the hip's ball and socket, and tails off at the thighbone's (femur's) lesser trochanter, not far from where your leg joins your hip. Physiologically, the psoas supports the internal organs and helps secure the pelvis. Its sleek body resting at our own body's central core, this muscle also literally connects our upper and lower halves. The psoas's head at the midspinal area resides near the central diaphragm—a muscular structure that moderates our breathing. Embedded in the psoas's "body" along the lower (lumbar) spine are several nerves that work with the diaphragm.

Granted, a few simple breaths and stretches alone will not renovate your house, but begin somewhere. When you inhale, let your lower belly relax, and as you exhale draw your belly in. The nerve network along your lower back's spine and the region where your fingers reside—at the pit of your gut—is often called your abdominal brain. Why? A lot happens here. The psoas meets the diaphragm, which moderates our respiration, and here much of our digestion occurs. Two thirds of our body's blood flows here. This area is the solar plexus, the *manipura cakra*, the city-of-jewel center, the energetic area of personal power, balanced will, and control of intense feelings. Here we have guts or have a weak stomach for confrontation; we "have a spine" and stand up to fear and doubt, or we get nauseous and bend over like Arjuna or Daphne. It's what the Japanese call the hara, literally "gut." Zen master Daiun Sogaku Harada said, "You have to realize that the center of the universe is your belly-cave."

So, this massive muscle called the psoas—the body's longest one, in fact—plays a pivotal role in the rhythms of our breathing, of our blood circulation, and, thus, of our body and imagination's responses to fear. With practice we can uncoil the psoas and change a potential psoas constrictor into a psoas elixir, a muscle that can work with us to release or at least re-direct our fears of writing and of exposing ourselves into giving ourselves the freedom to create and of mustering what Rollo May called "the courage to create." Poses such as **WARRIOR II** (*viribridāsana* II), **SIDE-ANGLE POSE** (*parsvakonāsana*), and some forward bends such as **EXTENDED EAST-STRETCH POSE** (*paschimāttanāsana*) help lengthen the psoas and give us room to breathe and move. We literally can create space in our bodies to breathe and for our cells to live so they don't, in a sense, suffer claustrophobia from living in a cramped, balled-up house.

ROOTS

Fear has its deep source. Patanjali notes that fear has its own *rasa*, its own quintessence, marrow (I.9). Transformation requires authentic movement toward and with that quality. So, as writers, if we genuinely wish to shape our fear, then we can view fear as a natural serpent that coils in our psyche, one that can be lured out of its basket and perchance taught to dance on cue rather than to strike unconsciously.

Lori, a writer, reached fear's roots. A talented dancer, technical writer, and fiction writer, Lori came to me as a writing coach for help. Writing mysteries, she told me, had been her dream, and now she sensed at last that this mystery novel—complete with sympathetic characters and intricate plot twists and fantastic settings—was ready for publication. For eight years she had worked on this novel, had attended writing conferences, pored over "the-craft-of-mystery-writing" articles and books, and had been a dedicated member of a writing group. I reviewed her preface and instantly noticed her ability to corral antsy words into beautifully choreographed sentences and plot lines. She is a writer, no doubt. So why does she need help?

"I'm afraid to send it off to an agent or publisher," Lori said, looking down at the floor like a little girl. Performance anxiety. All writers, even after publishing six books, get it. Like Daphne, Lori had been content to dwell for years in her dark lair, but the thought of offering her cherished manuscript to an agent mortified her. I assured her I could never help her overcome her fears, but possibly we could find ways to transform them. She was open to the idea of writing into her body as a way to identify and shift her fears' flow. We spread out a couple of yoga mats and blankets and got to work. We worked with the Apollo-Daphne myth to unearth the archetypal patterns of her fear, we brainstormed different personal fears, and then we coaxed her snakes.

And we got to the roots. In the process of our work through dialogue, visualization, bodywork, and writing, we discovered Lori's patterns of fear that stem from her lifelong need for approval as well as patterns of qualified praise. A sister to six gifted brothers, many of them older, she soon learned that all of her accomplishments—winning academic awards and scholarships, becoming a successful dancer, becoming a successful technical writer, having a happy marriage and charming son—were rarely good enough compared to those of her older siblings.

During our bodywork, Lori kept seeing a dancer standing in a rapidly flowing stream. Her feet stuck in the mud, the water flowed quickly and rose, so she flailed her arms like a whooping crane sending out an emergency call and a mating call in one. For a while she found peace in dancing from her hips up until gradually her winged embrace of empty space wedged her feet so she could dance both with and against the stream's current. After she sketched the images, she wrote a prose meditation upon these images, the liberation of her body from fear. "Analyze less," I suggested. "Feel more. Imagine more. As you write, follow one image at a time." Our intellect, in its mighty efforts to render fears impotent and invisible, often harms more than helps us. Imagination and intuition, however, frequently let us tame and transform fears.

Several months later, I ran into Lori. Not only had she mustered the courage to submit some of her short stories for publication, but two of three also had been accepted, and upon receiving another writer's advice about her novel she had decided to divide the long book into two shorter ones. She also had found an agent for it. The work we had done together, she said, had shifted her attitude and shifted her body's energy.

DRIVE TOWARD THE DIFFICULT

One intuitive way to inquire into your fear's origins is to list sayings, colloquialisms, quotations, and titles of works you've heard about that are related to fear. "We have nothing to fear but fear itself" and "Who's Afraid of Virginia Woolf?" will get you started. After listing fifteen or more, you can see if any patterns, such as common images or common attitudes, surface. You can take one or more of these sayings or quotations and write a prose piece in which you offer fresh insight into how to contend with fear. In your writing, avoid the word "fear." Or list everything you fear about writing and everything your Heckler tells you to avoid writing. Everything. Then, from the second-person point of view, write a playful list piece called "Ten Ways to Avoid Writing."

Sometimes we just need Krishna, perhaps literature's first writing coach, to kick us in the rear. When Arjuna wept on the battlefield, Krishna's first response was essentially, "Stop crying. Get up. Face the music, and live in dignity, not doubt." While time stood still, Krishna, though, also had infinite patience for Arjuna's deepest, most distressing questions about attachment, desire, conflicted feelings, and Yoga. Krishna became for Arjuna his Heckler's antagonist: his Confidant. The Confidant embodies the Heckler's most daunting antagonist: *shraddhā*. The usual translation as "faith" is misleading; the word encompasses in English qualities such as "confidence" and "mental repose." Our Inner Confidant(e), the force of *shraddhā*, supports us unconditionally yet lures us from our comforting safety spots to new places, possible clearings where we may even receive recognition for our work.

The Confidant inspires and guides us and doesn't let us get away with whining. We have work to do, and it's work that even our dearest loved ones often do not understand. With courage, steadfastness, and centeredness, we can face the battle that, we soon discover, is really no battle at all. We realize, too, that there's really nothing and no one to conquer. "When doubt disturbs your thoughts," Patanjali reminds us, "counter it with the opposite frame of mind" (II.33). We can convert the same energy that brings stifling doubt into invigorating confidence so we can face risk and uncertainty. The Heckler's opposite thought is the Confidant. Listen to it. Inhale confidence; exhale doubt.

Before fiction writer Andre Dubus died, he learned how to drive into fear. A fortuitous coincidence helped him move out of his comfortable mode of writing fiction and face the demons he had embodied for ten years after a crippling automobile accident. One night while helping a stranded driver on the side of a busy freeway, Dubus was struck by a car and lost the use of a leg. Although the driver never stopped, someone else did and called for help. Despite his daily agony in a wheelchair, he never wrote about his own situation. Too painful to face, he said, and so he stayed with fiction until ten years later some new neighbors moved in across the street. The woman, it turns out, was the one, the witness, who stopped to call for aid. Within a few weeks of getting to know her and her husband, Dubus finally faced his body, his pain, all of the demons he had embodied for ten years, and wrote his memoir. He said he suddenly felt "so possessed" to write about his experience—not to forget about or be done with it, because writing, he said, didn't rid him of anything. Instead, he just wanted "to go there" and "see if in that place there was any light."[3] Writing won't rid you of your fears. It can give you, though, ways to work with them.

We don't have to send fear back down more deeply into its hole; we can coax it out with our flute, let it spread its terrifyingly beautiful body before us, and see what it has to teach us. Sometimes, the best advice I can offer students about fear of writing is simple: Write. Drive into it. Fear is usually not a brick wall as much as a large mound of snow. It seems daunting and impassable, but if you keep your hands on the steering wheel, your wits alert, you can drive right through it. The best way I know how to keep driving is just to drive with little knowledge of what exactly is around the next bend.

Arjuna's driver, Krishna, gave Arjuna the best driving instructions I've ever read: "Self-possessed, resolute, act/without any thought of results,/open to success or failure./This equanimity is yoga" (2.48).[4] Replace the word act with write. And the next time the Heckler calls you to say you should be doing something more profitable or practical, switch the line to this pearl from Arjuna's Confidant: "It is better to perform your own duty poorly, than to perform someone else's duty perfectly; when you do what you should be doing, no pain will come to you" (3.35). The trick is to know that to act authentically is to act on your own authority and that writing is your duty to your authentic self.

TAKE A BREATH: LAUGH AT THE HECKLER
AND WRITE WITH EMBODIED CONFIDENCE

Intention:

When you work with your lower body in harmony with your upper body and heart, you can become an adept who frightens fear into obeisance. To embody confidence and faith (*shraddhā*) and to fend off the Heckler, try this practice for at least fifteen writing sessions.

Come into **MOUNTAIN POSE** (tadāsana), *focusing upon your feet first. Drop your weight so forcefully into your heels that no one could pick you up. If you can name one of your fears related to writing, do so. With eyes closed, take two full breaths and ask yourself, "What am I writing for?" Let that question pervade your whole body, knowing there's a core impulse for your writing. Allow the response to surface without force and to guide you. Then clarify that your specific intention is to keep the Heckler at bay and to write with confidence.*

Keeping full energy in your legs, bring your left foot back three to four feet and pivot your left foot diagonally forward at least forty-five degrees. Let your pelvis be open so that one sitting bone is almost behind the other. Adjust the width between your feet so you can maintain weight in the back heel without collapsing into your back arch. Draw your attention from heels to hips and bend your front knee. Let your knee line up over your ankle. Bring your arms straight up so your right arm is in front of you, your left behind, both palms down. Gaze over your right middle finger. This position is the skeletal form of **WARRIOR II POSE** (virabhadrāsana II). *The pose stretches your psoas, tones your abdominals, and increases respiration. If this pose strains you, keep* *your hands at your hips. It's imperative that you find the variation of this pose that stretches your psoas and groins yet also gives you a strong sense of "rootedness." Nothing can knock you over.*

Now, experience the internal form. Shrug your shoulders up and draw your shoulders back and down along your spine to let your heart open and support you in tandem with your lower body. On each of the next five inhalations, fill up your heart, and on each of the exhalations draw your attention to your belly. Close your eyes and imagine the in-breath coming down from your heart and the out-breath rising from your lower torso mix in your belly. After each exhalation, hold your breath for one or two seconds. Your heartful in-breath churns your fear. The belly's fire converts fear into confident action. Repeat this practice on the other side.

Then move to the desk and start writing. Write for at least one hour, and anytime the Heckler calls, inhale confidence into your heart and laugh out loud at the Heckler as you keep writing. Oh, hello, you might say. It's you again. Don't you ever get tired of this job? Thanks, but no thanks. What's stopping you?

Stay with this practice for at least seven to ten minutes a day before you write, for at least fifteen days or fifteen writing sessions. Fear is subtle. So, too, is changing fear's form. It's true that even sages get the blues and get laughed at, but they know how to laugh back and at themselves.

CHAPTER SIXTEEN

DOGS, LOVERS, AND OTHER THINGS THAT BITE: WRITING THE TRUTH

"TRUTH'LL NIP YOU in the butt, and you may not be any wiser for the teeth marks in your cheeks." That gem came from Lynne, a widow who used to live next door to me before I moved from Texas. Sixty-something, she'd have me over occasionally to bring in her groceries, clip her hedges, and "sit a spell." That particular day we were talking about relationships: her marriage that could be rather sweet and nutty, and my relationship at the time that, if adapted to a play, would've rivaled *Who's Afraid of Virginia Woolf?* for sheer bizarreness. She told me about her son's wife, an ambitious lawyer who color-coded her sweaters, went into rages when a bath towel wasn't folded properly, and insisted upon throwing out any leftover food for fear it might get bacteria in the refrigerator. While my guffaws sent me into fits, I suddenly grimaced and stopped. Lynne must've seen the pang of recognition of my own crazy relationship. It was then that she offered me her Texas brand of wisdom. "Just hope when it bites," she added, "it doesn't have rabies." I never was sure how to interpret truth as a rabid dog. It's moments like that, though, that make me miss the Lone Star State.

Truth in writing can bite, or at least it can provoke a physical response. Emily Dickinson has that line about how true poetry takes her head off (no wonder she wrote, "Tell all the Truth but tell it slant"), and Kafka supposedly said that "we ought to read only the kind of books that wound and stab us." I called a writer friend of mine one recent morning and asked her a light question to chew on over breakfast: "What's the most truthful writing you've ever read?" She paused, stumbled around the names of Tolstoy and Whitman, and said, "I'm really not sure, but I know it when I feel it. It can punch me in the gut while caressing the back of my neck." So, truth's a rabid dog, a murderer, and a seductive sadist. I know the feeling. While reading certain passages from, say, Salman Rushdie's *Midnight's Children* or Faulkner's *Go Down, Moses*, I've had to put the book down, catch my breath, and utter something profound, like "Holy shit." My temple throbs; my heart pounds. Truth can be sublime, at once beautiful and terrifying.

"So how do we write such neck-breaking, butt-biting truth?" a writer once asked. We're all susceptible to being spin doctors of our own emotions, experiences, and images. We can drum up hackneyed happy endings that would make John Hughes roll his eyes; we can go to the other extreme and rant like Al Sharpton without the rhetorical flair or one-liner wit; or we can dilute our genuine anger or passion into Hallmark homilies as if to put our prose on Prozac. And when we do so, we can hear our words' tinny quality that evokes no visceral response except a wince. And how, when the Heckler calls, can you keep moving toward the difficult and write the truth that must be written? Yes, how do we know when we're kidding ourselves, pretending to write the truth?

Sometimes, I think anyone's guess is as good as mine, that we're all writing in the dark and hoping against hope that some word will at least light a votive to get us down the next corridor without our bumping a toe and blurting an invective. Yet, my Yoga practice has given me a candle's worth of clarity on how to intuit truth as I write and read what I write. Yoga can awaken within us a deeper, more abiding sense of how our words can, in fact and in body, "ring true."

First, we have to agree upon what truth is—or at least what it is not—in writing. Truth in writing has less to do with factual honesty and more to do with emotional and imaginative honesty. Anyone who demands to know of a fiction writer, "Did this really happen?" misses the point about truth in writing. Truth in writing is something more intuitive that has to do with a work's ability to become timeless in its timeliness and universal in its particularity. Steinbeck's *The Grapes of Wrath*, for instance, centers upon the plight of migrant farmers during the Dust Bowl of the 1930s. Steinbeck, the ever-ready journalist, traveled among the farmers, "immersed" himself in his subject, and rendered with precision the details of Route 66, of families' social dynamics, and of the Southwest's terrain. Yet, he sensed something more significant in the people's plight than just the sum of details and facts, something that reflected the history of dispossessed people from the Hebrews onward. To feed this sense of something grand looming in their story, the agnostic author referenced the Old and New Testaments for guidance to rewrite the novel and to structure such an epic story. His venturous reflections upon humanity's perseverance that he weaves throughout the novel and its structure reflects a shift in the characters' humanity from being selfish and competitive to selfless and cooperative. Following his sense and not sticking with the facts led him to write a novel laden with truth.

Ideas more than facts leads us toward truth. First-time memoirists especially confuse facts with truth. The truth is in the making more than in the memory. Yes, James Frey, author of the best-selling and now infamous "memoir" *A Million Little Pieces*, flat out lied about salient facts regarding how he portrayed himself as well as his alcohol and drug recovery—facts that undermined the memoir's spirit of truth. Frey wittingly lied to make his protagonist appear as the macho rebel who tried to defy not only the law but also the entire Alcoholics Anonymous culture. So, yes, get salient facts straight. But that task alone won't lead you to writing the truth.

We can catch ourselves straining to write the truth. I know an aspiring poet who feels responsible to close her poems with messages. I understand the impulse. In fact, some poets react to what they perceive as other poets' sollipsistc obtuseness or surreal privacy by taking an extreme tact: Full transparency with a tightly wrought ending. The message can drown out the real truth, though. If you strain too hard to write Universal Truths, your writing may slip into clichéd themes, and a priest or rabbi may invade your voice as you pontificate upon love and beauty or the world's injustices. I have a "big Truth" voice with a booming tone like Charlton Heston as Moses that, usually, if I recognize it in time, can be halted before I subject my readers to its admonitions.

Novelist Richard Russo says he started his best-selling novel Bridge of Sighs with an idea. He wanted to write a novel that dealt with a particular small town's class and economic divisions. He knew that Division Street, that literally runs down the center of the town on which he based his fictional one, would play a role. He knew he wanted a polluted river to run through the middle of town. He knew he had things to say about these subjects, but what he wasn't sure.

To discover what you have to "say" and to render universals with truth, begin with particulars. Through details of dialogue, character, setting, situation, and story, fiction will unveil—surprisingly to you and to your readers—some inevitable sense of truth. Imagine you're writing a story about a demure, repressed character, Brian, and his spunky fiancée, Pamela. Over the dinner Brian has prepared, Pamela announces that she needs to "have some space to think about the future" and wants to travel for a few days with Mike, a guy she met at work and who has a charming summer home in Colorado where she and Mike can hang out, talk, help her sort through some things, you know. Brian, so utterly miffed, probably won't say much as he takes a bite of his stir-fry tatsoi. He may respond with "Maybe it needs more ginger or cloves. There's definitely something missing." If you have him break into a monologue or tirade about the misery of relationships and the fiasco of marriage as he flings his plate across the dining room, you're being emotionally dramatic but probably not emotionally honest with these particular characters, situation, dialogue, and story. (Although I know a guy whose mother kept the frying pan that his father flung against the wall in the plaster for two months so her husband could remember the one time he lost his cool.) From an honest attention to details, truth can emerge. Let it surprise you.

TRACKING TRUTH

"You'll feel it. You'll hear it," I say to writers. This vague response doesn't appease all of them because they're thirsty, and they want to feel and hear truth in their writing now. But this response moves us in the right direction.

Truth in Yoga resonates at the cellular level. Many-named in Sanskrit, the most common tag for truth is satya, worldly truth, the truth we manifest in our everyday life. In *Yoga-Sutra* II.36, Patanjali notes that when a yogi embodies this kind of truth "his words become so potent that whatever he says comes to realization."[1] *Satya* can pervade each breath, sound, word, gesture, and decision. "It is not our mind, but the inner voice of our cells which has the power to implement our intentions," yogi B.K.S. Iyengar notes.[2] So when our writing correlates directly with our body's deepest intentions as well as with an intuitive sense that our writing's particulars relate to something honest and universal, when we indisputably feel something "in our bones," we write toward truth.

This is a good time to revisit the act of setting an intention. The question "What am I writing for?" can connect us with a source beyond reason. Called "in-born knowledge" *(sahaja-jnāna)*, intuition is that unmediated—indisputable—knowledge of truth. It's that quality that lets us feel truth in our throat and in our gut. So when we ask ourselves, "What am I writing for?" the answer often is a fleeting apparition, a word darting by. Still, we aim to absorb the answer in every cell. We tune in our cells and trust that our actions, our writing, will line up accordingly. It'll take a while—years, maybe—to know what your truth is that you need to write. Even if you've been writing and publishing for years, it may take more time.

Truth in writing registers something universal and timeless. Many of us likewise sense an abiding force that keeps this world from spiraling out of control and keeps the planet from spinning off its axis. We sense a greater truth, maybe even an order to the cosmos beyond human perception. One name for this universal truth is *rita*. Because this truth is beyond human perception, we're given the faculty of intuition, *antar-jnāna* ("inner knowledge"), which helps us sense and "remember" the nature of everything as being inherently interconnected. Our reasoning alone—using the frontal lobe functions of breaking things down and dividing—won't always help us track truth. Yoga's practices, though, can stimulate this inner knowledge.

We can begin with the throat. I've been experimenting with how this word tunnel—which links our fiery, willful belly to our mouth—helps me and other writers hear the truth. The throat in part is metaphorical for the channel through which words pass. With too much clutter and obstruction, our words become distorted, our intentions detracted. We write muck.

There is something to this *cakra* stuff. The throat center, called the *vishuddi cakra*, houses energy for clear communication, courageous words, sacred speech. Shuddi means "to purify," specifically poisons, and if we purify our throat center, we can train our cells to register truth's notes. The first Hatha-Yogis intuited the throat's power, for the throat's thyroid is an antitoxin. When stimulated, the thyroid gland secretes the hormone thyroxine, which moderates our metabolism. The thyroid helps the parasympathetic nervous system's functioning, which in turn keeps our vital organs operating while also calming down our thoughts. With increased inner quietude, we're more open to hear within. The thyroid also moderates the rate of our cells' death and replenishment as well as muscle tissues' aging. Slow cell turnover and slow tissue decay lead to longevity. A natural elixir exists in our throat. A healthy, open throat, then, can clear the body's channels and give us clarity, that open certainty, that unhesitating indisputability that surfaces when we hear, feel, and write truth.

The **THROAT LOCK** *(kantha-bandha or jālandhara-bandha)* is a good starting place to appreciate the throat's importance for writing with truth. In a seated or standing position, you lengthen your spine and take at least two full breaths. As you inhale, you draw in your chin toward your collarbone notch and above your breastbone, and let the back of your neck lift upward as your shoulder blades drop. Doing so stretches your cervical spine and throat's back side. The lock position stimulates the thyroid and releases thyroxine, the "elixir." On the exhalation, you return your chin to its normal position. Repeat two more times to heighten your awareness of this area.

I know a writer who prays before she writes. She wants to connect to something more than that telemarketer voice. Some yogic lore contends that we have a bindu center at the top and back of our skull, a slight opening through which we receive the universe's answers to our queries about our existence, destiny, and so forth. Call it a cosmic antenna. The throat lock is believed to adjust this antenna. If that idea is a bit out there for you, just consider that the throat lock, if practiced consistently, does help your body listen to and respond to something more than your mind's daily chitchat.

Another easy way to quicken this center is through **VICTORIOUS BREATH** *(ujjayī-prāṇāyāma)*. This breath keeps your glottis and epiglottis healthy and clears the throat's channels. It also soothes your nerves and boosts energy by aerating the lungs and increasing cerebral blood flow. With calmness and alertness, we're in a position to write with truth. The crudest way to practice **VICTORIOUS BREATH** is by contracting the glottis and breathing from the throat instead of from the nostrils. You may hear a hissing "sa" as you inhale and a raspy "ha" as you exhale. To take the practice a step further, incorporate the **THROAT LOCK** by drawing in the chin after you inhale. The lock should help you feel breath caressing your throat's back and your mouth's roof, and it should help you hear your breath's "ocean voice" as it imitates the sounds of ocean waves. It also can heighten our ability to hear what's happening internally—essential for getting to the truth in our writing.

The throat center can be an ally when writing difficult sections of fiction or nonfiction. When poet and novelist Terry Wolverton rewrote a section of her memoir *Insurgent Muse: Life and Art at the Woman's Building* (City Lights, 2002), she knew she had to be truthful. The memoir includes not only historical background of the artists and writers with whom she worked while directing the Los Angeles Woman's Building during the 1970s; it also delves into stories about people she has loved and left, people she has hurt and who have hurt her. There was a lot of room for the book to offend, to hurt, to misrepresent. She told me in an interview, "I really wanted to make sure that my articulation was as open and clear as it possibly could be, and I needed to be a very clear channel in order to be honest and fair to the people that I was writing about." For forty mornings Wolverton, also a certified Kundalini Yoga teacher, practiced a Kundalini Yoga cleansing process called *kantha padma kriyā* (or, loosely, "the cleansing of the throat lotus")—a series of poses, visualizations, chants, and breathing that cleared her throat center. The process helped her check in with and act upon her intention, which was to tell the truth as accurately as she could present it. The energy and clarity she felt in her throat transferred to writing her memoir's especially difficult sections. When she found herself pausing for fear of hurting someone's feelings, she clarified her intention, heard what needed to be said, and got out of the way of the words that needed to emerge.

"Joan", an established writer with whom I have worked, has published six novels. She teaches creative writing full-time at a university. She can readily assess a student's story according to its voice, structure, or characterization. She knows craft. She knows how to write. She has written six well received novels. So why whould she call me? A few months ago, she had felt a rumbling in her abdominal region that originally triggered some deep memories that led her to realize it was time to write a memoir, her first memoir. It was time to write this story's truth. The story deals with her mentally challenged sister and the ways her parents raised the two siblings differently. The memoir delves into themes of parenting, intelligence, and identity, but writing the memoir, Joan knew, also would expose some deep wounds. How would she be able to stay with the project, meet the emotionally challenging parts of the memoir, and write the truth—all while still maintaining her marriage and her professorship?

Joan wanted a sequence and practice to help her move toward the difficult. After we spoke on the telephone, we designed a ten-minute practice she could integrate with her writing routine. It included work with the throat lock but also included practices that would stoke her belly's fire to help her persevere. We agreed to check in every six weeks or so. At first, the practice challenged her.

She wept a lot. Her stomach tied up in knots. Still, she observed her mind's habits of distracting her from the truth. While writing, she witnessed how her throat and gut tightened when she let some complex feelings surface. She made it through the dark nights.

Deep listening helps us hear truth's vibrations. "When people are speaking truth," poet Olga Broumas once told me, "there are different vibrations than when they are spinning their wheels. That's also something very audibly perceptual if someone brings their attention to it." To tune in to these vibrations requires us to hear our body's internal vibrations, the vibrations from which language emanates. Sound vibrations travel to the outer ear's tympanic membrane, which sends them to the middle ear's three bones called ossicles, which in turn amplify the sound vibrations so the inner ear can pick them up and convert them into electrical signals that travel to the brain.[3] But we can't hear everything the universe has to offer, as human ears on average pick up sound frequencies from twenty to twenty thousand or maybe thirty thousand hertz. Your dog, though, can hear frequencies as high as forty thousand, and that bat circling the trees out back in the dark can hear hums as high as a hundred thousand hertz. The simple fact that human ears have a limited capacity to pick up the universe's rhythms as compared even to certain animals should suggest that there is much more to reality and truth than what we can know with our cognitive senses.[4] Despite our outer ear's limitations, physicists are confirming that everything in the universe is held together with pulsing "strings." The "seers" of the *Rg Veda* intuited these universal vibrations centuries ago, well before the mechanistic tools of science could confirm their existence, so some mechanism in the inner ear's deep recesses helps us sense this truth's vibrations.

So sound out the truth with your throat and mouth-organ. In her poem "Artemis," Olga Broumas says her work with "tonguelike forms that curve round a throat" begins with "O, the O-/mega, horseshoe, the cave of sound." It begins with O indeed. The shape of the womb, the shape of lips as they let that O sound pass through "the cave of sound," O is also a combination of A and U, considered in Sanskrit as manifestations of the universe's most supreme sounds. Some songs, hymns, and mantras remind us of words' potency. When writing or when listening to what we've written, hum an "Amen," a verse of "Amazing Grace," "Atman" ("Self"), or "AUM"—all of which begin with the beginning sounds. When these words hum through your word tunnel, your *vishuddi cakra*, they can remind us of the truth we embody. The vibrations, especially the humming m sound, rouse the right hemisphere and calm your thoughts. A few bars of one of these chants can clear your throat of the muck. Revere your words. They can be truth's midwives.

THE GIFT OF TRUTH

In India I heard a story about truth and the goddess Vāc. In a time before "beforeness," a young goddess named Vāc, possessor of sacred speech, desired to give us mortals divinely charged language, but the Himalayan gods—not unlike their Olympian Greek neighbors who argued with the populist Prometheus—didn't want humans to have sacred speech. Vāc, distraught from the divine spat, fled to a forest, where she found refuge among the trees. The trees refused to extradite the sweet-sounding goddess unless the gods agreed that Vāc could endow humans with her linguistic gift. The gods gave in. So the "seers" of the *Ṛg Veda* attribute Vāc with inspiring them, and now musicians remember that their lutes and flutes carved from trees' bodies must be played with the breath of sacred speech, and writers create words published on trees' flesh and with words that also come from Vāc's defiant truthfulness (even when doing so defies popular opinion). Writing the truth the best we can is our gift.

It's a gift with a cost. In facing the struggle to write the truth, we in turn give this gift to others to persevere in expressing their own truth. Eugene O'Neill was tormented by the demons of his crazed acting family until he exorcised them by writing in the mid-twentieth century *A Long Day's Journey Into Night*, one of this country's first plays to unveil truths about manipulative parents, addictions, and the yearning for transcendence through art. O'Neill's courage emboldened the likes of Arthur Miller, who went on to write similarly unsettling plays such as *Death of a Salesman* and *All My Sons*, plays that disrupted the 1950s ideal of perfect nuclear families and the pursuit of our untainted American dreams. Miller's willingness to tell the truth encouraged the likes of Edward Albee, whose *Who's Afraid of Virginia Woolf?* shows how cruel and destructive relationships and language can be. Memoirists likewise have had to face authentic struggles to tell the truth about themselves, their families, and being human. Arabian poets such as Nizar Qabbani have ventured for decades to tell the truth about being human under state oppression. Even before feminism came into vogue, Qabbani used his role as popular poet to unveil the social stigmas imposed upon erotic relationships. His daring helped a generation of other Middle Eastern poets, men and women, write truthfully about desire and love. Writers risk exile, if not from their countries then from their religious and social communities as well as from their families. Their struggle, though, inspires us to face the truth and to speak out.

You're probably going to offend some people. Get ready. Writing truth isn't always kind or pleasant. A friend of mine grew nauseous over several days while writing the most difficult parts of her memoir. She kept using metaphors of "getting something out" and "purging" to describe what the process felt like. If your writing is coasting along your consciousness's bay without rock or wave, without a single idea that challenges your own or any of your readers' sensibilities or notions—in short, without much of an effect on you or them—then you might not be writing your truth. You have to write your truth. Sometimes, you have to write what simmers in the early morning hours in your imagination's background, waiting to be heard, and then what clamps you like a gila monster and makes you bowl over until you pay attention to it. Sound out the words, or let them sound you out. Stick with the honesty of details, first. The universe will follow.

Stand firm in the truth you write. Gandhi's specific form of political and spiritual resistance came to be tagged "firmness in truth," *satyagraha*.[5] Such whole-bodied resistance to complacency, to cliché, to simplistic writing, might be called the same.

All of this talk of truth can make us take ourselves too seriously. So, remember to laugh. I don't know which god or goddess gave us this gift, but I love humor that bites me with the truth too. I agree with Saint John that in the Beginning was the Word, but sometimes I have this queasy feeling in my gut that the Creator, being a clever writer, made the Word a Pun and that sometimes we just don't get it. Dogs and gods, they'll both sneak up on you.

TAKE A BREATH: WRITING THE TRUTH

Intention:
Try this practice to become more sensitive to feeling your writing's truth. Engage it when you need to write with emotional honesty. As with most practices in this book, it requires an authentic intention and persistent practice to recognize its effects.

Choose a seated pose with palms resting on knees. With sitting bones weighted in the ground and spine lengthened, focus on your breath and make space for your intention. When you feel openness, eyes closed or half-open, ask yourself quietly, "What am I writing for?" Tend to whatever words or images surface in response and let that response spread throughout your throat and into your body. Then, clarify that you intend to write a piece, whatever your subject, that stems from your own truth. Contract the back of your throat to breathe with the raspy victorious breath if it helps keep things clear of the Heckler's voice. Inhale, hearing your breath's hissing "sa," and exhale hearing your breath's raspy "ha." Then, repeat this way of breathing with your lips closed. On the next slow inhalation, retain your breath and bring the chin to the chest or collarbone.

Hold the inhalation for four seconds at first (longer with more practice). Then raise the head, drop the shoulders, and exhale slowly. Practice this throat lock practice (jālandhara-bandha) five times.

While you stimulate this level of sound, imagine how words can register deep notes within you. Visualize how the words you're going to write need to sound—not the visual images you've written but the words' sounds themselves, their "visible sound." If the vibra-

tions of what you want to write were to form a shape or picture, what would they look like? Shivering parsnips? An old man's hands whittling a flute?

Then begin to write. Write with a firm sense of truth. Keep breathing with the raspy victorious breath. You won't be fooled by the emotional spin doctor who tries, for instance, either to end every conflict with a bouquet of flowers or to render a scene so utterly dismally that your characters' theme song must be the Stones' "Paint It Black." You'll be wary of hiding the truth with disingenuous humor or of dragging the truth through muddy moroseness. Once you've drafted, you can delete or change those parts whose tone seems insincere, whose mood seems maudlin or melodramatic.

CHAPTER SEVENTEEN

WEB OF CONTRADICTIONS: WRITING THE SELF IN MEMOIR, POETRY, & FICTION

W E LOVE THE FIRST PERSON, at least this country's current reading habits suggest so. Memoirs and personal essays have had a renaissance of sorts. So, too, autobiographical and confessional poems (even if the autobiographies and confessions be partially fictional) have resurfaced prominently in literary journals, collections, and anthologies during the past twelve years. Why? Maybe our socially and politically tumultuous times send us to read about what we know—personal experience—as one theory goes. Maybe we're increasingly "self" absorbed (witness shifts in television programming toward more lurid talk shows and reality TV) and so choose to write primarily about ourselves and read primarily about people's personal experiences that mirror ours so we can project ourselves into a writer's world.

Possibly, though, we simply hunger to make and shape meaning. To essay (from the French essayer) is to attempt, to try out, to experiment. It is rarely to proselytize, to preach, to assert with absolute certainty. When writing personal essays—whether three pages or three hundred pages—we wander through our memories and our current impressions, and if we're lucky we happen upon a clearing, some small truth or insight that gives experience meaning. Fiction grants us certain freedoms because our characters can explore our own ideas and experiences at a personal distance, and poetry can play between the borders of nonfiction and fiction so that a speaker's experiences may or may not be literally the poet's any more than a fiction writer's. Each of these genres can be a vehicle for moving more deeply into the self's alleys and bays, its bistros and institutions.

Part of writing the truth includes exploring the truth of our self (or selves). Writing directly about the self or from our own experiences is tricky, though. A friend recently told me she wasn't sure her self merited so much attention in her writing. "How do I write about myself without being self-centered?" writers often ask. Self-absorption, self-aggrandizement (an ugly-sounding word), and self-delusion, these are potential traps of the ego. The first-person "I" becomes the hero, the brilliant narrator, the know-it-all speaker. But self-negation and self-loathing also stifle several writers I meet. These writers either avoid writing about themselves altogether, or when they do write about themselves their text reflects themselves in one dimension. It is possible to unravel some of these limitations.

WITNESS THE CHARACTER-SELF

The character on the page who shares your name is not you. It's a character on the page. I don't mean to sound like some smart aleck who holds up a print of Rene Magritte's painting of a pipe with the inscription beneath it that reads, *ceci n'est pas une pipe* (this is not a pipe). But the image is not the thing. The word is not the self. The character is not the author. A character in a memoir, poem, or novel who is most directly based on the author's impressions of himself I call the "character-self." When you the author can view the character-self with such distance, you begin to witness the character, so to speak.

The "witness" in Yoga or Buddhism refers to that quality that can observe thoughts passing through the mind without the mind latching onto and obsessing about them. It's no easy feat, this witnessing business, but it is a hallmark of a Yoga mind and of a self-aware writer's mind. You are less attached. In writing, we might call such witnessing "aesthetic distance." When you are less attached, you can begin to cultivate true compassion for this whole self as mirrored in a character or speaker.

Compassion is not gooey self-love. To cultivate compassion will not necessarily lead us to write sugary poetry appropriate for Mother's Day. Words of compassion often cut through obstructions and deliver truth with a prick, slice, slash, or slaying of a person's ego. I mean a certain quality of active compassion, karunā in Pali, that may distinguish a self-absorbed writer—no matter how fine the craft—from an emotionally mature writer. In *The Art of Fiction*, John Gardner discusses aspiring writers' "errors of the soul" and "errors of character" such as "lack of due warmth" and "sentimentality." These qualities reflect a novice writer's inability to treat emotional scenes maturely. Gardner suggests that writing teachers cannot "correct" these errors. "Correct," no, yet writing instructors can model how to write with active compassion that is neither cold nor saccharine sweet but authentic. Developing a writer's active compassion requires honesty with ourselves when writing memoirs, personal essays, poetry or fictional alter egos. Such honesty means we can embrace the full spectrum of our self—or selves—as complex and contradictory.

When a memoirist cannot view a character-self complexly, nonfiction suffers. When one memoirist published her story in the early 1990s about being a morally lost teenager hooked on antidepressants, she came across to many readers as being self-obsessed and neurotic. She aimed her anger at the "social system" that pressured this girl on one hand to succeed and on the other hand to cast herself as a beauty doll whose worth rested only in pleasing boys. Her tone, mostly whining and blaming, marred what could have been a powerful story about girls' struggles with these real and often conflicting pressures.

As writers it's a good idea to slay—or at least laugh at—the ego and to muster a complex perspective. A complex perspective means in part that we don't let character-selves become socially constructed clichés of "victim" or even of "hero" or "survivor." Casting a character-self solely as a victim ironically does not garner many readers' sympathy and compassion.

Consider, by contrast, Penny Wolfson's personal essay "Moonrise" from her book *Moonrise: One Family, Genetic Identity, and Muscular Dystrophy* (New York: St. Martin's Press, 2003), about her relationship with her teenage son who has muscular dystrophy. What could have been a self-centered essay about a woman's despair toward her son's illness, about her anger toward fate's irrational pickings, about her martyrdom in sacrificing her wants for her son's well-being, instead reads as a poignant, realistic depiction of a mother who tries as best she may to understand both her son's brilliance and his condition. Prone to collapsing from decayed bones, the son in one scene falls in a grocery store parking lot. As he calls out to his mother between gritted teeth to help him, she admits to herself and to us that what she feels is not pity or despair, but anger and resentment. She acknowledges her "terrible impatience" and wonders if she's a witch, a bad mother who can't have patience. Notes of such blemishing self-revelation register this essay's tone. Wolfson's neither pleased with nor condoning her anger; she's simply admitting it, and by admitting and wondering about it invites us as readers at once to have compassion for her and to admit to our own anger and frustration in such difficult situations.

Or take Nancy Mairs's revelatory memoir *Remembering the Bone House: An Erotics of Place and Space.* In her 1989 preface she acknowledges how her upbringing to be a polite young lady who remains silent on certain subjects—particularly of the body and things erotic—could easily lead her to self-censorship. She notes that such social conventions imposed on a woman can "foster feelings of shame that lead her to trivialize her own experience and prevent her from discovering the depth and complexity of her life." Mairs isn't silent or polite. For as she notes in the next sentence, "I've spoken as plainly and truthfully as the squirms and wriggles of the human psyche will permit."[1] F. Scott Fitzgerald's most illuminating writing may have been not his fiction but his nonfiction personal essays collected as *The Crack-Up*. Written during the 1930s, they offer a startlingly self-disclosing analysis of his self-absorbed mental breakdown. He reveals not only how every act toward another human being ultimately was motivated by self-preservation but also how he loathed people of various races, backgrounds, and classes. "All rather inhuman and undernourished, isn't it?" he writes at one point of his own condition. "Well, that, children, is the true sign of cracking up."[2] This way of writing about oneself so forthrightly, of course, also transfers to fiction. Updike's alter ego Henry Bech or Philip Roth's Portnoy are full of failings and inner contradictions. Accepting our character-self's blemishes is essential to developing characters with any real flesh that our readers would want to see more of.

Self-deprecation alone is not witnessing the character-self complexly. It's become almost expected for some young writers to assume an ironic, if not cynical, persona as they lampoon themselves, their family, and every facet of society the writer observes. An ironic persona indeed can be used in a striking way to expose just how absurd our lives can be, but it also can become a shield, a convenient dodge to avoid exploring our lives' gravitas. One writer, recently graduated from college and well steeped in all things ironic, attended one of my workshops and said her greatest breakthrough in the workshop was her ability for the first time to write seriously about herself and her family.

How can we knowingly admit our character-self's uncomfortable feelings and faults in sensitive scenes without making them seem pitiful? Understanding the nature of the self might help us witness the nature of the character-self.

WITNESSING PATTERNS

This complex yet individuated self in several Yoga texts is called *jiva* or *jīva-ātman*. It's described as being "bound" and entwined as a capricious animal. Most yogis in nondualistic Hatha-Yoga traditions ultimately seek to liberate the self in this world (jivan-mukta). As writers (and as yogis), our aims can be less ambitious at first. We can simply acknowledge this self's complex nature; liberation might follow. The self is fickle. Its mercurial nature, connected to the flickering psyche, often evades even the most astute seeker's net. Desire, fear, courage, love, vitriol, adoration, spite, pride, these emotions and attributes drive much of the shackled self's activity. Being bound in this twine of pain and pleasure is a central cause of the self's suffering.

Suffering is the source of conflict in stories, or at least in many of them. Characters suffer. "What is the nature and source of this character-self's suffering?" you might ask yourself. "What's unique about her existence in this entanglement of pleasure and pain?" "How does he cope with his own brand of suffering in his own way?" Camus's Meursault in the novel *L'Etranger* has a peculiarly detached way of coping, and his utter lack of emotion offers us an ambiguous glimpse into the heart of a character who, while trying to be authentic with his emotions, comes off as being emotionally stunted. Solzhenitsyn's Ivan Denisovich controls his psyche's attachments during a day of his life in a concentration camp so that while being trapped in a prison, his mind doesn't trap him. The heart of your story—fiction or nonfiction—similarly might explore these questions related to the the bound self's restlessness: "What does she think she lacks that she thinks she deeply wants?" "How will she set about getting it?" "What will get in her way?" "In the end will she get it?" Such questions can form the basis of a story's conflict, plot, and resolution.

Thoughts make up a considerable part of the self. Try to track some of your own thoughts for five minutes. Set a timer. Don't try to record them in detail—you'll never keep up with the whirl. Just note bits of the good, the bad, and the ugly. You want a brownie, you notice your back hurts, you want to glimpse God, the kids yelling on the sidewalk outside get on your nerves, then you think they're cute. Five minutes could produce just that much randomness. Now, you won't put all of those thoughts (I hope) into a piece related to your present situation, but if you're not already acknowledging and accepting how quirky, idiosyncratic, and unpredictable your thoughts are, then start.

Then, try the same exercise without getting attached to any of the thoughts. Just let them surface and let them pass. It's not easy. We writers especially love to obsess. If you can concentrate, though, and listen with your inner ear, you really can begin to witness some thoughts and then notice the repetetive patterns of your thoughts.

Witness your own stream of consciousness, and you can witness with some distance your character-self's consciousness. You can witness her repetetive ways of perceiving her father who listens to Hank Williams each night and weeps for her mother who left him fifteen years ago, her repetetive ways of over-reacting to her husband's dressing in white stockings in the winter, and so on, her inability to see clearly how she attracts the wrong kinds of men and the right kinds of women. Remember, though, you are not your character.

Explore consequences, too. In an extended story, a character-self might suffer from patterned actions and patterned consequences. They might be stuck in their personal Groundhog Day. Everything we think and do contributes to the path we take or are given. Such is a basic premise of karman—translated to "action." It also refers to the moral force of one's actions or thoughts. By moral force, I mean the consequences—preferable or not—from our thoughts and actions. The *Bhagavad-Gita* identifies three types of actions according to the self's intentions: those selfless actions that are aligned with noble intentions but have no attachment to outcome, those ego actions motivated by a search for a pleasurable outcome, and those careless actions performed without regard for the harm that could come from them. My guess is each of us acts upon all three, especially the first two categories (although I know a few reckless writers whose actions occasionally fall into the latter).

So whether writing into a past experience or a fictional scene, explore your character-self's motives. Imagine you're writing a short story about a character based on yourself who volunteers his time to offer free art lessons at a homeless shelter downtown. The character would like to think he's motivated by that Kantian ideal of goodwill, and you, the writer, find out that indeed the character is partly driven by a deep desire to help others find an avenue to express themselves through painting and drawing. But as the story unfolds, you discover that the character also wants to compensate for his otherwise self-absorbed life (as he views it). You also discover that he's trying to beef up his vita so he can apply for a grant that pays artists to offer "socially progressive" workshops. The lines between the first two categories of *karman*—selfless and ego-driven—are obscured. Now, if he started trying to seduce one of the women, it wouldn't be difficult to put that action into the latter category unless, of course, you present the characters as possibly "in love" (which might only serve to make the story overly dramatic instead of interesting). There's a danger, too, in oversimplifying a story—whether fiction or nonfiction—by simplistically stating that the artist, for example, just wanted to boost his vita. A story gets interesting (for you and for readers) when motives get mixed.

You don't need to psychoanalyze these actions or confess your character-self's debauchery. Your job as writer is to explore actions and their consequences as honestly as you can, and through such an exploration perhaps your writing implies a worldview or even a moral view without preaching to, asking forgiveness of, or simply shocking your readers.

Appreciate the self's smallness as well. It's tiny, really, made of minuscule, subatomic elements and of a series of wee moments. I heard a writing teacher of some repute tell a student that her writing would improve once she "went out into the world and had more experiences." This advice not only negated this woman's life, but it seems misdirected. We don't have to travel to Africa to hunt tigers or descend into a moral morass and take heroin in order to have a life worth writing about. If we focus only on exotica such as going to an ashram in India or on the common "big" life events such as getting married or divorced, or losing a parent, then their scale may tempt us as writers to examine the obvious external details of "what happened." Yet, any piece of writing worth reading and rereading is always more than a recount of what happened. Forget for now the cataclysmic earthquakes that we narrowly escaped—those "big" moments we think are "life defining"; the greater challenge of writing about yourself, in nonfiction or fiction, is to divine meaning in mundane moments.

To do so, I often ask writers to create a simple chart of their character-self's life map by making rows on a piece of paper that designate life phases. We label them 1–6 (years old), 7–12, 13–19, 20–29, 30–39, 40–49, et cetera. Then we jot down brief notes about moments that our character-self experienced during these periods. The notes can be as brief as "met hobo near train tracks," "fell out of tree," or "hummingbird moth landed on my foot." Your writing into a "small" moment prompts you to consider how subtly impressions are made upon your psyche and character.

Then, form a sutra self. A "sutra" is a thread. It's also an aphoristic bit of wisdom that is part of a series of aphorisms "threaded together." Hence, the *Yoga-Sutra*. In mapping such moments as described above, you'll probably notice patterns between or among them. One writer realized how frequently she had listed times when she had met a stranger—from when she was eight to when she was forty. That observation led her to write a compelling essay titled "Talk to Strangers: A Mother's Advice." Someone else noticed his obsession with Patsy Cline's and Ani di Franco's music (an odd pair that didn't appear on anyone else's map) and used that observation to form an essay, and another writer recognized how different kinds of cheeses played a part in his remembering romantic moments (which could've been, uh, cheesy, but he handled the connection well in a short story). In her memoir *Sleeping with Cats*, Marge Piercy loosely held together different parts of her delightfully crazy life according to the cats she owned, or that owned her, at different phases. Such a memoir's, personal essay's, series of poems', or short story's structure, then, may be seemingly fragmented as the writer threads a series of related anecdotes with commentary. The sutras' wisdom often surfaces for the writers while they're writing, threading, and rearranging the moments.

Honor your character-self's obsessions. You don't need to perpetuate the idea that all writers are neurotic and obsessive-compulsive, but surely your thoughts latch on to some crazed set of thoughts, habits, even trends, that no writer yet has explored fully. Nicholson Baker wrote a book-length essay not about his obsession with John Updike but about his feeling anxiously influenced by the senior writer. It's a wonderful study in quirky connections and threads, threads which often (but not always) offer some glimmer of self-understanding. Granted, much of Yoga is about quieting the inner chatter, which means that some writers might be out of a job—or at least completely "out of character"—but Yoga also is about accepting and witnessing those thoughts. This is compassion for the self of the highest order: not to yell at ourselves for talking so loudly inside our heads, but to acknowledge these thoughts and their oft-beguiling patterns. When we have aesthetic distance on such thoughts, then we can finesse them on the page.

Get a different point of view. Switch persons. The standard rule for memoir writing and personal essay writing has been to write in the first-person singular ("I," "me," "my," "mine."). Colson Whitehead's series of thirteen essays that comprise *The Colossus of New York* frequently shifts among first-person, second-person, and third-person points of view. When writing poetry, I especially experiment with second- and third-person for a couple of reasons: It frees me from feeling restricted to talking about the "facts" of what I think about myself, and doing so grants me distance, as if I'm witnessing the self as the words unfold on the page. Updike had his own character, his alter ego Henry Bech, interview him in an essay a few years ago. Jorge Luis Borges, always toying with notions of authorship, wrote a story called "Borges and I" in which the narrator sits down next to Borges and converses with him.

Adrienne Rich's poem "Integrity" explores the whole, complex self. Her self has come back to a shore, so to speak, with sun-scalded arms and with a beautiful understanding: that she has "selves." It's such a simple yet startling realization for her after so many years. Two selves she acknowledges especially, anger and tenderness that she says "breathe" in her "as angels, not polarities" woven from the same spider's body.[3] Rich acknowledges her complex self, her integral self (or selves). Images in the poem appear to surface from both the poet's memories and from her subtle imagination.

Writers in my workshops similarly have explored surprising and seemingly contradictory facets of themselves. "There is an ocean in me," one writer's piece begins. She then explores how she feels trapped in her mind's pond, unwilling to venture too far beyond the unknown. Another writer was surprised to explore two concepts that defined parts of her selves: teacher and whore. The word "whore," even more surprisingly, shares similar roots with "charity," so her whore self may be a teacher, and her teacher self a whore.

The ego can try to replay the same old songs of self. It often hides the self's subtle shades. Yoga, though, helps us bypass the ego's well-trod channels and replace instead of replay those songs.

TAKE A BREATH:
COMPASSION FOR THE INTEGRAL SELF

Intention:

Try this practice to gain fresh ideas for portraying the complexities of your seemingly contradictory self. You can use the insight gained for exploring facets of your self in a personal essay, memoir, short story, novel, or poem.

Several writers have had remarkable success in gleaning surprising insight into the self by engaging yogic breath work and postures while visualizing with the subtle imagination. The following **TAKE A BREATH** *exercise can further your self-exploration and your celebration of the self's myriad faces and shapes. This simple yet effective sequence makes it easy to practice on a regular basis. Every time you come back to this practice, the results may differ.*

I suggest you read through and try the following sequence one to three times before combining the movements with the inner concentration and visualization.

*You can review the illustrations for this sequence, which also includes two optional poses—***OPEN-HEARTED STANDING FORWARD BEND** *(hridaya-uttanāsana) and* **AWKWARD CHAIR POSE** *(utkatāsana). Use the sequence as a starting point for you to stimulate your subtle imagination when trying to explore your self in fresh ways.*

To prepare for this practice, come into **MOUNTAIN POSE** *(tadāsana) and for at least five breaths try to empty your thoughts and prepare to receive. Let go of preconceptions about yourself. With palms together at your heart, quietly ask yourself, "What am I writing for?" Inhale the response and let it circulate throughout your body. Let the response inform* *your self's actions. When ready, specify that you intend to gain fresh insight into the nature of your self's essential contradictions without self-censorship.*

Once you feel clarity about your intention, bend your elbows and hold your palms in front of you, elbow-height. Gaze at your dominant palm and fingers. See your palm as a mirror that reflects back to you images of yourself you consciously present to the rest of the world, the part of you that you hope others see. Take it all in. When ready, gaze at your other palm. This palm reflects those parts of yourself you don't always acknowledge, that you often try to hide from yourself and from others. Take it all in.

Close your eyes. What two words or images suddenly surface that each represent the right side and the left side of your self or selves? Be open to surprise, and let your body take in the words or images. With eyes still closed, inhale and extend your arms straight in front of you, palms facing away. In this offering **MOUNTAIN POSE** (pushpa tadāsana), *you extend both selves to the world. Your hands' and selves' back sides face you. How do these selves appear to others? When was a small moment that one or both of them appeared to others? Take it in for a few breaths.*

On an exhalation, open your arms straight to the side, shoulder-height into **EVEN-HEARTED MOUNTAIN POSE** (sama-hridayatādāsana). *Inhale, filling your heart space. Exhale, turn your head to the right hand, and breathe compassion from the heart through parted lips to this part of your self. Inhale, head to center, and exhale, repeating on the other side, and notice how it feels to extend compassion to each side.*

Exhale and bring your hands behind you, fingers interlaced, into **OPEN-HEARTED MOUNTAIN POSE** (hridaya-tādāsana).

Open your heart as you lift your hands, arms straight. Observe how the images or words come back together and play with one another behind your back. Perhaps parts of a memory surface in which these halves emerged within the same action or moment. Let pertinent details well up without analysis. Inhale fully and as you exhale bring together your hands, your selves, at your heart. Observe how these images relate again and perchance unite. Avoid forcing any reconciliation, though. You can continue your exploration with eyes closed by moving throough the next two pages.

Many writers continue this sequence one to three more times until ready to write. Once you have received information from your body, breath, and subtle imagination, draft a piece—either a prose piece, poem, or interior monologue—in which you explore at least two seemingly contradictory facets, two "angels," of your embodied self. You might situate your self in a specific memory and recount an incident in which these two selves emerged, or you might begin a reflective prose piece in which you poetically explore two seemingly contradictory facets of your self for fiction or nonfiction.

While you write, the journey's not over. See what writing itself unveils. You can begin with a palpable image, and weave in particular details. Heed the rhythms of your heart and of your breath as you write. Metaphors should unfold naturally and subtly. Finally, avoid trying to reconcile the two parts too easily.

CHAPTER EIGHTEEN

STORIES OF SCARS AND DEEP MEMORIES: WRITING BEYOND TRAUMA

MY THIRD EYE IS SCARRED. Dented. Or at least the skin region where my third eye resides once was rent. I don't remember exactly what happened, but one summer night, when I was seventeen and drank too much whiskey, I nodded asleep while driving, veered to the left on a quiet street, and crashed into someone's parked Cadillac. My forehead smashed into and cracked the windshield, and a piece of broken glass lodged itself between my eyebrows. My car—my old Toyota Corolla, the first and last car my father bought me—was totaled. Luckily, my friend Jodie had followed my weaving car on the way home. He had tried to wrest my car keys from my hands, but I had refused. A lot of whiskey combined with my stubborn seventeen-year-old self made for an intolerable friend, but Jodie stayed by my side. "Listen, you have to wake up your father," he had told me. It was after two in the morning. He told me the name of the road and the neighborhood where we had left my wrecked car and asked if I knew how to get back there. I nodded, hugged my friend, and apologized for being such a jerk.

My father—sprawled, crashed, on his bed—looked like a hibernating bear. Sobering up quickly, I pulled the sympathy card by stooping to his eye level as I shook him so that when he would open his eyes he'd see my face caked with blood. Even drunk and dazed from a car crash, I could be manipulative. It worked for a moment. At first, I whimpered; then, I confessed.

Terror and anger must have rushed through my father. He must have seen himself. Not only a spawn of himself but himself twenty-six years younger and just as lost and uncontrollable in a drunken forest. He likely had been trying to sleep off his own meeting with Jack Daniel and his cronies. At that moment, standing before an irresponsible and ungrateful teenage son, he probably didn't remember teaching me at nine years old how to mix his whiskey-and-waters during his all-night poker games and praising me with a chuckle when I lay heavy on the whiskey. Eight years after that first bartending lesson, I genuinely thought that being a man in part meant drinking a lot and keeping your wits. I had mastered the drinking part but had failed the wits bit of the formula. I'm not sure which of these facts—that I drank a great deal or that I had lost control of the steering wheel or that I mirrored him so clearly—angered him most. He would punish me mostly by not letting me have another car and by insisting that I learn to handle my liquor. When I rub that spot now I still remember the reckless spirit I have inherited and have domesticated that I not end up lost and alone on a dead-end road. But this dent at my third eye also reminds me of my uniquely fractured imagination, that I often see reality through a shattered windshield, a windshield that at once distorts vision like a kaleidoscope and distills light's reflections like a snowflake. Where some people see ugliness, I often see a story.

We all have scars and bodily oddities. Bunions that stick out the insides of my feet look like sixth toes. My ring finger's knuckle still swells from an argument several years ago when a friend (still a friend) yanked my finger back and out of joint. And skin still scabs on my belly button from a bad picking habit started when I was four years old. Whether inherited or accumulated, our bodies' scars, scabs, and beautiful irregularities harbor stories rich for the telling. Our scars remind us of foibles and fights, of accidents and adventures. Our "irregularities"—our nose that others call a ski slope, our feet petite and narrow like a geisha's, our birthmark on our thigh that looks like a profile of Lincoln—bespeak our unique brand of being in our bodies. No need to pack on the concealer to hide our wrinkles. Another aspect of extending compassion to the self is to explore the physical body itself—the blood and guts and especially the wounds, the scars, and anything anyone else might call a "physical oddity."

I have worked with courageous writers who have been raped, molested by their fathers and grandfathers, beaten by their wives. Yet, each of them has found ways to write through and beyond trauma. They have explored and made meaning of their experiences in fiction, non-fiction, and poetry beyond resorting to cultural clichés. Authentic writing moves us beyond such conditioned responses and demands we explore our unique experiences with fresh if not complex insight. It asks that we consider tragedy more than trauma, myth more than fact. By discovering the complex patterns of how and why we and our characters each are uniquely scarred or shaped, we can reimagine our bodies as guiding reservoirs of creativity.

This kind of exploration makes several writers squirm. They've become accustomed to forgetting this physical body with aching joints, swollen ankles, a marked cheek, an untrustworthy uterus, a gimp eye. But Yoga and authentic writing are not about denying or transcending the body. You come to Yoga and to writing from where you are. If your neck is stiff, it's stiff. If your back aches from a ski accident in 1983, so be it. Yoga and authentic writing each ask us to accept where we are, and where we are has largely to do with where our physical bodies are. Our physical bodies are part and parcel of who we are and of who our characters are. So taking a journey into the physical body is a journey into the self's most palpable map.

Our flesh's marks—our divets, birthmarks, pimple potholes, skin tracks, and "irregularities"—belie our memories of mishaps and bed stories of who we are and who we've been. Sensory data itself traveling along our spine often leaves traces. When we hit our heads or jam our thumbs, the sensory stimulation that registers pain reaches the interior part of the brain called the thalamus and along the way makes subtle imprints on parts of the body. The sensory stimuli that help us determine where we are and how we move in space reach the cerebral cortex and leave distinct impressions on parts of the body. It's as if our "accidents" leave internal scars—or at least internal tracks of memory.

When our neck whips in a car crash or our skin welts from wasp stings, then our instincts heighten, our breath quickens. Our altering breath imprints our cellular structure slightly, subtly. Less dramatic breaths—as you watch your cat lap milk or feathery snowflakes float to the ground—still impress. At each cell's center, a nucleus contains forty-six chromosomes that map part of the body's genetic code and a part of who we are or how we view our self. Since at each cell's nucleus or center reside some of our genetic stuff, it's as if each breath potentially plays with who we are and who we will become. These stimuli in turn register with our body's previous sensory experiences, so that our body's memory in part shapes our perceptions of any present experience. Mindful movement, breath work, and visualization can bring some of these impressions out of storage.

As writers we can find much fodder for our writing if we delve into our scars, wounds, and other bodily oddities. Doing so can grant us wisdom about our own or our characters' histories and motivations, their physical reality in relation to their psychic reality. Ugliness, scars, and bodily oddities often drive the fates of fictional characters. Cyrano de Bergerac's nose, of course, helped him foster a quick wit and a sharp tongue that at once could pierce the hearts of his enemies and pluck the heart of his unrequited love. There's also Hugo's Quasimodo, who despite or because of his humbling hunchback, swings for Esmerelda's love. Essayists have found their scars and bodily oddities to be deep fodder for digging too: Esmerelda Santiago maps her skin marks and dots ("Skin"), Floyd Skloot offers startling revelations about having "an insult to the brain" ("Gray Area: Thinking with a Damaged Brain"), and Phillip Lopate exposes several parts of himself including his eyebrows that grow together, his various scars, and even his penis, which has two peeing holes and "has the personality of a cat" ("Portrait of My Body"). None of these essayists' work I would describe, incidentally, as solipsistic or pure navel-gazing. Their respective idiosyncratic "irregularities" become springboards for reflecting universally upon identity, appearance, memory, love, self.

BEYOND TRAUMA: THE TRAGIC, COMIC, AND MYTHIC LAYERS

Authentic writing moves beyond the traumatic into the tragic, the comic, and possibly the mythic. Some made-for-television movies and popular psychology books, despite good intentions, may perpetuate simplistic categories of trauma: "victim" or "survivor." Trauma is not tragedy. It's not enough as a writer only to render the facts that something bad happened to your or a character's body (and psyche). Authentic writing is more than retelling what happened. In trauma writing, a writer may see only one cause. The cause may be something outside of one's self (an automobile accident, an abusive parent or spouse, a natural disaster), or it may be some single point of self-blame (carelessness, cowardice, stubbornness). A tragic view mixes both and more. We explore complexly how a person's fate stems from a mix of personal decisions and personal dominant qualities as well as outside forces of other people's and society's influence. We venture to wonder about larger factors perhaps of "divine plan" or of chance (depending on your beliefs and still avoiding being preachy). In such a complex account, when a protagonist constantly faces mishap, sorrow, and ultimately ruin—in light of, if not despite, seemingly noble personal attributes—then your story may be a tragedy, a complex worldview of self and world.

But complexity can be comic too. The comic mixes with the tragic. Shakespeare brings in his fools to remind us of our absurdities and frailties. If something ridiculous happened simultaneously or in relation to the event you're recounting (or inventing), include it. In Mark Twain's bleak novella *The Tragedy of Pudd'nhead Wilson*, a plantation owner's baby is born on the same day as his light-skinned slave's baby. The slave switches the babies' beds, an act that propels a series of comic and mostly tragic consequences. The slave's baby, treated as a plantation owner's son (even by his mother), grows up to be a morally wretched and wounded individual who loses his inheritance to gambling and drinking and who sells his mother down the river for some money. Yet, Twain's dark sense of humor, especially through the witticisms of the title character "Pudd'nhead Wilson," keeps the novel from being weighted with too much gravity. Francine Prose's self-deprecating sense of humor also provides comic relief in her essay "The Nose" in which she recalls the first time she realized in sixth grade she was tagged "the kid with the big nose." Similarly, a student explored, with initial discomfort, how one of her breasts is notably smaller than the other. Recounting with horror and amusement how a former boyfriend used to ridicule her, she gave her readers a glimpse into one person's ability to celebrate her unique form. Not every scar, wound, or oddity may lend itself to wit, but a light tone and self-revelation, without becoming solely therapeutic and overly self-analytical, can make some writing both delightful and insightful.

The mythic dimension also moves some writing beyond trauma. Each of us lives a mythic life. When the meaning of our lives exceeds rational cause-effect explanations and enters the realm of story and of patterns, of coincidence and chance and fate and synchronicity, of symbol and of metaphor, scars become more than sore spots of resentment or embarrassment; they become wellsprings of meaning and of magic. Visit a museum, for instance, and you will notice how various parts of the body are represented in different sections. Oriental, African, and American Indian art portray the human body in mysterious and mythic ways. Joseph Campbell's series *The Masks of God* spans the gamut from Oriental to Occidental to what he called Primitive Mythology. These tales remind us that our bodies are repositories of ancient stories that link us as human beings on a level beyond the rational and analytical. We can go back to Achilles' famous heel, accidentally not dipped in the River Lethe (the River of Forgetfulness), to recall how physical wounds can shape our fate, but your own character's body also contains a symbolic and mythic dimension.

STEADY NAVIGATION

Poet Afaa Michael Weaver did not have an easy start as an adult poet. As reviewed in a feature in *Poets & Writers*, Weaver at nineteen left college to marry his pregnant girlfriend. Their son, Michael, died at ten months old of complications related to Downs syndrome. The death sent Weaver into a depression that contributed to his marriage ending five years later. Still, Weaver wrote, and in the writing began to confront, as the feature notes, "an earlier trauma—incest."

Weaver was abused as a boy for over a decade. While acknowledging that he is, of course, "an incest survivor" and that this identity has informed his poetry, some of it directly, Weaver does not over-identify with the trauma he has suffered. "I don't subscribe to the theory," he says in the interview, "that artists are created through trauma."[1]

He has always been, he says, a poet. For over twenty years, Weaver has persisted as a serious poet, publishing nine books of poetry and earning awards such as the National Endownment for the Arts Creative Writing Fellowship. Yet, he has not received full attention and recognition for his persistence and accomplishment. Such a life would send many writers packing, questioning their choices and talent. But Weaver has found since 1979 a way to navigate his depression and the hardships his journey has brought him.

Each morning Weaver meditates and often moves through a series of Chinese standing meditations—Xing Yi Quan. A poet who can read, write, and translate Chinese, Weaver says the Chinese meditation and movement not only have helped him deal with his trauma but also have helped calm his mind so he can move forward with his writing.[2]

Yoga's tools similarly are the perfect pick axes and ropes to access and navigate these deeper terrains. Moving through a series of Yoga poses while harnessing slow, deep breaths can relax the body's defenses and the protective ego's defenses. The frontal cortex's analytical mode quiets. The emotional hindbrain, where powerful emotional memories are "stored" so to speak, can be stimulated. Writers often experience an ease of accessing deep memories and deep, surprising images that proffer them fodder and intuitive insight for their stories and poems. Such a relaxed body and mind can invite writers to explore cause and effect, the brunt of conflicts, and meaning in surprising, intuitive ways. They often can do so without feeling overwhelmed by the raw spots the journey exposes.

I have witnessed Yoga work its ways repeatedly with writers of all sorts. At one retreat, an author explored similar layers to reconsider the gist of her first memoir's story, a story that involved her husband's sudden death in their kitchen, her post-mortem discovery of his rampant affairs with several women, and her fall-out and eventual rebirth. Yoga, among other things, helped her keep moving through these difficult memories without resorting to cliché. Over a couple of years, she lifted a potentially traumatic story of "what happened" to a powerful and often humorous reflection upon personal choice, identity, and freedom. The memoir will be published soon. A surgeon and essayist, Renee Rossi, wrote this sketch called "Soft Spots" during a Yoga as Muse workshop:

> When I was a child playing hide and seek, I hid behind the couch below a large, framed Maurice Utrillo canvas—an impressionistic blend of Europeans walking down some cobblestone street lined with brownstones. I think it was late autumn. The frame came down on the centerpiece of my head with a crunch, the crunch of a depressed skull fracture. I might have said, "Look now, Mother, I've reopened my fontanelle," as I now bore the prescient knowledge of all those Europeans. My dent proved itself a font for new ideas, the flat spot to balance a book bag on the way home from school, obviating the need for study, and later, the vent of the volcano of my body at puberty.
>
> A few years back I flew in the air in a rollover accident. When the car hit the ground, my skull was compressed like an accordion between earth and floorboards. I was glad for my vent hole; shedding the hair in clumps right over it to make room for the new stream of molten lava issuing forth from the pain of my mother's death a few days before. I was reborn out of the spout in my crown, Athena, the wisdom-warrior, strong woman-child of Zeus, alone to face the world without my mother.

Her seemingly detached tone and her playful use of a surgeon's diction grants her a perspective that doesn't reduce the piece to emotional trauma. The connections between these two memories didn't surface in Renee until she moved through some yoga poses and heeded her subtle imagination. While working with her breath and imagination, the allusion to Athena suddenly surfaced and, blending with the fact of her mother's death, fits the piece's tone and focus.

Artist Frida Kahlo suffered a life-altering, body-impairing trolley accident when she was a young woman. In the film Frida, as Frida and her soon-to-be husband Diego Rivera begin to make love for the first time, she stops him. "I have a scar," she says. "Let's see." He slides her dress down and looks along her lower back, where a six-inch scar from her trolley accident makes tracks on her back and spine. "You're perfect," he says, and kisses her back and its tracks. Sure, the accident traumatized her body and her psyche and ultimately shaped her rage, her art, and her early death. But her story wasn't all trauma. She created a life rich with love and pain, of pleasure and revelation, and from her life she created a series of dreamlike canvases that give us glimpses into humanity's mythic body.

We can begin our own journey into our character's physical body by kissing it and acknowledging its unique perfection.

TAKE A BREATH: HONOR YOUR CHARACTER'S SCARS AND ODDITIES

Intention:

This practice will stimulate your cellular memory and your subtle imagination so you can explore either your or a character's physical body. You might try the practice in three sessions as designated or in one session.

From **ADAMANTINE POSE** (vajrāsana) *or a seated pose of your choice, lengthen your spine and take at least two full breaths. When you've calmed some of your chatter, ask yourself, "What am I writing for?" The answer will circulate throughout your cellular* *body and inform how you explore your character's physical and mythic body. Then, clarify that you intend to pursue the nature and significance of a character's scar, wound, or oddity.*

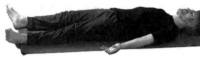

With eyes closed, come onto your hands and knees into **CAT POSE** *(marjarāsana). Exhale and arch your upper back as your tailbone drops toward the ground. Inhale and bring your back into a straight table back. Repeat this movement between exhaling and arching with inhaling and straightening four more times. Then exhale as you curve your spine sideways to the left by looking back toward your right hip. Then repeat on the other side. This movement rouses the stored sensory stimuli and impressions along your central nervous system.*

When ready, come into **CORPSE POSE** *(savāsana) by resting on your back, your knees bent if you wish, elbows toward your torso, your palms for now toward the ceiling. Breathe steadily and slowly.*

#1: THE PHYSICAL LAYER: *Using either your physical imagination or one hand, scan your body for scars, wounds, or irregularities: train-track ridges in your skin from a surgery, that healed yet still visible scar that forms a kiva in the skin below your left eye. Rather than being ashamed of this place, honor it. With your imagination, notice this place's shape, texture, hue. Move over it from every possible angle, and notice with appreciation every tiny ridge, mound, valley, or creek. Either begin writing or continue.*

#2: THE TRAGIC LAYER: *Extend your exhalations for four to six slow seconds, and imagine the breath illuminating your body's hallways. Walk your breath along your spine and to the place you're exploring. As you continue to breathe deeply, ask your imagination and body the following: What happened that led to the scar? How old was the character? Where was he or she? Who else was involved? How did the character carry her or his body at* *the time? Consider consequences: What happened as a result of this scar or as a result of the incident that rendered the scar? What other incidents in the character's life before or after this scar might relate? How did elements of society, nature, chance play into this event? What prevalent trait of the self might have led to this event? Don't force answers. These questions help you approach a story's storage room, but answering them alone may not give you a full story. Either begin writing or continue.*

#3: **THE MYTHIC LAYER:** *Then begin to imagine this physical body in a larger context. As you continue with your slow breathing, imagine this body in a sea of human bodies. Each body floats like a boat—a ship, canoe, paddleboat, sailboat—across this vast sea. This one body's unique shape links in some mythic way to this sea. These questions might help you imagine the body in the context of human beings' beautiful mythic struggle (or dance) with their own and others' vulnerabilities, clashes, disappointments, and mistakes: How does this scar and this incident define part of the character's uniqueness? What does it look like—a shield? a bridge?—that could symbolize the self or the self's journey? What other stories from literature, fairy tales, mythologies, or legends might give light to your story's meaning? What does the scar and its story or stories reveal about the tenuous nature of being human?*

When you've allowed some impressions to surface sufficiently, begin writing. You can begin with description. Locate its unique hues. Aim for particularity. Don't settle for "red" or "purple." Precise descriptive diction grants your body part its deserved uniqueness. Then, explore its metaphorical reality. Fashion its shape in words by letting loose your childlike mind of associations and metaphors. Does it look like an animal? A thing? A place in nature or in a city? A type of building? A temple? A passageway? Sketch the scar—as it is or metaphorically. Find the shape in your subtle imagination that shows how the scar and its metaphor are one.

Being open to wonder as you draft, heed any unexpected connections or telling images that might stand in for explicit analysis. You need not overanalyze. Be subtle by describing another story, artwork, fairy tale, or myth that might connect. If it applies unevenly, all the better. The comparison will potentially be even more particular. As you explore the story, be patient. Authentic writing and active compassion do not lead to simplistic forgiveness. They lead to acknowledging an incident in all of its complexities and trying to portray those complexities as truthfully as possible. Refrain from easy answers; aim for truthfulness.

CHAPTER NINETEEN

COMPASSION FOR THE GOOD, THE BAD, AND THE DOWNRIGHT DEPRAVED

S OME WRITERS ARE GODDESSES and gods. Maybe I'm overstating the point. Granted, no photo of Balzac or Faulkner sits on my altar. It's not their aura or their magnum opus that inspires my awe. It's their capacity to characterize that makes them divine. Their ability to form authentic characters whose hearts and minds and bodies I otherwise would never inhabit puts them in the company of the androgynous figure Avalokiteshvara, which translates to "He (or She) Who Hears the Outcries (Sounds) of the World." So struck and moved by hearing and seeing humanity's cacophony of suffering, this essential Buddhist figure sprouted a thousand arms and hands—with an eye in each palm—to help not only hurting humans caught in their own hells, but suffering animals as well.

Faulkner mentions it in his Nobel Prize Acceptance Speech, Morrison deems it essential, and Maxine Hong Kingston says it's the single most important trait for a writer to possess. Compassion. You don't have to be Mother Teresa to write authentically (no doubt that a writer can appear gracious and loving in her pages and near depraved and loathsome in her daily interactions). Yet, ultimately, to sustain your practice of writing authentic fiction, nonfiction, or poetry, you can work to develop active compassion, *karunā*, for other beings, especially—and here's the kicker—for those "characters" who don't reciprocate your feelings, for those wholesome ones who just flat out get on your nerves, and for those characters whose very existence challenges your patience and desire to contain your judgment.

Ten years ago, I may not have understood how Yoga could improve not only a writer's relationships with her mother but also her novel. But now I'm not surprised. One writer I met in a Yoga as Muse workshop told me how she no longer dreads talking on the telephone to her mother. "I actually try to listen to her." Dorie even imagines what her mother is doing on the other end of the line—rubbing her stiff wrists, staring at the muted daily news that only heightens her fear of the world. Especially whenever Dorie's mother begins her harping refrains about Dorie's failed marriage, her dead-end job, or her "wayward" twenty-something children, Dorie tries to feel the sensations in her mother's aching back from forty years of living on a farm in Maine with her husband, now dead, and her four sons and one daughter—or the algetic wrist and hip, broken from a recent fall off the front porch when a squirrel startled her. "Little my mother complains about really gets to me much anymore," Dorie said, "except when she starts in about how much weight I'm gaining. Then, I'm just ready to hang up." She laughs. "But I'm practicing, and it's helping me write my novel." The protagonist of Dorie's novel is based upon her mother.

Dorie trains her body and imagination to embody compassion while writing by harnessing her breath, setting an intention to nurture her compassion as a novelist, and moving through a series of simple poses designed to energize the heart region. "It's a way of training my unconscious while I write," she told me, a training she says helps her "crawl into the skin" of her often miserable yet endearing protagonist. As a result of Dorie's practice, several of her characters have become more rounded, her narrator's point of view more complicated, even unreliable in a way that has deepened the plot. She even feels more at ease when moving into emotionally charged scenes. The habit sounds simple—practice compassion—but any writer who has tried to extend compassion toward a character of fiction or nonfiction whom she deems difficult, even reprehensible, knows it's far from easy.

But a Yoga practice has helped me, Dorie, and numerous other writers feel more versatile when portraying characters of any shade of personality. Patanjali's *Yoga-Sutra* I.33 speaks directly to this practice: "When you're friendly toward those who are happier than you, compassionate toward those who have so much pain they cannot extend compassion to you, joy toward those whose accomplishments exceed yours, and indifference to those who make mistakes, your mind becomes tranquil." Yes, and you merit sainthood, too, you're probably thinking. Yet if we wish to write authentic fiction, nonfiction, and poetry that informs our hearts of what it means to be human, we need to extend compassion not just to ourselves and to our own physical bodies—as we explored in previous chapters—but also toward those characters who live in suffering. Just as working with the heart region helps us view ourselves more complexly and with compassion, so our heart region and our imagination can guide us in literally embodying compassion for our characters, corrupt or charismatic.

The heart—the literal one, not the symbolic—holds power for writers. Current science validates Yoga's ancient wisdom. Our hearts are wired with neural networks so complex that some people call the heart another brain.[1] Our nerve-charged hearts emit an electromagnetic field of energy—a literal domain of energy produced from and surrounding the heart. What's unusual about the heart's electromagnetic field is how far it reaches—fifteen feet or more. The heartbeat's waves, for instance, can be graphed on a machine called an ECG (electrocardiograph) similar to how our brain's waves can be graphed on a machine called an EEG (electro-encephalograph). Its charge apparently is so strong that an ECG placed within three feet of you can measure your heart's waves and energy field without being directly hooked up to your physical body. That is, your charged heart casts off energy around you. Literally. Your body inhabits that field. Literally.

The work of HeartMath Institute—a research center in Boulder Creek, California—has been verifying what yogis have been teaching for centuries: that when our thoughts correlate with our physical heart, we shift our physical energy. After thirty years of research, scientists at HeartMath have been helping people especially who suffer from anxiety by taking them through a simple process: When a person recognizes anxious thoughts surfacing, she shifts her mind's focus to the heart region, slows down her exhalations, and imagines a peaceful scene. Not only do such a person's brain waves, as measured by an EEG, slow down to the alpha-wave rhythms—the rhythms of one-pointed concentration as discussed earlier in this book—but the brain waves' graph also mirrors with startling similarity the heart waves' graph as measured on an ECG. The brain and the heart synchronize, and the person's anxiety dissipates as she or he feels not only more at ease but also more connected with all around her or him. It's no wonder that texts such as the *Shiva-Sutra* advise us that "when a person shifts her thoughts to the heart, she experiences unity" (1.15). In yogic terms, we take our attention as writers to the essential heart center, what is called the *anāhata-cakra*.

So, it takes practice, but as writers we have the stuff of compassion and of powerful writing both within us and around us. I have met liberal-minded child beaters and women haters, conservative-minded pedophiles and prostitutes, corporate crooks and petty thieves, warmhearted hunters and cold-blooded vegans, heroin addicts and sex addicts, hypocritical priests and abusive gurus. They live in Dallas. They live in Woodstock. They live on Texas prairies, the Himalayan nooks, the Australian outback. Money-centered cities or art-centered towns, it doesn't matter. The human heart's shades and shadows live and move everywhere. And such is the stuff of good (or at least memorable and enlightening, though not necessarily enlightened) characters.

I agree with Faulkner: Give me a drunk, unreliable, unrepentant woman over a chaste one anytime. At least in literature. Faulkner says in his Writers at Work interview with *The Paris Review* that one of his favorite characters is Dickens's Sarah Gamp: "a drunkard, an opportunist, unreliable," he says, "most of her character was bad, but at least it was character." Indeed. So much so we call a person of such ill repute a "gamp" now in her honor. Think of the most powerful characters you've ever encountered. They're often ones who challenge your heart's boundaries. I prefer to read about corrupt characters over unblemished saints and gurus, not because I hover over the carcasses of the depraved but because literature, with less-than-perfect protagonists, often slyly expands my heart's walls to let these social orphans in to rest and chat a spell. Dostoyevsky's Raskolnikov, Nabokov's Humbert Humbert, Joyce Carol Oates's maniacal, sadistic surburban mothers, or Truman Capote's cold-blooded murderers—these characters' interior monologues and sordid acts take me into the oft-ignored crags of humanity's caves. While wedged like a spelunker in a writer's discomforting pages, I may have no choice but to see myself in the sharp-toothed stalagmites of a character's heinous deeds.

A couple of years ago, I was reading aloud to my wife Toni Morrison's first published novel, *The Bluest Eye*. The novel's opening descriptions prompt pity for the little girl Pecola, who desires to be everything that she is not: white and blond with blue eyes. The perspective of the novel's second section shifts, though, as we follow her father Cholly Breedlove's upbringing as he drifts from home to home, as white men humiliate him in his first sexual experience, as he attempts, despite his hard boyhood, to live as an adult in a romantically musical rhythm, and as he loses his music to marriage, daily drudgery, and drink. Once the reader has accepted Cholly into his heart, the story returns to his life as a father. As I read aloud to my wife the beginning of a pivotal scene between Cholly and Pecola in their kitchen, I paused and said, "I don't think I can read the next part aloud. I'm afraid I know what's about to happen." I had recalled a vague, brief reference in the book's opening pages to Pecola having her father's baby. Now, over 150 pages and a widened heart later, I read the next two pages, put the book and my head down, and just sighed, not knowing how I felt. Cholly raped his daughter. "He fucked her," Morrison writes. Anger, pity, confusion, swirled in my reader's heart. Pecola had entered my heart from the beginning, but by this scene so had Cholly. And he stayed there. The bastard stayed there.

Many characters enter and dwell in my heart not because I see myself as them, nor because I aspire to be like them, but simply because they are human, all too human.

Forget being a guru. Writers aren't gurus or preachers. Guru means "remover of darkness," whereas writers often bring us into the darkness of the human condition. Novelist Hubert Selby (author of *Last Exit to Brooklyn*) once told me that writers must embrace the darkness of their own hearts and of others' hearts. And once you move characters into the darkness, you don't necessarily lift them out of the inferno with some miraculous visit by an angel. Novelist Rosellen Brown has written about her bemusement with readers and critics who expect some of her morally messy and confused characters to "lift themselves up" from their morass and make a tidy fablelike ending. About the characters she creates, Brown writes that, rather than make smooth-edged dolls, "if I let their texture stay rough and their responses dangerously lifelike, I dare to think I might have resonant characters pocked and shadowed with complexity."[2] Without a willing understanding of the human heart's frailties and complexities, we'll weave thin characters better left for Lifetime movies.

Of course, even good characters need our full compassion. If we're portraying otherwise noble characters, we must be willing to render their mistakes and wicked thoughts with as much compassion as when we handle their kindness and generosity. Too much goodness is as unbelievable as too much evil. Arthur Miller once said that we like characters such as the flawed John Proctor (the protagonist in his play *The Crucible*) because we can more readily identify with a blemished character than with a seemingly perfect one. Not to allow an otherwise admirable character to fail or have flaws is like insisting a spouse or child not have a misstep. If you're working with a character you like, you'll find out soon enough the nature, if not the names, of his blemishes. It's like falling in love with somebody. With time, he'll start irritating you with his limited perception of women or how trapped he is in identifying himself with his job or how he can't seem to follow an idea to its logical conclusion.

Practicing Yoga can alter our writer's heart indelibly. For the sake of testing things our for yourself, try this. In a seated position, cross your arms and crouch forward, your midback arched. Note what it feels like to protect and to close your heart. Note what singular word or image surfaces that describes how writing from this position would feel. Then bring your arms out and either to the sides or all of the way behind you. What one word or image surfaces to describe how writing from this position would feel? Students often respond with words such as "locked versus free" or "crowded versus open" respectively. But others will respond with "safe versus vulnerable" or "protected versus dangerous" to describe the same positions. Either response, of course, is valid, but it's a quick way to assess how you feel about living and writing with an open heart.

Another approach is to levy the judgment. Come into cramped heart position again by crossing your arms and crouching forward, your midback arched. Note what it feels like to protect and to close your heart. Staying hunched over, close your eyes and imagine your heart as a shrinking room with walls closing in like a medieval dungeon. Feel the sensations of your heart shrinking. Is your breath skipping and constricting? Does your head hurt? Do you feel safe? Strong? Weak? See and feel the character or person enter this closed-in room, and notice how it feels when he or she enters. View the character through a one-way window as you preside over him or her like a chief judge. Let the walls continue to close enough to restrict most of her or his movement. As if through a sound system, levy all of your criticism and judgments on this character. Let loose your litany of admonitions and accusations. When ready, address your judgment to the character. Do you feel relief or even more tension in your body, mind, heart, and imagination? This practice usually brings mixed responses from writers. Some of them feel relieved; others, drained. Writing from this place can be exhausting because we're fighting our characters, and it takes far more energy to write a novel or memoir in which we're full of rage and judgment than full of clear compassion.

Acknowledge that every character suffers—even the seemingly cheery ones whose successes get on your nerves as much as the depraved ones who challenge our morality. *Dukha*, suffering, is a condition of having a vitiated heart, Bernard Bouanchaud notes in his commentaries of the *Yoga-Sutra*. Why does your character suffer? What does she lack or think she lacks? What has happened to her, and how has she responded in such a way as to induce her own suffering? What is she attached to? How does it physically feel to inhabit his suffering body? As you begin to play out your character's actions, thoughts, and scenes with an open heart, you almost accidentally develop compassion for him. You must let him do things that you wouldn't want him to do but he nonetheless must do and learn for himself. When we can begin to inhabit the hearts of our characters nonjudgmentally, when we can inhabit their painful, knotted bodies, hear their thoughts, and hear the world through their clouded ears, we are practicing one of a writer's most remarkable gifts: compassion.

Memoirists might resist these practices more than fiction writers. A character—often a difficult parent, a spouse or former partner—is too "real" and close to be imagined richly. One traditional meditation practice that works for such writers is, first, to imagine a dear friend or mother figure, someone who has nurtured you or been a source of selfless support. You imagine that person in your heart for several minutes. Then, imagine the difficult or corrupt character—the mother or father, the former lover, abusive stranger—as that friend or mother figure in your heart. This step won't be easy for most of us, which is why it requires practice. Alice Walker wrote in a recent essay that a variation of this meditation—called metta (lovingkindness) meditation—sustained her not only through a divorce but also through writing three novels, including *The Color Purple* (a novel that portrays corrupt characters with far more compassion and complexity, incidentally, than does the movie version). Embodying compassion requires consistent effort if we genuinely wish it to emanate from us as we write (and live).

The interior monologue may be the best literary form to support this practice for writers of all genres. Not always a stream-of-consciousness form, an interior monologue is told from the character's first-person point of view. We the reader are privy to the character's thoughts, perceptions, conceptions, secrets, and longings. We see her own corner of reality as she rails to us against her pregnant daughter and the rest of the corrupted world or as he confesses to us his desires for the young girl down the road. Interior monologues provide structure for Faulkner's *As I Lay Dying*, James Kelman's Booker Prize–winning *How Late it Was,*

How Late, and Kingsolver's *The Poisonwood Bible*. We respectively enter the bodies and minds of poor, perplexed Mississippians, a down-and-out and blind alcoholic in Scotland, and four girls and a mother from Georgia uprooted to Africa. Sandra Cisneros uses the form throughout much of the short story collection *Woman Hollering Creek*. The form invites us into the neighborhood mostly of Hispanic girls and women whose varied background and travails Cisneros renders with equal compassion. German Romantic author Friedrich Schiller wrote in 1801 that the person who lacks a full education of humanity's complexities "never sees others in himself, but only himself in others." Writing in the first-person interior monologue can educate you to bring those difficult others into your self.

If writing nonfiction, you also can experiment with the interior monologue. Tammy Nelson, author of *Getting the Sex You Want* and with whom I worked in Connecticut, took a risk when she extended compassion (for the first time, she said) to her mother. Each time she had tried to write about her mother she found her tone strained and point of view limited. We went through a process that allowed her to explore her mother's perspective and body, as well as to hear her mother's voice distinctly. Here's an excerpt from the interior monologue she drafted at the workshop:

> He's coming to see me and this sweet newborn baby clutched to my breast. Orange light bleeds through the hospital blinds onto my blankets. "When he comes we mustn't tell him." The newborn bundle of soft, pink, mottled flesh squirms closer to the smell of a full breast but doesn't answer. "If he knows the truth he won't come back for us," I whisper. Its forehead so smooth, its wisps of fine, black hair too. Will he notice? Will he mind? What if he says, "This baby doesn't look like me?" What will I say to him? It's 1962. I'm an independent woman. I'll be OK without a husband. Won't I? Oh, my body aches. Oh, God, this C-section wound, a gaping, stitched hole from my pubis to navel. Such a hole in me. He'll never know. But maybe the doctor knows. I wonder if he knows I'm a nurse. And that my breasts were firm and beautiful before this baby, before they were filled to exploding with milk that threatens to pull

them down to my knees. What if no one wants me ever again? What if I miss my chance and am alone now with my sagging breasts and this screaming baby. Why is she screaming? I raise the pillows and press the button for the nurse. Please God, someone, come and take this baby. She won't stop crying and my belly hurts and my breasts are leaking and where is my husband. Is anyone coming to see me?

Tammy's knowledge of her own birth to a woman who committed adultery provides the setting and inspiration, but her imagination and heart fuel the monologue. Placing the mother character in a specific situation anchored Tammy's imaginative compassion and allowed her to begin viewing a crucial situation from someone else's body, mind, and heart.

If you need inspiration from people less close than your family, take your practice away from the desk and mat. During the next week, become aware of strangers. Zero in on one person. Without stalking, watch him or her. If you're at a restaurant, note how he eats and speaks and twitches. If you're on the subway, note what she's wearing, what he's reading, how she smells (if you're that close). Record in your mind all of the facts. Then, when no one's looking, record in your notebook the facts and imagine the character. That is, without giving way to stereotypical assumptions, imagine the person's name, her earliest memory, his deepest desire, her most relished secret, where he has a tattoo, her most reviled song, what he says when he talks to himself. The Lakota tribe has a saying that has kept me in good stead for years: Imagine your life richly. Give it a twist: Imagine a stranger's life richly. You could develop worse habits.

Sing the unloved's song. Rilke wrote a series of song-poems, each from the point of view of society's downtrodden—a fool, a drunkard, a prostitute. Like an Emile Zola novel, these songs of the destitute offer truthful, endearing glimpses of how certain members of our society might feel and think. Edgar Lee Masters's *Spoon River Anthology* is a more benign collection of poems, each told from the point of view of a town's deceased citizen looking back on his or her life. W. D. Snodgrass took a bold leap of compassion when in his book *Füehrer Bunker* he wrote a series of poems from the perspectives of various well-known Nazis, including Eva Braun, Hitler's mistress. Whether the unloved be a misunderstood relative, a despised politician, or a mother who drowned her children, write a poem or prose piece from her or his perspective. Tell us about the objects that matter most to her, find and repeat the refrain that defines his way of life, reveal her deepest longings, expose her secrets that help us understand her. Avoid sentimentality. Be ruthless if you think the person may be ruthless with herself. Be actively compassionate, not sweet. Play with whether the person's "song" would be composed in rhyme, in couplets, in chaotic and uneven lines, or in a prose poem. Let the form, in other words, reflect the person. Such an act of writing is an act of *karuṇā*.

For the writer, isolated, self-consuming and self-consumed, her work can be imprisoned and imprisoning. When work flows, though, from a source of love, when it unites with what we love, when work is love, then our hands come together. They celebrate, reach out, and applaud human beings for all of their frailty, strength, and victory.

TAKE A BREATH:
MAKE ROOM FOR THE DIFFICULT

Intention:
This practice helps you imagine and embody a difficult character. Practice the Yoga sequence a few times first and then integrate it with the writing.

Stand in **STANDING POSE** (tadāsana). *With a firm connection to the ground, take at least two full breaths. When ready, establish your twofold intention by asking yourself, "What am I writing for?" Inhale the response up into your heart space. Then, clarify your intention to imagine and to embody a difficult character.*

Eyes closed with attention on the heart space, see this character or person in a situation (imagined or remem-

bered). *Observe any details or images of the scene that surface as if they were recurring in your heart. See the room's surroundings if it's an interior space. Notice the air's texture. Scan the character's body from crown to feet. Notice what truly unique features this character's body possesses. Just tend patiently to what glimmers or flashes surface.*

Keeping eyes closed, inhale deeply into the heart space. With each inhalation, imagine your heart's walls begin to expand. On an inhalation, lift your arms straight out in front of you and then to the sides in **EVEN-HEARTED MOUNTAIN POSE** *(sama-hyridaya-tādāsana). Feel the hands reach out as you discover what this character wants. Try to articulate what this deep want is and how his or her body reflects that want.*

Eyes closed, move your arms into **OPEN-HEARTED MOUNTAIN POSE** *(hridaya-tadasana) by bringing your arms behind your back and interlacing your fingers. Try to bring your palms toward one another and straighten your arms as you lift your hands toward the ceiling. Open your heart and face toward the ceiling. Take three to five full breaths and bring the arms down. Repeat three times, each time imagining your heart's walls making room for this difficult character or person.*

On an inhalation, release your hands and cross your arms to hug yourself. In this pose, begin to embody this character and begin to see the scenery from the character's point of view. How does this body feel? How does it move in this scene? How does this body help or hinder the character in getting what he or she wants?

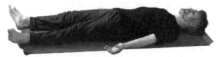

Come out of the pose and rest on your back in **CORPSE POSE** *(savāsana). Then listen. What does this character have to say? Let the unique timbre and music of the voice strike your heart's unstruck cord. What is she thinking? How do his thought*

patterns flow or skip? What images keep surfacing, haunting, or soothing?

Then, write. With sensuous imagery and particularity, describe the scene from the person or character's point of view. Try to capture his or her unique way of speaking, the colloquialisms, the rhythms, the favorite words. Don't let the character reveal everything to your readers all at once. What we explored about dialogue's ability to reveal earlier in this book applies as well to interior monologues. Continue to be surprised as you write, and refrain from betraying your own judgments of the character's actions or personality. Aim to take your reader somewhere new—into this character's head, heart, and body.

CHAPTER TWENTY

Be Careful What You Hate:
From Anger to Satire

Yogi and Buddhist Sylvia Boorstein once said that practicing compassion never means that we can't be angry. Since you're a human being and writer with convictions, surely there's some human behavior that rankles your skin and sends your sweetness bones packing for a while. Writers I know are often angry. War rumbles on, jobs evaporate, Americans sleepwalk—these are common litanies I hear. Because I practice and teach Yoga, writers sometimes cower when I press them more on what ticks them off as if I think "anger is bad, bad, bad."

"Good for you for being mad," I say. "You have convictions. Something matters to you." Then they'll blush and mutter some neorelativist apology of "Well, I'm not perfect either, but, but." Of course you're not perfect, and it's just this falling short of perfection that so outrages us sometimes. So once they get over the common discomfort of actually acknowledging they're angry, we talk about satire. I spent, or misspent, my youth on *Mad* magazine, Monty Python, and Mark Twain. When I was sixteen, awakening to human beings' utter contradictions and hypocrisies, I thrived on sarcasm, puns, innuendoes, subtle put-downs, and sheer fabrications and distortions of the facts. Satire gave me and my friends soft armor to wear in a world we found increasingly strange, unreliable, and hostile.

Satire lets us convert anger into authentic writing. Some variation of anger—a feeling of injustice, righteous indignation, disgust, or contempt toward some facet of being human—fans the fire of many inflammatory satirists. Satire is criticism driven most often by wit that can form a whole piece or can serve part of larger work. And hypocrisy and ignorance remain its two most common subjects (we seem to provide one another with endless amounts of material). Some of Yoga's practices and principles not only can help you confront and convert that anger; they also can keep your satire from becoming mean-spirited sarcasm.

Before we explore satire, consider the other options of "working" with anger: letting it fly or ignoring it. You probably sense or know what anger does to your body. We tag habitually angry people as "tightly wound" for a reason. Anger signals the sympathetic nervous system to stimulate the adrenal gland, which releases adrenaline and cortisol, which in turn constrict muscles, especially in the stomach, shoulders, neck, and jaw—all places where our bodies prepare the troops for defense or attack. Our bodies, from our midriff to our neck, tighten. This hormone release and muscle constriction shortens our breath and flushes our flesh. No coincidence that the English word anger is kin to the Old English *enge*, "to narrow" and, more tellingly, to the Latin *angere*, "to strangle." Habitual anger narrows our arteries and chokes our voice. And the mind on anger? "The mind is its own place, and in itself/Can make a Heaven of Hell, a Hell of Heaven," John Milton wrote in *Paradise Lost*. No wonder, then, that numerous yogic texts deem anger (*krodha*) as one of hell's main gates (meaning one's mental hell and not a steamy underground club where the morally decadent are locked in and subjected to AC/DC perennially playing "Hell's Bells"). Anger (*krodha* in Sanskrit), especially excessive and chronic anger, no doubt obstructs concentration and thus meditation. When boiling mad, we can't think straight. Or think at all. We become disoriented and confused. We lose our way.

Writing with rage, anger's most extreme mask, often leads to incoherent rants that, we usually hope, we don't have the foolhardiness to submit for publication even if to our loved one's collection of personal notes. Like fury, rage sends us over the top, over the edge, down into our darkest lair where who knows what creatures will come out in our full-moon midnights. We become traffic vigilantes. We toss our spouse's strewn dirty clothes into the street. We are "mad," indeed. With anger so deeply embedded, a writer likely will have difficulty breaking this broncolike emotion into artful writing.

But suppressing the demon altogether only irritates it. Left unattended, this volatile emotion can creep through the body like a dangerous imp, playing tricks in the house of the culprit's mind. You can stew and steam, releasing your frightful diatribes about the woes of humanity only occasionally as you drive your children to school. Or you may sense you're enraged at something or someone but cannot name the target, much less aim accurately. Writing done with repressed anger can become distorted and manipulative, the demon disguising the intention.

So, authentic writing isn't necessarily about just venting steam to make ourselves feel better while everyone else around us feels drenched and beaten from our hurricane release, nor is it about keeping our polite mouths shut when we know something's wrong and unjust, if not absurd. Authentic writing includes identifying the level of our anger, finding the broad target of our anger, and finding the most effective way to transform that anger into art.

Satire is a middle way between diatribe and repression.

With satire, there are no sacred cows—not even in India or in Yoga. Yoga helps us embrace life's paradoxes. Indeed. "To create a new self, we must destroy an old one." "Soaring requires rootedness." "You have to heat up to enjoy cooling down." A shrewd yoga teacher I used to know was always espousing these kinds of aphorisms that, if he were on a roll, could lead to a brain-numbing homily. His hair casting an aniline sheen, he was noble in a creepy sort of way and so earnest, if not smarmy, that he could've moonlighted by selling stolen Bibles to widows (especially attractive widows). This guy had special powers, all right. He'd waltz into class wearing all white, waving his wand of incense, his supercilious eyes half-hidden by his eyelids, a gesture that assured us of his spiritually superior serenity.

Then, this New Age Elmer Gantry would wrap his legs in lotus, glance around the room, and land his eyes on a young female student dutifully clad in her minimalist yoga gear. ("Less is more," I think was another of his mantras. What a wit this guy was.) While the student would swoon and blush beneath his gaze, he would say, his voice echoing through the studio like that of Shiva himself, some pearls of wisdom such as "Yoga is about divine union, about the feminine and the masculine merging together in ecstasy." In the same breath in which he would pronounce to us the virtues of chaste thought and action, he would add that, however, if you just so happened to meet an advanced yogi, then you could take a leap of, say, seven years of spiritual training by making love to such a teacher. Seven years of spiritual training in a torrid hour—now, there's a salesman. By the end of class, he'd have the student's phone number for, I'm sure, a private session of spiritual leapfrog. He was always making generous gestures like that with his time and energy. You know, he doesn't have to give those privates, as one student reminded me when I suggested possible impropriety. Yeah, I'd never thought of it that way. What magnanimity.

So, here's where writers become uneasy when we talk about satire. They realize that not only are they going to acknowledge and convert their anger, but they're also going to offend someone (a usual sign of successful satire). Yet, once they get started on listing what bugs them in this world, their fears for a while disappear, and I have to interrupt the rants of those very writers who previously seemed like reticent mice before their red eyes pop out.

Satire's angry voices often rise out of irritation or indignation. Irritation scratches our back the wrong way. To be vexed or irked is more like "pre-anger," a prelude to the big acts. So during the next week, track what bugs you. Slow drivers, fast drivers, messy people, tidy people, weather changes that foil our plans and parades, smug people, shy people, misbehaving children (someone else's, of course), misbehaving computers (your own, of course), or anything that disrupts our creative flow can nettle us. List at least ten human behaviors or societal trends that irritate you. Refrain from limiting your focus to just one person—such as a roommate, family member, or politician. Instead, focus on the behavior that can be generalized. For instance, if your husband drives you bonkers when he circles a packed parking lot for five minutes to wait for a spot near the store to open, use your husband as an example of the larger human behavior (because your husband isn't the only one with this peculiar condition). From your list, choose a topic that really rouses your ire but also seems like fun to explore.

If you're not merely irritated but indignant, your target may supersede your personal irritations or neuroses. The rage is "out" of and beyond your self; it is outrage, not inrage. Emotions of injustice, unfairness, or shamefulness on a personal, social, or political level fuel this potent writing. Say, hypothetically, if when unwarranted war is on the brink of breaking out and only one lone bird among a democracy's senators sings out with eloquent indignation and only a few writers can muster the wits and time and wherewithal to be heard, then you may be alarmed and indignant. (Just to give a hypothetical.) A few students have a harder time with this list because they realize a moral judgment against one or another sort of behavior is inherent in the majority of these topics. Yet, most of us have a gnawing feeling that something is not right in the world, that some imbalance and injustice does exist that genuinely bothers us. All-too-human enough to be shaken from our own bliss, we're sensitive to others' suffering. We even grieve. For the English anger also comes from the Old Norse word angr, "grief." Don't be afraid to touch even what's most sacred to you and most taboo to others to criticize.

These topics aren't easy to acknowledge or to explore. Yoga poses and breathwork, though, provide ways to do so. If you drop and circle your lower jaw, you'll probably notice by the degree of your jaw's tightness whether or not you clench your teeth, an indicator of unconscious anger and tension. Your neck muscles, directly influenced by the jaw, also betray where we ball up. Drop attention a little lower to your chest. There, around our heart, because of restricted breathing that anger induces, we store quite a bit of frustration. So, poses that help stretch and open up these areas can work like release valves that both relieve and frighten writers because we don't always realize just how much anger inhabits our bodies. Yoga students have broken out in tears while practicing back bends—poses that, because of how they open the thoracic spine and chest area, could be called "heart openers." Often, these tears are mixed with anger, confusion, and relief. With an ongoing practice, though, of Yoga poses and breathwork, you can learn to identify your anger and convert it into something else rather than let it dictate your thoughts and reactions. Your body becomes an ally in greater self-understanding, an aid in any writing but especially in a form as potentially tricky as satire.

Once you've acknowledged and chosen a subject, you then can choose an existing form to buttress your satire. Eulogies, for one. Or obituaries. Ellen Goodman writes a clever mock eulogy and mock obituary of "The Company Man," a generic EveryBusinessMan who forfeited everything else in his life—his marriage, his children, his friends—to be loyal to his company, which, in the end, merely saw him as a well-behaved cog. Goodman assumes the somber tone and journalistic format of an obituary so convincingly, peppering it with just the right details and fabricated dialogue, that she will fool any careless reader who may see merit in such corporate sacrifice. Imagine that an imaginary person who embodies your wrath's target has died. How would you sum up the quality of that life? What legacy? Have at it.

You also can don a mask. Assume the perspective of the very group of people whose behavior you loathe or at least deem morally repugnant. Crawl into the skin of one of them, and talk from that person's point of view (while, of course, revealing that point of view's inanity, as you see it). It's a frightening prospect, isn't it? Imagine how it would feel to spoof Hitler in his own words. Or the white guy in Texas who dragged the African-American man James Byrd behind his pickup. You can see the risk. Not only might your thought patterns, sentences, and images—in short, your "voice"—get confused with a bigot, serial killer, corporate bamboozler, war propagandist, or whoever your target may be. Your greatest challenge is to strike the right tone that communicates to your audience your intent—namely to show the idiocy, absurdity, or moral depravity of whoever's belief system or worldview you're mimicking. With the wrong tone, your readers will think you're coarse, insensitive, or brutish (when in fact these may be the very qualities you're aiming to expose). So, take a risk, but you don't have to begin by crawling into the skin of the world's Louis Farrakhans or David Dukes.

Start with a group of people more benign. Like the jaded privileged youth who like to "slum" by doing "working-class" things. This group is loosely the focus of the persona monologue of "I'll Try Anything with a Detached Air of Superiority," written by the staff of the satirical magazine *The Onion*. The title sums up this twenty-something group's "philosophy." Beginning with "I'm a pretty sophisticated, well-educated person," it details for us how she (I assume for some reason it's a she but could easily be a he) ventures to bowling parties, professional football games, and even rummage sales to whoop it up among the hoi polloi—but always with bemusement, as if the working class are a novelty, like someone from another nationality on exhibit. Her attempts to analyze herself and to poise herself as having a sophisticated sensibility are summed up in these lines toward the end: "If you can do such things and still maintain your sense of haughty superiority, you've done more than merely lived. You've tasted the sickly sweet nectar that life has to offer and said, 'I am above this. I am better than this. This is beneath me, but I will still do it because I'm open minded enough to try anything and look down my nose at it at least once.'"[1] I can hear a grating pseudo–Boston Brahmin tone trying to cover an otherwise snotty little-girl voice that rationalizes and self-promotes her daring "class adventures." People with this attitude may irk you, but this piece at least may help you laugh, if only with scorn.

So your persona can be a caricature voice representative of a loathsome group, or it can be a mockery of a single person's voice. It can appear in your fiction, nonfiction, or poetry—no matter. Let's say, hypothetically, there was a high public political figure whose grammar and diction sounded embarrassingly like that of a fourth-grader whose views on family, work, and foreign policy have been steeped on Dynasty and The A-Team. Let's say that same figure tried to deflect criticism of his (or her!) illiteracy. It wouldn't be difficult for you to invent a line this person might say such as "I know there are lots of people out there that value intellectuables and say I use malpractices in my speech. But I really see, don't see, the connection between having a big vocation—er, vacation, uh, vocabulary—and my job." Can you imagine such a person?

Then try looking at yourself. Dave Eggers, Nick Hornby, Neal Pollack, and possibly self-deprecating jokesters such as David Sedaris and David Rakoff are Ironic Young Men (or Ironic Johns, not to be confused with Robert Bly) who have roughed up this country's pages and airwaves with their bald, edgy wit. Having mastered the personal narrative form in fiction and nonfiction, they take as their targets their closest friends, relatives, and—a key trait—themselves. If these writers are angry at anything, it's people who take themselves too seriously. Dave Eggers—whose *A Heartbreaking Work of Staggering Genius* mocked almost every facet of the ever-popular memoir while still telling a story full of pathos—has a mission to slaughter every grazing sacred cow among the literati while still poking fun at his own ambitions. If uneasy with piercing others' egos, start with your own. Come on. You have at least a tad of self-importance worth pricking.

Your other risk in all satire—far more common, unfortunately, than a writer's misstep—is poor reading. Many readers, especially of the self-important sort, just don't get irony, wit, and satire. A high school teacher told me that some of her students still get up in arms over Jonathan Swift's "A Modest Proposal." One student wrote her a sincere note saying that, in essence, "during these times when reports of child abuse have risen, I don't think we should be reading something, no matter how historically relevant, that advocates eating babies." Such misreading cost former Dallas newspaper columnist Joe Bob Briggs his job in the 1980s when he wrote a spoof on the song "We are the World," the popular song, most of whose proceeds went to help starving children, sung by a medley of rock stars. Among the do-good celebs were Michael Jackson, Cyndi Lauper, and Bob Dylan. The journalist's piece poked fun of the celebrities' personal quirks and pretensions, but several readers took umbrage because they considered the project too earnest. When the writer refused to apologize, since he was spoofing the song, not being serious, he resigned.

To avoid this sort of misreading, clue your readers in with your language. Sure, you can begin with the mock-formal tone of a scholar examining the cultural phenomenon of increasingly stupider television shows being viewed (and written) by people with college degrees, or of a scientist reviewing a study of a new epidemic of cultural amnesia, or of an anthropologist observing, say, a tribe of the CowHomeBoys, those white adolescent males from predominantly rural and suburban neighborhoods who feel like they're living on the edge by wearing hooded sweatshirts, putting a Band-Aid on their nose, and blurting lines to each other that they've snagged from rap music. But then have some fun with your tongue. Exaggerate to the point of near-absurdity that pushes your readers almost to the point of disbelief. Pun if it fits. Mix in unabashed metaphors that zap the target with plain language, or pepper in words my mother would deem "from the sewer" with le mot juste. In satire, you can have a tossed salad of tones and diction levels, but be ready to give your readers more than a few leaves of iceberg lettuce and some tomato slices dressed in French. Trust that your readers will have more taste and will be surprisingly satiated by your tongue-tickling wordplay. Such play should remind most careful readers that at least to some extent, despite an authentic intention, your tongue is in your cheek.

When writing satire, it's essential to be clear about your intention. Satire, perhaps more than other kinds of writing, is distinguished by intention (although some of the young Ironist Johns love to mix intentions and keep you guessing at every sentence). Simple sarcasm intends to hurt, burn, or tear down a target rather than to provoke someone. Likewise, humor alone aims to entertain and not to provoke. Perhaps it helps you to consider how you want your readers to respond. If you wish them to wince at your words' force and then to loathe the target, then you may be writing something critical but not satirical. If you want your words to make your readers chuckle without the least bit of resistance or disturbance, then comedy may be your métier. But if you want your readers to laugh with a bit of dissonance, either from seeing themselves in your subject or from having their moral birdcage rattled, then your intent is satire. And what the self-deprecating Dorothy Parker says of wit applies to satire (which was her intended application): "Wit has truth in it; wisecracking is simply calisthenics with words." So when you sense something in your writing sounds cruel, remind yourself of your intention. Ask yourself what truth you're trying to reveal (and what falsehood to lay bare).

Hate alone doesn't drive satire, but don't discount its force. Now, you may think this talk of hatred very unyogilike. Not so. Remember our earlier discussion about paradox? Try this one: Intense hatred of God can liberate you. At least according to one interpretation of a legend from an ancient Yoga text called the *Bhagavata-Purana*. According to one account of the legend, a king named Shushupala despised the god Vishnu. His utter hatred for the god worked on his mind like a meditation; because he thought so much of Visnu in his hatred, he united with the divine. There is an obscure and controversial practice, then, called "yoga of hatred" (*dvesha-yoga*), in which a practitioner learns to fear the divine by having an impassioned hatred for the divine. The awe-inspiring emotions prompt a blissful union.

So be careful what you hate. You just might actually hate it enough to merge with it. For instance, a certain political figure toward whom I occasionally harbor animosity reappears in my dreams. In my waking life, my tongue can't stop lashing this easy target for my own "unresolved" hostility toward arrogant, ignorant people with too much power. At night, though, my unconscious is telling me something else. In one dream, the former governor ran into my house to warn me of an army of tornadoes headed my way. I was annoyed, yet surprised, even thankful. A year ago, I dreamt I worked for this same politician, who is now in a higher office, as one of his most respected writers and advisors. In the dream, I fell out of his favor although I deeply desired to please the head honcho. The big boss also recently helped me cross a street in New York City. Amid the city squalor, we chatted about the weather, our families, our mutual friends. The sunlight glowed behind his head. I smiled. I was quite sure that if he asked me to have a beer while we chatted about foreign policy, I'd join him. We'd become buddies. The dreams keep mixing up my feelings. In my waking life, he's my enemy; in my dream life, he's my ally. Do I detest him or love him? Is there something in him in me? If you can become what you hate, I expect to wake up one morning in his body in his bed beside his wife. I shall smile at her and recite a poem by Walt Whitman or Sam Hamill, and then I'll prepare for a press conference about bombs made of poems, poem-bombs that will explode with metaphors and music that will be dropped on the capital of a nation whose leader threatens to stifle his people's imaginative freedom. United we dream. There's an essay brewing there that I haven't dared to write yet.

What we writers hate and what we love with fervor are often the same. And most of us know that quite often the target of our love is also the target of our anger, as our lovers and spouses can attest. But becoming acquainted with our hatred and anger helps us as writers to know our intentions for writing pieces fueled by such fire. More than anger, hatred is easy to deny. Don't gloat in cruel hatred, but at least acknowledge what in this world you genuinely despise personally, politically, spiritually, socially. Words you abhor. Textures you hate. People's behavior. Kinds of people, if you dare admit it. Experiences. Trends. Films. Songs. Perhaps in the delight of writing about what you hate, you'll come to love some of it.

To dare to write satire is, finally, dare I say it, an act of compassion. It's better to acknowledge, shape, and communicate these feelings than to stay muzzled in a room all your own. Not just because writing satire's healthy for you. It's healthy for all of us. Writing satire implies you still have hope. You're putting it out there because you sense it might provoke people to think, maybe even change their attitudes or behavior. It implies you believe in your convictions, your voice, your wit, and wit helps us cope. When we express anger with wit, laughter relaxes tight jaws and necks as well as mutes anger's shout.

Throughout parts of India, yogis called "crazy adepts" engage the full spectrum of human beings' emotional life. On cue, they can weep or guffaw, act horny or prudish, tremble and cower or stand tall with puffed chest. As people—even gurus—try to continue with their serious business, these clowns mock them. At the most serious sacred ceremonies, people laugh. Such double-sided consciousness embodies the seriousness of laughter that satire prompts. These crazy adepts—not unlike Hopi clowns or Buddhist clowns or satirists—remind us of our foibles and foolishness.

Learn to be a crazy adept writer. Crazy adept writers understand the unwieldy nature of their emotional demons and learn how to shape these emotions artfully. Crazy adepts also risk looking like fools. Anne Sexton once wrote, "As a writer one has to take the chance of being a fool. That perhaps requires the greatest courage." I love that. And respect it.

TAKE A BREATH: FROM ANGER TO WIT

Intention

Focus upon some human behavior that makes you irritated or indignant. This practice can help you raise your anger to the surface so you can move it to witty writing.

Begin in **MOUNTAIN POSE** (tadāsana). *Stand approximately six to eight inches away from a wall. Once you've taken at least two complete breaths, ask yourself, "What am I writing for?" The response can be revealing, particularly when working with satire for the first time. Then specify that for this session you aim to begin a draft of a satirical piece or section of a piece.*

When ready, inhale and lift your arms out to each side into **EVEN-HEARTED POSE** (sama-hridayāsana), *arms straight and with your fingers folded inward and your thumbs stretched up and back. Follow this movement: Exhale, thumbs forward. Inhale, thumbs up. Exhale, thumbs backward. Inhale, thumbs up. Repeat. And repeat. And repeat. For at least five minutes. Yes, five. You should feel irritation in your neck and shoul-*

ders. This variation of a practice common among kundalini prac- titioners I find remarkably irritating—which is part of its alchem- ical work.

Then, still standing six to eight inches away from a wall, with a lengthened torso, inhale and stretch your arms straight overhead and back, arching your back and bringing your fingertips to the wall. Keep your hips forward. Exhale and return to MOUNTAIN POSE. Repeat. As you bring your fingertips to the wall, keep your hips over your ankles so your mid- back will bend and your chest will open. If you're more flexible, you can move your heels farther away from the wall. If you feel okay, repeat three more times and then re- main with your fingertips at the wall and lift your heart toward the ceiling.

Finally, take your hands to your hips and keep your heart open. Take a deep inhala- tion, and on each of your next two exhala- tions, extend your tongue out toward your chin as far as it will reach, direct your eyes upward, and from your feet and root center upward roar out an "AHH" as loud as you can, letting your grief or irritation or anger vibrate through your body, across the room, and off of the nearest mountain. This isn't a variation of Reichian therapy. It's a way to rouse your throat center, to relieve your neck and jaws of tension, and to laugh at yourself. Did you look at yourself in the mirror? Did you hear yourself?

Write with your whole body. With vibrations still moving through your neck, chest, and back, begin writing when you're ready. Your narrator might begin with a description of physical sensations and then move outward to the subject of your ire. The words might lead your narrator to a memory, an incident, an image. Begin playfully describing someone behaving the way that irritates you. What you *write may come from an actual memory or a hypothetical incident. Begin with the specific and then follow the specific to a general humorous essay about this irritation or indignation. Notice if with irritated jaws and shoulders your syntax seems jumpy, your imagination slightly skewed if not wicked. Have fun with this piece and assume, like a crazy adept, a different tone or persona if you're not accustomed to voicing your irritation. Gradually, you'll discover a point, a focus, maybe even a humorous solution that will help you revise the piece if you wish. But as you write, enjoy riding the passion of your contempt. Write with a strong spine.*

IV

LOOKING BACK AND LOOKING FORWARD

CHAPTER TWENTY-ONE

EATING LEAVES AND OTHER WAYS TO RE-VISION FOR FORM

W HEN DIANNE ACKERMAN DESCRIBES her first flight lesson, she relates it to our human longing to step back and see the earth as a whole, to observe how rivers feed into oceans, how factories and mountains feed into rivers. The same is true for writers. You learn to dwell well in the details, but you also want to be able to step back and look at a whole piece of your writing to see how one section relates to, feeds into, plays off of another or how a poem's stanzas, a story's scenes, or a book's chapters may need resequencing. This ability to envision a piece of writing as a whole and to rework it accordingly with both intuition and analysis is to re-vision, an awkward verb form I prefer to distinguish it from the more particular and minute steps of revising. To re-vision well, we should consider the nature of form. Without form, Flaubert said, there is no art.

Everything—be it a sonnet, a sonata, a sentence, a snowflake, a baseball pitch, a memorable kiss—has a form. Even oak tree leaves, each of which may come from the same tree, have a beautiful, distinct form. Generally, the leaves' shapes, like the shapes of human bodies, appear the same, uniform. Yet, within each leaf resides a slightly distinct pattern.

Such is true, too, of Yoga poses (*āsanas*)—perhaps the most recognizable aspect of Yoga in the West. Some writers come to Yoga thinking that each pose has a Form, some Platonic ideal toward which each of us with a serious practice must and should strive. True, certain universal principles exist for aligning the spine in each pose that help us practice with safety and depth, and, yes, it can be beautiful to watch a veteran yogi flow from one exquisite pose to the next. Yet, we can deepen our experience with Yoga if we realize that each person—whose physical temple has a different history, shape, and internal working—need not strike a pose in exactly the same way as everyone else. We can appreciate tradition's forms without being stifled by uniformity or conformity.

A yoga pose is a form, a *rūpa* in Sanskrit. *Rūpa* refers not only to the body and to physical beauty, but also to a physical "sign," that is, a sort of message from the gods. An authentic yoga pose stems from a yogi's genuine intention as well as from the yogi finding the organic variation of the pose that suits his or her body at the time of practice. By "organic," I mean that the pose may be fluid instead of static; it should feel natural and composed, not imposed. There's also something beautiful in watching a beginner find her own variation of a pose that suits her body and spirit for any given time.

So it goes with writing and learning to re-vision. With a genuine intention, we let a form, at once fluid and organic, emerge from the needs of any given writing at any given time. For the form of a story, essay, or poem can be rigid, simplistic, and predictable, or it can be elegant, intricate, subtle, and unique. At a superficial glance, many complex texts may appear to possess similar external structures or no artful structure whatsoever; yet, they often embody unique shapes whose intricacies—whose inner form—escape the untrained eye, mind, and imagination.

If we've become lost in our first drafts (which, ideally, I think we should) and even in our second, third, fourth, and fifth drafts, at some point we need to step back and view our writing from afar. How do we see a piece as a whole, and how do we begin to re-vision? Since an organic form feels alive, not static, first, think about your piece's movement. In *The Essay: Theory and Pedagogy for an Active Form*, Paul Heilker of Virginia Tech reminds us of the authentic essay's "kinetic" form. To write an essay, Heilker notes, is to be in perpetual motion like that of a dancer or a golfer's swing (or, I should add, a yogi's flow): "[T]he essay is kineticism incarnate—the embodiment of perpetual mobility, motion, and movement."[1] The same is true, though, of a charged poem or story. Our ideas, images, and words carry us (and the reader) through the piece with some anticipation and exhilaration that we don't always know where we're going next, and yet we sense that when the piece is complete it is a beautiful whole, however rough or loose its edges.

One key to considering movement is the reader's experience. Although we sense what we like in what we read, sometimes we can't put our finger on why one book works magic on us and another flops. Much of the magic on the reader has to do with movement, how a piece shifts, progresses, surprises, and weaves along the way. Form shapes much of how readers experience a text, and readers' experiences with texts—their surprises, their predictions, their connection-making, their emotional shifts—often help determine whether or not a text is effective (that is, whether or not a text "affects" readers). How does a piece move a reader's intellect, heart, and/or imagination? It takes a lot of rewriting to make a piece appear effortless. Through re-visioning, then, we give our readers something exquisite and well-crafted that still feels organic.

TOOLS TO RE-VISION

Take a piece of your writing and think about its beginning, middle, and end. With my students, we get out our drafts, reread them to ourselves, and then read them to one or two other people in class, and consider these matters.

Beginnings: A beginning should be an entryway at once compelling enough for the reader to enter and subtle enough for the careful reader later to learn just why that beginning was so appropriate. When Hemingway showed Fitzgerald one of his early drafts of what became *The Sun Also Rises*, Fitzgerald recommended he cut the first forty thousand words, which mostly provided exposition related to Jake Barnes's experiences in World War I, and begin the story in the fictional present in Paris. Hemingway took his advice, and the novel catapulted Hemingway into fame as literature's new golden boy of the 1920s. Notice if you're beginning in a safe and dull place, or if you're starting a poem, scene, or chapter with a reliable "trick" you learned years ago in a writing workshop. Maybe in your first two or four pages you're warming up your engine and don't get going until page five. Scrap the first four pages. A friend of mine poured out his soul to write his first novel, some six hundred–plus pages. His agent told him that in six hundred pages he basically had an excellent twelve-page short story. My friend pulled the best part of the manuscript and burned the rest.

Middles: Your middle shouldn't idle; it should keep your reader revved. A sign of a dull middle is if you're staying methodically on subject and on schedule. Notice if you're halfway through and you haven't been surprised once by anything that's surfaced in your imagination or language. If you're falling asleep as you read what you've written, imagine how your readers will respond. Or maybe you're holding your breath because you're writing so rapidly just to get finished. The other extreme may be that you've digressed so much and gotten so lost that the piece's energy and movement are too scattered to sustain even the most patient reader's attention.

Endings: Beware if you wrap up everything in floral designed paper, if you force your characters to make up, if the sun always comes out. Or maybe you don your philosopher-theologian hat with the equivalent of a two-page appendix that explains your clever symbolism. (I actually heard a writer at a reading take pains to interpret all of his poem's symbols.) Not every loose end has to be tied, not every symbol explicated. For the tragic-minded fiction writers, beware of killing your characters at the end or having them commit suicide unless you really mean it, that is, unless like Camus or Kate Chopin you consider suicide an important existential question. Otherwise, your readers may feel cheated.

I know these signs well. They're all bad habits I've had and that still hang around. Beginning writers get scared, so they rely on these things. Seasoned writers get lazy. In both cases, it's easier to travel down a reliable road clearly mapped and demarcated than to detour down a nameless gravel road. Yet, it is exactly at a dead end that you might find an unmarked forest holding many surprises.

The "magical movement" inherent in several forms stems from their organic nature, something that appears at once natural and artfully, if not effortlessly, composed. There's an art to executing most yoga poses. It's why they seem somehow so natural and feel so right to the body. Yogis create poses in part by knowledge and by experimentation, trying out forms to see how each one affects the body-mind. When something works, they stay with the pose until they refine it without it becoming rigid. Similarly, in writing there are boundless organic shapes that can help us imagine and re-vision how parts of our writing can be reformed. So once we've picked up on and identified problems with our writing's form, I give writers ideas for "mapping" their stories and poems. I have them consider and imagine unconventional, organic maps that I hope will help them create their writing's unique form.

Take the letter S. Imagine the top of the S as your story's beginning, which employs a memorable image or anecdote. Then, you seem to curve away from the subject—down the back of the S—until your story's middle refers again to the opening image or anecdote and, then, slides down the story's belly in another apparent digression and, ultimately, closes with a renewed reference to the opening image or anecdote. Such structures demand the reader be patient and enjoy the storyteller's circuitous path as a sort of literary odyssey in which the reader is not going to return to Ithaca by the most efficient route. Odysseus, after all, was a journeyer, not a tourist. Something in the peregrination, the gods know, builds character—and delights writers and readers.

Then there's the DNA story form. A DNA strand is composed of three molecules that entwine around one another and, in their mutual individuality, form a single unit. Similarly, in Hatha-Yoga, we have an image of the subtle body that works as an analogy for this form. A single line of energy runs approximately up the spine while two other core and complementary lines of energy begin on opposite sides of the spine's base and spiral up either side of the spine. They intersect one another at certain key points near the midline until all three meet at the third eye. In DNA stories, two or three substories, themes, or images begin separately yet seem to be remotely related as they occasionally intersect. Two or more characters, in parallel storylines, may fatefully meet one another. In the introduction to Barry Lopez's *Arctic Dreams*, he begins with two compelling memories—one of bowing to a nest of plovers, the other of seeing the gravestone of an Arctic explorer while back in the United States. He explores the two memories at first independently; then, gradually, you sense how the two intersect and come together in Lopez's new dreams for the Arctic, his dreams of our being humble enough to bow to the earth even while we explore new terrain. The two strands unite.

Past and present can flip-flop and meet too. The chapters in Margaret Atwood's novel *Cat's Eye* alternate between the protagonist's past and her present. An artist, the protagonist is haunted by childhood memories of an older girl who bullied and tortured her while seemingly remaining her friend. Her past unites with her present life when her childhood "friend" appears at the protagonist's art opening. It makes for a compelling climax. This movement back and forth keeps readers—and you the writer—guessing how the parts may or may not come together. Atwood peppers in comments by the protagonist's physicist brother about physics and time bending, to reflect, of course, upon the novel's exquisite form.

To sense how the movement of one of your stories affects your readers' imagination, film it. Imagine you were to film parts of the writing with a wide-angled, regular-angled, or zoom-in lens. The zoom-in lens applies to those parts of your story in which you hone in on the details, the filaments of Ella's eyelashes or the texture of tortillas cooked on an open stove. The zoom-in lens can be a writer's primary lens—as in the work of Proust or Nicholson Baker. The regular-angle lens applies to action and narration. The wide-angle lens applies to all of those scenes in which you offer some contextual perspective, such as describing a whole town in which a character lives or when your narrator gives historical or personal background information. The wide-angle also applies to those parts in which your narrator reflects upon "the big picture," the big ideas in your piece. For most stories and poems, these musings are woven amid the zoom-in details and regular-lens action. It's a visual cliché in movies for the camera, once the last words are spoken, the last human gesture made, to pull back and give us a bird's-eye view of the city in which our hapless or happy characters have been contending with life's drama.

You don't need to overanalyze your piece's perspective, and I suggest you not color-code parts of your story according to zoom-in, regular-angle, and wide-angle sections, else you'll spend precious time coloring more than writing. With a sensibility to "lenses," though, you can guide your reader's imagination.

The other way you build internal movement is through repeating or associating key words or images or incidents. These repetitions, like color strands in a tapestry, unify a complex text. They hold together an essay, story, or poem's parts more subtly than paragraphs or stanzas. Usually, you don't do this knowingly at first. A ladybug keeps appearing in certain scenes, and before you know it, the dotted bug has invaded several parts of your story or poem. Why is this insect or just the word "ladybug" bugging you to be repeated? That question propels you to re-vision. Readers enjoy piecing together these beads, although they don't have to amount to heavy symbolism. (And writers such as Thomas Pynchon and filmmakers such as David Lynch love to toy with our symbol-making minds.) So review your draft and note how some words and images have naturally been repeated or naturally associate with one another. You likely will have a medley of associated words. Your job now is to play with how best to emphasize these key words and images without being heavy handed.

Reread a story, essay, or poem whose movement you want to map—yours or someone else's (I like to map writers' works to figure out how the parts hold together). Note how it begins, how that first sentence or line invites you in to sit and listen, to be engaged, to be puzzled and delighted. Flip to the end. An editor of a journal I know says whenever he goes through his stack of short story submissions, he reads the first paragraph. If the first paragraph has made a compelling enough invitation to read further, then he moves directly to the last scene. If there's a compelling enough relationship and progression from beginning to end, then he'll bother to read the middle. So notice how the beginning and end relate. What's happened to the character? What similar words or images appear in both places, suggesting some subtle movement? John Cheever's short story "Reunion" begins with "The last time I saw my father was in Grand Central Station," which seems innocent enough until we compare it with the closing sentence: "'Good-bye, Daddy,' I said, and I went down the stairs and got my train, and that was the last time I saw my father."[2] Last means final, not previous. Similarly, Gary Soto's essay "The Pie," which recounts how as a boy he stole a slice of apple pie, begins, "I knew enough about hell to stop me from stealing," and ends with "I knew sin was what you take and didn't give back."[3] There's been a shift in the boy's thinking and in his knowledge—a key word in this clever contemporary morality tale that plays off of Eve taking from the Tree of Knowledge.

If you're really lost in your draft, try defining your piece's purpose. Ask yourself, *What are you trying to get at and explore in this piece? What do you intend for your readers to think, to feel, to reconsider, to experience by this work's end?* Granted, many of us aren't sure what the heck we're trying to do when drafting except dodge being clueless, and the intentions we set early in a writing project, of course, change by the time we finish a piece days, weeks, months later. But answering these two questions clearly can give you perspective on your piece's whole form because then you can assess how well or not your beginning, middle, and end meet that purpose. Some people may think that these questions should come earlier—maybe even during the drafting stage. I would agree if you're writing journalistic or strictly expository prose (and if you're on a looming deadline). But these questions, while vital, can short-circuit the more organic ways of finding a form.

If necessary, get out the scissors. Or their equivalent for long works—index cards. Cut up sections of a draft and rearrange its parts. See how one section might create more interesting tension when rubbed against another. See how a bit of fragmentation or disjointedness might suit the piece better than seamless fluidity. Omit a section, and see if the piece is better for the excision. Go directly to the part that you think is cutest, the most precious, even the most clever. Cut it. You'll be glad you did. Believe me. Index cards I use for longer essays and books. I write topics and tentative titles on the cards and flip-flop and rearrange, gauging which one is best for the beginning, the best sequencing of one to the next, and the best for the ending. In fact, I did this very thing for this chapter. After writing several drafts, I wrote fourteen topics on fourteen cards, laid them out on my worktable, and played with their order like puzzle pieces. My imagination likes the physical manipulation.

THE THIRD EYE & CREATIVE INCUBATION

Let your stories, images, ideas, and drafts sit for a while. John Gardner said he would place a drafted story in a drawer for a year, and if after a year the story merited more work, he'd consider revising it. Time gave him perspective on the manuscript's shape and the language's texture. Would that most of us had such patience and persistence. When Richard Ford realizes the muse isn't visiting, he doesn't fret; he watches SportsCenter and forgets about her. He advocates taking breaks so he can consider whether what he's written is worth keeping or scrapping and so he can reward himself for some grueling (but, he warns, not overly difficult) work. Too, the ritual of taking a break allows a writer to follow the example of his subject and live in the world. Similarly, Paul West has written about that dreamy place where writers float he calls "The Castle of Indolence." Give in to it, he says. These moments of not working often proffer the freshest, most surprising ideas.

We need not escape to an island or lock ourselves up in a New England cabin to incubate. Instead, some tools of Yoga help us withdraw from our external senses so we can fine tune the inner senses. Deliberately withdrawing from the external senses is called *pratyahara*, what Patanjali calls the fifth limb of yoga. Sensory withdrawal prepares yogis for concentration, meditation, and bliss. We can practice this limb for a few minutes in our own study or bedroom. Doing so may help us rest in the silky coat of those ideas we want to birth in a new form. Stepping back and reseeing our writing may require that, for a while at least, we stop looking at it so logically with our normal eyes.

Writer Dame Edith Sitwell, according to Diane Ackerman's *A Natural History of the Senses*, used to close herself up in a coffin for a few hours before writing. Try it. Wait for night. Draw the blinds. Take a notepad and pen and turn out the lights. Light a candle. Use earplugs if you have them. Then, find the variation of the form that suits your body at this moment.

A heightened intuition mixed with clarity of intention can help us with all of these practices for re-vision—from mapping movement, to cutting up, to incubating. Intuitive insight occurs not when the brain is lazy but when certain parts of the defensive hind brain, responsible for our fight-or-flight response, quiets, and parts of the creative brain, such as the frontal lobe, are active. We can alter this brain activity by harnessing our outer senses as well as by shifting the body's position to increase cerebral blood flow. When we alter our body appropriately, we can shift our outer and inner vision so that we have the insight to re-vision.

While living in a cabin in the Berkshires a few summers ago, I reached down to plug in my desk lamp and noticed what I thought were at first huge dust balls collected around the laptop's plug. Shaped like silken garlic cloves, two half-finger long rock-climber tents lay suspended from the precipice of the computer plug and outlet. Outdoors, any one of the thousands of trees might have made a suitable resting space for this caterpillar and his friend, but they chose instead to come indoors and wrap themselves where we humans have channeled virtual fire. I wanted to imagine then, without wrenching the moment of its overt symbolism, some reciprocal charge from the energy being stored in those cocoons and the energy being stored at the cord's other end.

On the main doorway's threshold, a half dozen or so cocoons were nestled too. Cocoons on the threshold. Inside these pupal caves, their jaws shift into long, curled tongues, their short antenanne grow longer, and from their backs emerge four large wings. One night, as I fed the woodstove old sheets of this manuscript, I imagined the converted words and leaves, the pulpy slivers, transmuting with my imagination and subtle body and spinning out of the small smokestack a billowy, silken cocoon that feeds down the roof, slithers over the windows, and wraps me in a satin oasis. There I would stay for as long as needed, in complete retreat with these strange images and impulses and ideas that often usurp my willful mind's and body's banana republic, their poem-grenades and story-bombs sabotaging my conscious desire to keep things orderly and logical. The window covers would give me just enough translucence to nourish me and just enough opacity to keep me looking in, looking in, looking in. What shape shifting could I perform, I wondered. Cristo (the artist of grand wrapping) couldn't make a better artist's studio.

A kids' book on bugs says that these worms probably have gone through three to five instars, stages of molting and transforming. Each time, they eat so much they literally grow too big for their skin, which busts at their backs' seams and gives them a new range of colors, bumps, and hair. They are horizontal pillars of patience.

In this way, caterpillars are a writer's insect. For after eating leaves for weeks, they inch their way with utter instinct in search of some warm, safe spot to settle for a few weeks, to spin themselves into a web, to retreat. And then they wait. They incubate. They eat up images and ideas until their bodies burst.

It seems worth pointing out here that musician, former surgeon, and founder of New York City's Polarity Therapy Institute John Beaulieu once showed me a diagram of where in the skull the pituitary gland, the gland the third eye stimulates, sits. It's housed in a groove of the sphenoid bone. The diagram, with no stretch of the imagination, clearly resembles a butterfly or moth, complete with four wings, spots on the wings, and eyes at the optic foramen. A butterfly imprint on our skull.

TAKE A BREATH #1: CLOSE YOUR WINDOWS

Friendly Warning:
If you have untreated blood-pressure issues or heart problems, please do not try the breath retention part of this practice. You can practice closing all of the other "gates" except your nostrils.

Benefits: This practice relaxes the sense organs and quickly calms the analytical mind. This particular practice, according to one study in Scandanavia, also has been correlated with releasing nitric oxide—the neurochemical responsible for deep happiness and also associated with deep intuitive experiences.

Intention:

Engage this practice to stimulate your third eye to receive insight for re-visioning a piece's form.

While in a comfortable seated position at or away from your desk, focus on your breath. Place each thumb in your ear, each index finger atop each eyelid, and each middle finger's tip along the outside of each nostril. For this variation, the other two fingers can rest near the mouth. Other students prefer to rest on their backs and use an eye pillow and earplugs. Take a deep inhalation, hold the inhalation, and let your middle fingers close your nostrils. Hold here for as long as you're comfortable. It may only be a few seconds at first. Repeat at least three times. As you do so, notice how shutting off light from your eyelids, closing your eyes, and even shutting off the sound of your breath heightens your stillness.

Then, without retaining your breath, inhale slowly and as you exhale hum with lips closed. It will sound as if bumblebees are making honey in your skull-hive. Repeat two to four more times.

Then, rest your hands on your thighs and move your eyeballs up toward your third eye and try to imagine the shape of your story, essay, or poem in question. If a sudden image surprisingly surfaces, either stay with it, or open your eyes and note it or sketch it. If nothing surfaces, imagine you're taking a trip through your writing. How does the journey begin? How does the entry feel? What key image or concept designates the opening? How does the journey progress to the next part? And to the next? What key images or concepts keep recurring? How does one feed into the next? Follow the path that your writing has laid out or wants to lay out in your memory. If you have difficulty remembering certain parts, don't fret. Take the forgetting as a possible sign for re-visioning something more memorable. Notice how it feels to arrive at the end of the path. As you look back, can you see the beginning? Have you looped back near where you started? Or is there no going back?

When ready, open your eyes and roughly sketch or jot down notes from this experience.

TAKE A BREATH #2: INVERT YOUR VISION

Friendly Warning:
Remember, the idea is to find the form that fits your body at any given time and not to force your body to fit a form. If none of these variations feels right for your body, then recline in CORPSE POSE (*savāsana*). If you've been practicing for a while and have some flexibility in your neck and cervical spine, see the illustrations for two more advanced variations using **REVERSED ATTITUDE GESTURE** or **SHOULDER STAND**.

Benefits: The practice of **REVERSED ATTITUDE GESTURE** (viparīta-karanī mudrā) *and its variations is not so much to turn your work upside down as it is to shift your body's regular flow and help you relax your senses, especially your eyes, so you can improve your inner vision. Options 2 and 3 below also increase cerebral blood flow and can slow down your brain waves—both physiological traits of creative activity. Each of these pos* *es is believed to shift vital energy back toward the brain and is known to cool down the sympathetic nervous system as well, allowing the defensive part of our brains to rest and the creative parts of our brain to awaken.*

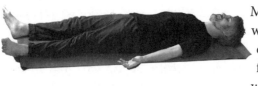

Intention:
Move into this pose when it's time to with-draw and gain ease-ful insight into your writing's form.

Variation #1: **CORPSE POSE** *(savāsana). Rest on your back, knees bent or straight. Let your arms rest to the sides, palms face up. Breathe from your belly's base.*

Variation #2: **LEGS UP THE WALL.** *For this popular variation of* **REVERSED ATTITUDE GESTURE,** *come to a wall, rest on your left side, and push your tush against the wall while still on your side. Once you feel both buttocks against the wall, come onto your back as your legs climb the wall. If this po-sition feels uncomfortable, then place a folded blanket with a three-foot length six inches away from the wall on which your back can rest, and let your buttocks hang off the edge of the blanket. Let your back body melt into the ground as your legs rest and your blood flow shifts.*

Once you've found the variation that feels most relaxing yet stimulating, close your eyes and keep your focus on your breath. Anytime you smell, hear, or even feel something, let go of paying too much attention to it and instead draw your eyeballs up toward your third eye as you guide your breath from your third eye down and back up your spine. As thoughts or images surface, also try to let go of them. Try doing so for at least two minutes. Then, breathe less and less distinctly. Don't worry about deep breathing. Aim for soft yet satisfying (not deep) breaths. Take breaths whose undu-lations are so indistinct you can't hear yourself breathe and can barely feel your body moving with your breath. Try doing so for another two minutes.

This practice is challenging at first and may not get any easier for a while. Here's a suggested schedule for using the practice fifteen times to let a draft incubate:

First–Fifth Sessions: Get comfortable with the practice. Get comfortable with letting go of thinking about your draft and with focusing less and less on your senses and thoughts. You might do so for only five minutes at a time.

Sixth–Tenth Sessions: Try to lengthen the practice by five minutes. Notice if any sessions become easier for you. During this stage, observe any changes in the quality of your mind and body as you draft pieces other than the one you're incubating. Are you less distracted? More receptive? If not, don't fret. Aim for a caterpillar's patience.

Eleventh–Fifteenth Sessions: In these last sessions, your third eye may grant you some insight into the nature of what needs re-visioning in your draft. As you move deeply into withdrawing from your senses during these sessions, keep open to an image that may relate integrally to your draft.

But remember this: Refrain from expecting anything, grand or small, to happen. In fact, the insight may come between sessions while you're planting cherry tomatoes in your garden, while you're sailing, or while you're walking your dog. Insight may actually come during the seventh session or even during the third one. But just try not to force the moth or butterfly to emerge too soon. Each practice can set the conditions for insight to surface.

CHAPTER TWENTY-TWO

LETTING GO OF DELUSION AND CONTROL: REVISE!

A T LAST YOU'VE FINISHED drafting your novel. You've even "re-visioned" parts of it into good shape and form. But you're not through yet. You still must revise. I meet writers in almost every class and workshop who harbor antipathy toward revising. Why? What keeps us from revising? Some beginning writers resist revising because of the "Tainting the Pristine Moment Syndrome." Based on the Jack Kerouac idea that real writing rolls onto the page in a transcendent, exalted moment when a writer levitates from her chair while drafting, this argument claims that to revise an otherwise "inspired" poem or story taints its authenticity. Legends of writers composing novels in six weeks in a frenzied flurry often feed this idea and ultimately starve beginning writers from understanding the years of crafting that may have preceded that six-weeks performance. This notion of the first draft as the final, authentic draft keeps writers who otherwise have talent from producing work worth reading and re-reading. My Texas friend calls this syndrome the "Whatever I Shit is Gold Syndrome."

Some of us shutter at anything that smacks of criticism. A few writers who have approached me as a potential editor share past experiences that they treat as wounds. The over-bearing teacher, the cruel writing professor, the poet who ripped a young writer's poem in a workshop, the editor who shredded a manuscript. I assure them that most of us who have weathered workshops and graduate programs have had or witnessed such moments. Parts of my old poems once lay scattered across university room floors; they have become, I'm sure, engrained as part of the cold lino-leum. We don't let criticism stop us, though. If we did, we'd have no books to read. Some younger and beginning writers I meet and work with simply do not yet have the perspective, acumen, and detachment to revise well. They want to revise, they tell me; they simply don't know where to begin.

Each part of the writing process has its valuable place. In draft-ing, you create characters, get lost in fresh ideas, and discover your story's heart. You are an artist. In re-visioning, you re-imagine your writing's structure, incubate on its shape, and make global changes. You are a designer. In revising, you hone in on, prune, double-check, and correct your manuscript's details. You are a caretaker. To revise and to edit your manuscript can be an act of respect for your creation and a gift for potential readers.

I say the following from experience: Much resistance to revising stems from delusion and refusal to let go of control. Delusion, of course, is when we have a false judgment or opinion about some-thing—in this case, our writing. *Bhranti-darshana* in Sanskrit translates loosely to "living in delusion" or "having mistaken no-tions." Patanjali lists it in Sutra I.30 as being a major obstacle to a yogi's path of self-realization. I know this concept intimately because I've embodied its various forms for years and continue to do so. If you readily use any of the following defenses to yourself (all too familiar to me) or to someone editing your writing, beware of delusion:

- "X just doesn't understand my writing style." [X could be a trusted friend, editor, spouse/partner]
- "But that's the story's funniest/cleverest/most original line/image/example!"
- "I've been writing/publishing for ten years; I know what I'm doing."
- "I graduated from X; I know what I'm doing."
- "I was inspired when I wrote that; I can't touch it, or I'll taint it."

Related to delusion is demanding control of our writing. "I am the author; thus, I am the authority" sums up this mentality.

Don't fret, though. Limited self-understanding and false self-conceptions simply are part of being human. Thankfully, we can reflect upon our writing's qualities, we can reassess our writing, and we can refine our craft. To let go of delusion and control requires in part cultivating discernment. In Yoga, discernment is called viveka, the ability to separate what factors in one's life contribute to self-realization from those that do not. A yogi chooses and omits activities, habits, and external elements accordingly. A writer's discernment might seem less daunting, for it is a disciplined process of distinguishing which words, phrases, or sentences work and do not work in a piece of writing. Having discernment can exercise your intellect and sharpen your craft. As you grow more confident in handling your craft's finer details, you rely more on your own authority.

My writing process is not simply linear as in moving smoothly from drafting to re-visioning to revising, nor is it for most writers I know. Granted, I do prepare myself for a revising and editing session differently from a drafting session. In a drafting session, I'm wandering, sauntering, moving through forward bends or other poses that will induce my subtle imagination to open up some fresh ideas and images and metaphors. My open-minded drafting buddy goads me to do what I wish. My editing taskmaster, though, is a no-nonsense and rather persnickety female figure, a necessary foil to my frolicking drafting buddy. She knows we have work to do and not always much time in which to finish it. My drafting buddy generates ideas; my editing taskmaster helps me choose, cut, and replace. So when I revise, I want to be alert, not dreamy. I have a clear path and mission. Usually, because my drafts tend to be bloated and weedy, my mission is to slay, slice, and prune—slay my drafting ego that may wish to hold on to precious parts of my writing, slice the excess words and sentences, and prune the wordy phrases. I become a linguistic hunter and gardener.

Yet, for me drafting and revising often overlap, and my process is more recursive than linear. Sometimes I write and rewrite several sentences as each one comes out—a series of steps and back steps, creations and erasures, on the word-processing screen—as if to steal the proper timbre or tone. My taskmaster nudges her way in with questions: This word or that word? Begin this sentence here? Place this phrase where? What are my options? I'm rewriting this very paragraph's sentences as I'm drafting them. My taskmaster wants to protect me from making a fool of myself, whereas my drafting buddy encourages me to do so, but I get nowhere without both of them.

I share with writers and students other things I do to develop a discerning attitude when revising is my mission. A few standing yoga poses, back bends, and particular breath work can increase cerebral blood flow and ensnare the wandering mind to stay on discernment's path. Refine, refine, refine often is my mantra. Once I get my body and mind in agreement with the task before me, I print out a draft (my taskmaster likes to mark things up). Sometimes I stand up and read a draft aloud. Whether sitting or standing, this practice of reading aloud can help you hear almost instantly the clunky sentence structures and inappropriate or imprecise word choices. You'll hear the foggy nonsense that you and your drafting buddy thought was, a week ago, the most brilliant thing ever written.

In the early stages of editing, you might recruit someone you trust just to listen without commenting. James Thurber, an avid reviser never satisfied with his first drafts, said his wife was his best editor. When reading his early drafts she would say, referring to his attempts at humor, something like "Thurber! This stuff is high school nonsense." When I begin editing, I don't want that kind of feedback yet, but having another attentive person present can make you more aware of a potential audience. It directs your writer's mind toward communicating with or affecting someone. Sometimes when I read aloud a sentence that I think is funny to my wife, she will remain silent and then say, in a near-motherly tone, "Jeffrey." My taskmaster nods and makes a small x and ? in the margin, and I read on.

In these read-aloud sessions, you might feel like a happy weeder in a neglected garden, near giddy when drawing lines through rows of words and marking X's through paragraphs. I underline sentences whose structure needs revisiting. Next to paragraphs that need rewriting I draw vertical lines in the margins and make a brief note—more color, less color, more examples, fewer examples. A circled word tells me later I need to find a more precise or appropriate word or that I need to check its meaning. You have to find, of course, what works for you, but whatever you do, tend to the details.

An essential point of business is words. Choose the right word. It helps to know a word's denotation—its literal, agreed-upon meaning—and its connotation. Connotations are a word's shades of meaning, the associations that readers register with words. Take the various synonyms for "thin": skinny, gaunt, scrawny, svelte, slim, sleek, reedy, twiggy, stalky, lanky, puny, meager, cadaverous. Each option's literal meaning hovers loosely around the field of "thin," yet nearly each option's shade of meaning can signal a completely different effect. If you want to suggest that a character appears like a walking corpse, then *cadaverous* is your word, but if you want your character's body frame to conjure the image of a feline form, graceful and elegant, then *svelte* is your word. Be careful of unintended connotations. Recently, I compared the joys of drafting to walking through a hemlock forest. The comparison came from my own satisfaction in being surrounded by hemlocks that have made, in the past hundred years, a revival in the Catskills. An editor, though, reminded me of many people's association of hemlock with poison. She was right, and the risk of a missed association wasn't worth it, so I changed it to the more commonly positive association of "evergreen forest."

A select verb can invigorate a sentence and your message's connotations, but not just any verb will suffice. Choices for describing the manner of a vociferous character's speech, for example, include *harangue, babble, ramble, elucidate, gibber, expatiate*. Of course, *elucidate* stands out from the pack as being the kindest in connotation due in part to its root, the Latin lucidus, "bright." To elucidate is to "shed light" on a subject. *Expatiate* rightfully sounds the most neutral, as it means "to speak or write thoroughly." *Babble, ramble,* and *gibber* have similar negative connotations of the relative who will not cut to the chase so the rest of us can eat our dinner, but each word has a slightly different denotation. *Babble* is sheer nonsense, the sort that makes the most diplomatic among us bite our tongue in amazement that the speaker's jaw doesn't come unhinged from being overworked. *Ramble,* like the Rambler automobile of the 1950s, suggests a way of talking at once leisurely and digressive. To *gibber* can be to talk nonsensically, but it also can describe speech purposefully vague or pretentious.

Now, one person's view of a "rambling" speech may be another person's view of sheer "babble," while what one person considers to be a careful "elucidation" may be to another person nothing more than a "harangue." But you're the writer, and you're the one who gets to have fun playing with point of view, character, and purpose.

Imagine you're writing a story about a woman named Elizabeth who is dying from an unknown cause. Your narrator is a man who purports to love her, and here is your first effort for him to describe her appearance:

> Her **frame covered** by **thin epidermis**, Elizabeth appeared unhealthy.

This description sounds almost comical in part because of the use of the formal word epidermis. Frame also sounds oddly neutral or suggestive of a building's structure, not a loved one's body. Maybe that's your intention. Maybe this character remains throughout the first part of the story emotionally detached and aloof from the reality that Elizabeth is dying. But maybe you were just having trouble choosing the right words. A rewrite might read as follows:

> Her **skeleton draped** by **translucent flesh**, Elizabeth might have disintegrated in the breeze.

This description is still a bit stiff, but more emotive (if not more affected) not only for the hyperbole that closes the sentence but also for the diction. It also implies the character's emotional attachment and creates for the reader a far more vivid and emotionally charged image of Elizabeth than does the first description. It would make an interesting story if at times the narrator's emotions seemed affected and disingenuous.

Economy matters too. Whereas my drafting buddy can spend words freely, my taskmaster budgets everything—especially the number of words I can use. At this stage her pruning shears and her gleaming smile come out. "Less is more," she parrots like the Mies van der Rohe of writing. Among my numerous pruning tools, a favorite is to discern the wicked *whiches* from the good *whiches*. The *which* in the following sentence can go without losing meaning:

> Ben works in the Zenith building, ~~which is~~ the tallest building in downtown Phoenix.

You also often can cut a phrase to a word or two. Take the following first draft of a sentence from this very paragraph:

> **Drafting buddy's version:** I have any number of tricks to share for pruning, but one of my favorites is to discern the wicked whiches from the good whiches.

> **Taskmaster's first version:** I have numerous tricks for pruning, but a favorite is to discern the wicked whiches from the good whiches.

> **Taskmaster's current version:** Among my numerous pruning tools, a favorite is to discern the wicked whiches from the good whiches.

Numerous replaces any *number* of, and a *favorite* butts out *one of my favorites*. The phrase to share is implied, so it can go. Revising saves me six or more words in one sentence. Multiply six by however many wordy sentences your first draft contains, and you realize that a hefty thousand-word story or essay could become a lean seven hundred words. It's not uncommon for a magazine editor to ask me to cut a 728-word piece down to 500 words because of space constraints. Despite my attachments to certain parts of the writing, I comply quickly often to an editor's surprise.

The more careful the practice, the easier this part of the writing may become—if you can let go of delusion and control. Take these two sentences, for example, from a student's story that express the same basic idea:

1. Eleanor, who is a woman noted for her ability to be able to make rudely bold and demanding business executives soften with her small talk and to make really angry clients feel less angry, was a perfect candidate for the customer service desk at Bulworth Associates. (Forty-six words.)

2. Eleanor's warm soft-talking could melt the most brazen executive and defuse the most incensed client. No doubt, she was a perfect candidate for Bulworth Associates' customer service desk. (Twenty-eight words.)

Delusion would justify that the first sentence is thorough and substantive. Actually, it's long winded, redundant, and clunky—yet structurally typical of many first drafts. With a few revisions of word choice and sentence structure, the second sentence not only saves your readers' time; it also gives the idea more force and, thus, effect than the first version. The metaphors of *warm* and *melt* give you a more vivid sense of the power Eleanor's voice possesses and may even help you imagine how she'd sound when handling an ornery client. Breaking up the first sentence into two sentences and including the more colloquial *no doubt* also makes the voice less formal than the first. You'd be hard pressed to justify not revising that first sentence.

Yet—and this point is essential—clarity and economy are not incontestable aesthetic virtues (although Strunk and White zealots and die-hard followers of Raymond Carver's fiction and 1980's writing workshops may argue otherwise). I relish, for reasons of philosophy and disposition, artful digressions and expansive poetry and prose—all elements of writing that may test readers' patience. One writer with whom I have worked for over two years often questions my choices for a clipped sentence when she is aiming for a more colloquial voice. Our exchange itself is important because she is making choices. You have to decide, ultimately, whether revising a sentence for fewer words subtracts from the sentence's voice, music, and overall effect. But as in all cases, beware of pleading "poetic license" to justify poor writing (and laziness when revising).

Joe, a yoga teacher I know, takes his students through the same pose four different ways. He lets them feel the pose one way that, without discernment, might seem right. Then he shows them another way of coming into the pose that, through contrast, lets them experience how much better some simple adjustments can make experiencing the pose. Then he'll have them press into their left big toe mound, for instance, while stretching, say, a hip extensor and then shifting their right shoulder three inches to the left. Joe's refinements of a pose mirror how writers must approach part of their writing. Of course, spending this kind of energy on every move in Yoga would make the practice tedious just as it would in writing. But refinement and discernment deepen your appreciation of details. Such discernment is part of letting go of our attachment to words on the page.

"Letting go" does sound like "newage." "Newage" is what one writer—and long-time Yoga pilgrim—calls the language of New Age that often reduces complex experiences to bumper sticker addages. Still, Yoga practice has helped me be less attached to the words that unfold on the page. I move through a sequence of postures, breathwork, and meditation every morning. The daily meditation practice calms my thoughts enough to let me witness how they surface in patterns during the day when I am not sitting.

"I have a few observations," my wife says of a short story I'm writing. I bristle. I can actually feel my jaw tighten and my shoulders slightly lift. *What does she know? Why is she so damned critical? Is she trying to prove herself?* I can be the worst student of sorts. And yet, even without her knowing it, I am having this subtle conversation in my head during the few seconds between when she says "I have a few observations" and when I say something in response. There is a voice, call it the witness, that sort of chuckles at my patterned defenses. I recognize them for what they are—instincts to protect—and then I hear the witness say something to those defensive patterns like, "Oh, shut up and listen." Your witness might be a gentle grandmother, but my defensive ego often needs a five-star general to make it perk up and shut up. I look at my wife with soft eyes, drop my shoulders, take a deep inhalation, and say, "Okay, let's hear your observations." For her care and attention, I am always thankful— even if that gratitude gets obscured sometimes by crankiness.

To revise your work is to respect your writing as well as your potential readers. It is to acknowledge the art of "getting it right," whether "it" be the tone, image, word choice, phrasing, or sentence structure. If you're unwilling to tend to your writing's details, you're treating your own writing too cheaply, as if it's expendable and forgettable. Recently, I waited on a plane before takeoff for over thirty minutes while the mechanics checked and double-checked the plane's wiring and engines. The man next to me complained. "Another delay! Don't these people know we have schedules to keep? They're just clueless." I understood his response. Delays are irritating, and before taking off on a flight I'd like to think I were in control when really I'm anything but. But to this flustered man I suggested that if we have to wait another thirty minutes to assure the plane flies right and safely, then I don't mind at all. He didn't respond and checked his watch. If you want your writing to get off the ground, if you want it to soar, and if you want your readers to come back to your writing, tend to the details. Revise.

TAKE A BREATH: HONE THE BLADE

Intention:

If you either are blocked about revising a piece of your writing or if you just need aid developing discernment, try this practice.

Benefits: The following practice, **SUN BREATHING** *(surya bhedana pranayama), stimulates the sympathetic nervous system as well as the brain's left hemisphere. It often results in writers feeling slightly more alert and clear-headed.*

Vi in viveka *(discernment) means "to separate." Try to separate yourself from words on the page. Come into a comfortable seated position of your choice. Let your spine grow long as you close your eyes. After two or more slow breaths, ask yourself, "What am I writing?" Connect this response to the more specific task of revising your work. Then, clarify that you intend to cultivate an objective discernment to help you prune, clip, even omit parts of your writing.*

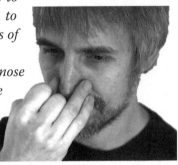

Lift your right hand to your nose and fold your index and middle fingers to your thumbpad as if in preparation for **ALTERNATE NOSTRIL BREATHING.** *With your ring finger closing off your left nostril, breathe in only through your right nostril. Then use your thumb to close your right nostril, and open your left nostril. Breathe out through the left nostril. Repeat this breathing pattern—in through the right and out through the left—nine more times.*

Sit quietly for up to ten more soft breaths. Feel your mind clear and alert. Feel your mind as having the quality of pruning sheers or a sword. I am clear. I am clearing.

Open your eyes. Move to your writing. Let the mind cut and clear. Let it be quick at times. Trust the tool. Do so for the work.

CHAPTER TWENTY-THREE

FRIENDLY WARNINGS OF
INAUTHENTICITY

MY VERY FIRST PUBLIC READING initiated me in the temptations of inauthenticity. In my early twenties, I was just starting to publish my poetry and read some of it at open-mike events. Someone asked me if I would like to be one of three poets featured at a special reading. I was flattered. This seemed like big stuff. When I found out who the other two poets were, though, I froze. One was an older guy known for his slam-style poetry and the other was a young, sexy woman—both of them the most popular poets among the mostly youthful poetry scene because of their bold and clever sex-driven poems. Plus, they had snazzy names like Belle and Devo. I had no erotic poem, or hip name for that matter, to compare or compete. I was in my ascetic abstinence stage, then, and my sexiest poem explored the passion of making popcorn.

It was my first reading, and I feared coming off as the pathetic, sexless poet. I had two weeks before the reading to change that, and in two weeks I managed to write three erotic poems drawn from pure imagination. One was about a guy who, while having sex, can't stop comparing his girlfriend's navel to divine metaphors. The poems were clever but corny, to say the least, and latent with gratuitous references designed not only to titillate but also to make me look like a hot-blooded American male poet who could compete with the hottest poets in town.

The reading occurred at a quiet coffee shop located in a mostly conservative neighborhood and frequented mostly by sweater-

and khaki-clad adults. The host introduced us, and the format upon which we agreed was for each of us to read one poem and continue to circulate in this manner. I went first and started with a poem about bridges in Texas. Belle and Devo followed with similar placid pieces. The latté-drinking couple at the table in front seemed pleased. Then, as I read one of the erotic pieces, the same couple suddenly looked as if they were watching a John Hughes film that had become a raunchy skin flick. When I finished, Belle pulled out and read a poem about faking an orgasm, complete with sound effects and gyrating hips. I read yet another erotic poem, and a few poems later, while we poets seemed engrossed in a linguistic ménage-à-trois, the coffee shop was nearly empty, and the proprietor threatened not to let the host return. Devo shook my hand and said he had a new respect for me. Belle said she should have married me instead of the drip she'd recently hitched. I went home feeling like a completely successful fraud. I made myself some popcorn and went to bed alone.

The heart of inauthenticity is not acting upon what you know at your core to be true. In most instances, only you will know if you're being inauthentic when you write, but we can heed a few "indicators" of inauthenticity. They're reminders for myself as much as they can be for you.

Much of inauthenticity has to do with trying to fit in or to "reach an audience." Editors at commercial publishing houses understandably are hard-pressed to find audiences for the writers whose works they champion, and many writers are encouraged if not implored to be find ingenius ways to gather their own audiences. This fact became obvious at a recent conference that offered numerous panels of editors, agents, and authors. On one panel, Chuck Adams, editor at Algonquin Books, discussed how his priority often is to determine whether or not a book has a potential audience of, say, 30,000. His colleague on this particular panel, Dawn Davis of Amistad, also said she wants to know what an author is "going to bring to the table. I do want to know—and I hate to say it—but I do want to know what is the author's platform."

"Platform" is the dreaded but inevitable word that creeps up at almost every writers' conference that addresses publishing.

"Platform" includes all of the ways that a writer reaches out to and sustains a growing audience without a publisher's assistance. I often imagine a writer who wants his book to be published so it can be read (and so he can make some money from his writing). So he finds an empty warehouse. When he's not writing, he's spending his time buying material from WritersDepot and reading manuals to help him build a stage. Then he creates a catchy name for the warehouse to make it sound like a place for people who like writers and readings and artsy kind of stuff to gather, creates a hip website, creates funky fliers, and tells all of his hip friends about the place, and gets a crowd to gather on Friday nights so he can stand on the platform and read his stuff. He has created his audience.

There's nothing wrong by itself with a writer doing some leg work to find her audience, her true audience. Writers have been doing so long before the "p-word" infiltrated publishing buzz-speak. Still, it comes back to that one simple question, "What am I writing for?" If you're writing solely to please an audience or writing to fit in at a certain publishing house, you are not being true to your own voice.

After all of the panel's lectures on audiences and platforms, Chuck Adams advised writers in the audience, "But always write from your heart. Write what you know you must write and how you must write." Once you hone your craft and persist, then you can find the audience for your work.

Similarly, catch yourself if you're editing part of your work so as not to offend somebody. If it's essential to your story that your characters have sex, that they're addicted to heroin, or that they say "fuck" all of the time, let them. Your job is to present your characters as truthfully as possible. Sanitizing is not truthfulness or authenticity—regardless of what a parent might have told you. On the other hand, if you've lived in upstate New York most of your life and you're tired of your characters talking about the weather and church and carpentry, you don't have to create a crack-shooting sex fiend with a foul mouth just to be "gritty" or "realistic." Booker Prize–winner James Kelman's characters say "fuck" three times in a sentence because, as Kelman says, *fuck* to his Scottish characters is a comma. To Kelman, language is language is language, and distinctions such as standard language, dialect, colloquialisms, or vulgarities contribute to class inequities. When you have that kind of perspective, the *fucks* are fitting, not gratuitous.

Sometimes beginning writers, particularly younger ones, so want to thwart conventions that they equate authenticity with raw emotion. I know one young poet who, every time he reads a poem, yells and screams, repeating something like "What have you done to our planet, you bastards?!" Such raw emotion in writing is dramatic, if not histrionic, but doesn't always lead to authenticity.

To write authentically is to write from your own authority, and so many matters of writing without authenticity relate to denying your own authority and deferring to someone else's. This "listening to your own authority" is tricky, especially for the MFA students with whom I work. Teachers, professors, and other writers can be seductive in their authority—the more charismatic, the more persuasive. I know of one college writing teacher whose colorful talks on the hazards of writing conventions and craft enchant his students. Appealing to the rebellious teenager in all of us, he likes to posit himself as an iconoclast—particularly when he slashes his students' writing. It's his way or no way, one of his former students once told me. This particular student said that for nearly two years she would write with the sole intention of pleasing her teacher. If she could please him, then she knew she would be a good writer. It's easy to fool ourselves into thinking so.

You can learn from such teachers, but if you find yourself following every word that writer says despite your own thoughts, then you're giving your authority away. It's one thing to be a writing apprentice (an honorable yet underrated role in our country); it's another to be a lackey. An apprentice, while receptive and open, should be full of questions, tinged with curiosity and healthy skepticism, and willing, of course, to essay things. I've been fortunate to have teachers—in Yoga and in writing—who aimed ultimately to wean me away from them and whose intention was to try to make me my own best teacher. So if you find yourself in a writing class in which the instructor is unbending in entertaining differing yet legitimate views about writing and seems hell bent on thrusting a singular agenda—namely on gathering his or her disciples—run.

You don't have time to waste with egomaniacs. (The same loosely applies, incidentally, when seeking a yoga teacher.).

When you're in a writing group, ego dynamics can surface in even more complex ways. Check in with yourself when writing a story, poem, or essay that you know you're going to share with your writing group. The anticipation of having your piece read and critiqued can alter what and how you write. Say you're crafting a scene between your character Betty and her new coworker Alex. You're having one of those rare moments when you're completely absorbed in the scene, and the sexual tension between them is mounting subtly. Something else is happening, too, in the scene with language—you're playing with the jargon of their financial-consulting lingo and the language of lovers. Just when you think the scene is flowing, you remember Andrea from your writing group. She's been publishing her stories steadily and recently has assumed queen-bee status in your writing group. She hates scenes or plots related to love or sex. Boring, she says. Andrea's always talking about "layering" and "contextualizing" with other subjects like history and physics. You don't really get what she's up to, but you feel you should. Soon you notice you're questioning Betty and Alex's relationship in your story. Maybe you should throw in some physics or history references somehow—the history of bending time with financial consulting?—to "layer" the story.

This compromising we do unknowingly. We substitute a professor's authority with another person's authority. If you genuinely want to write a story in which the characters may have an intimate relationship, or there may be tension that suggests they want to have sex but aren't sure about the whole love thing, then go for it. Make it as authentic as you can. At your next writing group meeting, if Andrea begins one of her "layering" sermons, hear her out. Maybe she'll say something that makes sense this time. But when she's finished and everyone else has finished commenting, you can do one of three things: First, concur and perhaps recognize some validity to some of the comments. Second, let Andrea and the rest of the group know that writers will never exhaust the complexities of relationships and that you intend to continue exploring how to render freshly these complexities. Or, if you think that comment will only goad Andrea into another hour's worth of lecturing, you can smile and genuinely thank everyone for his or her comments and move on. Being in a writing group should help you see your writing and writing craft in general afresh. So welcome comments by trusted teachers and fellow writers without negating your own authenticity.

It can be challenging for Yoga to break down the ego for those of us who are trained and mentored by writers with strong egos. Some of us have been trained to compete, to seek recognition as validation, to win contests and awards, to get pats on the head from other notorious writers and editors, to be told "Good boy!" and "Good girl!"—puppies all of us.

But for those of us who persist with a practice Yoga can do its thing on a writer's ego. It can speed up not-striving. It can slow down anxiety. It can speed up gratitude. It can slow down envy.

Almost everything I've suggested in this chapter, if not in every other chapter, goes back to being clear about your intentions. A yogi obsessed mainly with trying to stretch out her hamstrings so she can perform intricate poses and make her students ooh and ahh is no more authentic in intention than the writer who seeks mainly to get his name in print so his friends can read with envy. Returning every day not only to the question of what you are writing for but also to smaller questions such as why you're including one scene in your story or why you're writing about a particular subject helps keep you authentic. It's an ongoing part of the journey.

CHAPTER TWENTY-FOUR

FOR WRITERS WHO ALREADY PRACTICE YOGA

I F YOU'VE BEEN PRACTICING YOGA for a a few years or more, you might have a good-sized tool belt of yoga poses, breath work, and principles. You might even have a regular home practice. So how do you engage these upaya, these "skillful means" in ways that make sense for you as a writer on a daily basis?

Begin with creating your own "writing flow" of poses, breath work, visualization, and/or meditation that seems most compatible with your writing process. The general guidelines that follow later in this chapter can help you be creative. Learn what you need as a writer, and try out the tools to build a strong personal writing laboratory: your body-mind-imagination. For me, an embodied writing process, again, includes these elements in this order at least five times a week:

- Setting a Twofold Writing Intention:
  What am I writing for?
  a specific statement of my focus for a particular writing session

- practicing Yoga (poses, breathwork, meditation) for fifteen to sixty minutes to manifest that intention

- writing for at least three hours a session with frequent awareness of my breath, body, thoughts, and imagination (If three hours a session seems too long, you begin with where you're at: thirty minutes, sixty minutes).

This process works for me. Although I work best with a regular flow of poses and breath work, I daily vary from this flow according to whatever ache, sensation, or mood surfaces. Sometimes, I surrender to the mat and stop pushing the flow to sense what pose naturally needs to follow.

Work with what challenges you in your writing. Acknowledge what's difficult in your writing, and dare to employ the Yoga tools that help you work with, although not "fix," that challenge. I heard yogi Rodney Yee once say that he could distinguish beginners, intermediate students, and advanced students accordingly: Beginners, eager to learn anything, will try any and all poses and practices. Intermediate students, savvy to their own limitations, will practice only those poses that they can do well and will avoid the other ones. Advanced students, also aware of their limitations, deliberately practice those very poses that challenge them.

If you've been writing and practicing Yoga for a while, move toward the difficult. It could be your most important habit to cultivate as a writer. You probably know your physical, emotional, spiritual, and creative limitations. (Don't we all? Don't remind me, you say.) When I made this suggestion to a group of writers in California, one woman rolled her eyes, smiled, and said, "You know, I've had enough difficulty in my life. I'm at a stage in which I don't think I need to move toward it because it moves toward me." I know what she means. Busted relationships, disappointing jobs, betrayed friendships, broken bones, a slew of rejection letters, and collapsed organs can be part and parcel of our daily difficulties, so why move toward it as if stepping onto the middle of a freeway? I'm suggesting we recognize and work with—rather than try to ignore and overcompensate for—the limitations of our creative writing and our writing life. I've had to work with the limitations of my erratic mind that loves to play, my delusions of grandeur and my pity parties (sometimes in the same day), as well as my proclivity for happy endings. The beauty of having a regular "advanced" Yoga practice as a writer is that you develop such a large repertoire to work with those limitations that after a while you may not even recognize a challenge as a challenge but simply as a creative problem to work with.

Here are some ideas and general guidelines when considering how different poses affect the body-mind-imagination. I've had to simplify some of the explanations for the sake of space, but these guidelines I hope will be enough to prod you to test out for yourself how your breath, your body, and your mind can indeed be your muse.

STANDING POSES, BALANCING POSES, CONCENTRATION, AND PRESENCE

Standing poses facilitate **concentration** and **presence**. By drawing attention downward and away from our heads, we can quiet the chatter. These poses remind us of our physical connection to the ground (and flighty writers whom I know beg for grounding), which in turn helps us remain aware of this body and material world. Since we have numerous nerve endings in the feet, these poses also naturally quicken other body parts and organs. Poses such as **MOUNTAIN POSE, EVEN-HEARTED MOUNTAIN POSE,** and **WARRIOR II POSE** aid diaphragmatic breathing, as well, which quiets the brain and the sympathetic nervous system. **EXTENDED SIDE-ANGLE POSE** (*utthita parsvakonāsana*) so stretches the torso that it also increases your breath capacity and aids the digestive system—boons to concentration. (Note: **ADAMANTINE/KNEEL-ING POSE** *(vajrāsana)* also stimulates several important nerve and energy points in the feet and legs, which makes it an excellent pose to open and close a sequence for heightened concentration.)

STANDING BALANCING POSES aid **concentration**. If you want to develop a sequence for **concentration** before writing, try to include at least one balancing pose. With some standing poses' benefits, balancing poses can deepen your concentration because more parts of the brain are stimulated. Choose a balance pose such as **TREE POSES** *(vrksāsana),* **WARRIOR III POSE** *(viribridāsana III),* **EAGLE POSE** *(garudāsana),* or **HALF-MOON POSE** *(ardha chandrāsana)* with which you already are familiar and comfortable. The more accustomed your body is to the pose, the more your fretful thoughts and hastened breath can relax while your brain remains stimulated.

BACK BENDS AND EMOTIONS

In the early morning and midafternoon, sometimes we need a jolt of energy. **BACK BENDS,** such as **COBRA POSE** *(bujanghāsana),* **LOCUST POSE** *(shalabhāsana),* **UPWARD FACING DOG POSE** *(urdvha mukha svanāsana),* or **CAMEL POSE** *(ustrāsana)*—generate intense energy and can be allies for **perseverance** and working with intense emotions such as **fear, passion,** or **anger.** They counter drowsiness and muddled thinking by rousing our sympathetic nervous system, encouraging energizing thoracic breathing (that is, breathing in the chest area), stimulating beta brain wave activity, and preparing us for action. They also open our heart region and break down our emotional armor. So, while some students become a bit cranky, irritable, if not mad, during back bend sequences, they also prepare their bodies and imaginations for **compassion**. Of course, if you've been practicing Yoga for a while, you know that they're best practiced not only with caution and after some warm-up but also in tandem with other kinds of poses, especially forward bends, which have a reverse effect on the brain, mind, and imagination.

ABDOMINALS AND PERSEVERANCE

Practices that work the **abdominal** (that is, stomach) muscles also help you develop long-term **perseverance**. Whereas back bends kick in quick energy, **ABDOMINAL POSES** build a long-term reservoir of inner heat. **LEG LIFTS**, if executed safely with the back flat on the ground, increase blood oxygen. The **SOARING LOCK** *(uddiyana-bandha)* in which you lift your abdominals is one of the most efficient ways to generate long-term heat. It's also possibly the only Hatha-Yoga practice that stretches the diaphragm. **SHINING SKULL CLEANSING BREATH** *(kappala-bhati-kriyā)* not only stimulates the abdominal muscles and digestive organs but also rouses the brain approximately three to seven times more quickly. These practices increase blood oxygen, steroids, glucose, and adrenaline in addition to toning our abdominal muscles, so sixty rounds of **SHINING SKULL CLEANSING BREATH** followed by three minutes of the **SOARING LOCK** before each writing session can shift your outlook and stamina. Again, be cautious and know your body. If you have a history of high blood pressure, avoid these types of practices. If you have an ulcer or hernia, best to consult a holistic physician.

CONCENTRATION AND PERSEVERANCE SEQUENCE

After I set my twofold writing intention, I flow through my daily morning sequence that I created for **concentration** and **perseverance**. It takes all of eight to ten minutes and usually sets me on my way for three hours of sustained writing. The sequence is outlined and illustrated in the Chapter Four's last TAKE A BREATH exercise. This skeletal flow gives my body-mind-imagination a familiar sequence, from which I then deviate according to what I know or intuit of my writing needs. This sequence, a foundation in many of my Yoga as Muse workshops, has helped numerous writers develop their own embodied writing process.

FORWARD BENDS, INVERSIONS, AND IMAGERY

FORWARD BENDS, such as **STANDING FORWARD BEND, DOWNWARD FACING DOG,** and **BACK EXTENSION POSE,** stretch the lower back and hamstrings as well as increase hip flexibility, so we can sit—on our meditation cushions or at our desk—for longer periods of time without strain. They also calm the sympathetic nervous system as well as the autonomic nervous system. These poses, mixed with back bends, help me work with intense emotions of anger and fear, respectively, so they, too, become manageable muses instead of hindrances.

I find forward bends especially stimulate my subtle imagination, that embodied reservoir of fresh imagery and ideas. When I begin a first draft or feel my writing lacking fertile imagery or ideas, I induce a dreamy "theta brain" state of mind that stimulates my subtle imagination. To do so, I flow through a series of poses that then finishes with back extension pose for three to five minutes, **KNEE-TO-CHIN POSE** (*janu sirsāsana*)—not illustrated—and then move to **SHOULDER STAND** (*sarvangāsana*) for seven minutes, practice three minutes of **ALTERNATE NOSTRIL BREATHING** (*nādī-sodhana* *prānāyāma)*, and finish with five to seven minutes in **LYING RELEASE/CORPSE POSE** *(savāsana)*. Twenty to thirty minutes of working with my muse in forward bends and shoulder stand usually grants me hours of richer writing.

While being cautious of your neck and cervical spine and avoiding these poses altogether if you have high blood pressure, consider these options, for instance, for the TAKE A BREATH exercise in Chapter 20:

Variation #3: **REVERSED ATTITUDE GESTURE** *(viparitakarani mudrā)*. You may place a blanket underneath you for extra padding in this pose. To come into this pose from resting on your back, press your hands, palms down, as well as the forearms against the floor, and use your arms and your abdominals (stomach muscles) to lift your legs, knees straight and feet together for better control. Keeping your arms on the floor, bend your elbows, and place your hands under your pelvis for support. Your thighs and legs can be at an angle so that your feet come over your head until you get accustomed to this pose, or your legs and thighs can be vertical and perpendicular to the floor. This pose places considerable weight on the forearms, and so you may find it too difficult, but it's a good preparation for shoulder stand and is a pose honored in the Hatha-Yoga-Pradipika as one of the most essential poses for maintaining the brain's vital energy. It also places less blood pressure in the neck and chest than the standard shoulder stand and in fact releases constrictions in the neck's vessels, which lets more blood flow to the brain.[1]

Variation #4: **SHOULDER STAND** *(sarvangāsana).* From lying on your back, roll your shoulder blades back toward one another, bend your knees, and, using the hands to support the pelvis, lift your hips overhead. Place your hands near your rear against your lower back and wrap your thumbs around your sides. Your body may be at a 140-degree angle or so at first. If your neck and chest are comfortable here, you can experiment with moving your hands farther toward your upper back as your torso gradually straightens. Remember to listen to what your body needs and not to what your will insists that you think you should do to achieve some ideal Form.

HUMMING AND HEARING

HUMMING or **CHANTING** rouses the brain, the throat, and our cells. The practice helps us hear with our **inner ear,** a vital trait for any writer who must spend hours talking to herself and who also must tend to the cadences of her words, lines, and sentences. My mother sent me a photograph of her singing at church. Joy rippled through her body. In this way, she chants at the level she's comfortable. Whereas Mantra-Yoga is a far more intricate system in practice and principle—just try humming. Even singing a non-sense song is a start to help you hear how words vibrate in your body and in your readers' inner ears.

LETTING GO

Finally, let go of intentions. This book begins with and sustains a focus on setting an intention. The book's focus also has explored Yoga in service of writing. The sweetness of practicing Yoga, though, is to practice Yoga. Get to the mat just to see what happens or what doesn't happen. More than one student has told me she feels most at home or most herself when on the mat. Yoga teachers can lose sight of this unconditional practice just as writing teachers can forget the joy of writing to write, for more than one writer likewise has told me he feels most at home and most himself when on the page. So write to enjoy this crazy thing we do, that we still love despite the agony it sometimes brings. And you know, usually it's not writing itself that brings agony so much as our expectations of it or because of the sorrow-laden rooms it takes us to.

The more I understand about Yoga, the more I realize I do not know or understand. But the more I study and the more I try things out for myself, the more I learn about my own writing process, my own crazy congress that tries to legislate my thoughts and actions and feelings, my own pernicious Heckler, and this wonderful ally that has been with me since I was a long-haired, towheaded boy climbing trees in Fort Worth: my imagination.

Don't stop with this book. Continue to explore for yourself how your practice feeds your creative process. Send me a note about what works for you and what you're discovering for your own process.

And be patient. Nothing so counters our American desire for transformation than our assumption that we can drive through and order bliss with our happy meal. Yoga is no panacea for writing woes. But if you're persistent, if you do in fact give yourself at least a five-week plan and try some of the practices and principles for at least fifteen consecutive writing sessions, you will notice some changes in your body-mind-imagination. Though Yoga still won't make writing easier per se, it can make writing all the richer and you all the more resourceful on your path to write authentically.

CHAPTER TWENTY-FIVE

A WRITERS' *SAT-SANGA*

WRITERS DO NOT EXIST in a vaccuum. Put another way, I heard Richard Nash, publisher of Soft Skull say at a conference, "The idea that writing occurs mostly in an attic or closet alone somewhere is horse shit." His point was that writers need to participate in their culture and get to know their world and even one another. An aspiring writer I know refuses to seek help. He has struggled for years to figure out how to craft and finish his short stories and essays. He has read books, honed sentence structures, knows precise diction. He's taken a few writing courses, too. But the idea of joining a writer's group or of seeking an editor's or coach's assistance galls him. "Hemingway and Fitzgerald didn't join writer's groups," he often scoffs. "No," I say, "They just sent their manuscripts to other trusted writers (to one another for a while), and Hemingway and Fitzgerald simply had the best editor a writer could have during the twentieth century—Maxwell Perkins." We have this conversation once or twice a year. My friend the aspiring writer still scoffs and still aspires, alone. When I last spoke with him, he still had not finished a story or essay.

I was invited to hold a seminar at a university's MFA in Creative Writing residency. I knew no one on faculty there although I had recognized the name of one of the professors, a poet whose sultry voice and mode of delivery I had heard some fifteen years earlier. His gentle sensual voice held in his tall and broad physique made many women poets swoon, I swear. He had been hailed as the next great thing. And his delivery was, indeed, great, and his imagination wild. I had been impressed, too, when he went on to publish three more poetry collections and then to teach at writing centers and universities on other coasts and in other places that back then seemed far, far away. I would keep an eye out for him, I decided, once at the MFA residency. The morning before my seminar, I ate breakfast alone in the hotel lobby. In crept a man. It had to be him. Although tall and still broad fifteen years later, he slouched into the hotel chair and ate a bowl of yoghurt by himself. I got up the nerve to introduce myself. He seemed grateful for the company. I mentioned a few common friends' names.

"Yeah, yeah," he said, "You're doing the writing and yoga thing, right?" He lit up. "Yeah, I might try to go to your seminar," he said. "I need all the help I can get. I haven't written anything much in six or more years." I was sort of shocked but nodded. He had taken a teaching job in a part of the country he didn't much care for, he said, but he moved to where the work was, and with the teaching load plus a series of personal setbacks—among them a divorce—he just has not been able to focus on his writing.

We writers can be guarded. Aspiring writers want to "tough it out" alone. Established writers can hide behind the titles, awards, and positions that suggest, falsely, that they have this writing thing all figured out.

Yoga, actually more than any writing workshop, has connected me to other people. My Yoga practice helps me open up and give— as well as receive—from the heart. My Yoga teachers created for me an environment of support characterized by clear communication and compassion, free for the most part from words of cruelty, narcissism, or passive-aggression. Which is not to say that the yogis I know—teachers or students—don't have their ego issues. They do, of course. Within these yoga communities, I've known randy single mothers, flustered business executives, women and men who left their corporate jobs, young men and women fresh out of college seeking to deepen their soul's education. Tattooed girls and CPA men. Politically, we were liberal and conservative, green as well as red-white-and-blue capitalist. Yet, because each of us students shared the same intention (to transform how we lived in our bodies and in this world) and the same set of tools to manifest that intention (the principles and practices of yoga), we loosely could be called a community of like-hearted individuals—what in Sanskrit is called a *sat-sanga.*

Imagine an authentic writers' *sat-sanga,* a place where we writers can communicate with one another on a basis of clarity, truthfulness, and compassion. It is a place where we can gather on our journey, sit a spell, share our experiences, and receive some helpful advice and perspective on our work—our writing. It is a place not unlike the inns that welcomed sojourners centuries ago—a sanctuary of diverse camaraderie and conviviality. This spirit emerges at Yoga As Muse retreats and workshops. A group of writers inevitably clicks. One staunch individualist meets another. Soon, three independent-minded writers hover in a room's corner and read their works aloud to one another. By the week's end, all ten or fifteen or twenty writers want each other's contact information to stay in touch.

At the end of most Yoga As Muse retreats, writers agree to stay in touch via email. They each set their fifteen-day intentions and then their five-week intentions. At the end of fifteen days and five weeks, they each send a message that describes their progress or lack of progress on their various projects and share what they're learning about Yoga As Muse at home. They commiserate. They celebrate. They advise. They sympathize.

One group of writers sends each other messages each five weeks. Usually one or two writers will remember the timeframe and send a message, and within a day or two the other writers follow suit. Invariably, the vagaries of being human become part and parcel of the practice. Carol works to finish her novel while tending to her troubled teenage son. Diane has discovered a new shape for her memoir while tending to her aging mother. Darlene seeks ways that Yoga might help her leave her emotionally taxing job of twenty years to find a simpler line of work that will give her more time to write.

You can create your own writers' *sat-sanga.* A virtual *sat-sanga* can begin as easily as exchanging e-mails with one another. You'll probably want to clarify some guidelines and some commitments to one another (explained later in this chapter). If you're going to meet face-to-face, so much the better. Decide upon a regular time and place to meet. A common coffee shop or diner or bookstore (with a tolerant staff) or library room can be the best route, because no one feels pressured to host the group at his or her house. One group I know of meets in a college classroom on Sunday afternoons when the building is virtually unoccupied. The regularity also often increases each member's commitment level.

But then I'd advise you in a few areas. First, be clear with one another about the group's intention. When I consult with writers who wish to begin their own groups, I often suggest they gather to offer one another support that is both truthful and compassionate. These tenets mean that when a writer genuinely feel that a person's writing is not working well to serve her own writing intention, it's the other writer's duty to respond tactfully yet truthfully. Each writer, however, must aim to understand and have compassion for another writer's intention and focus on his or her writing life or career. If some writers only want positive feedback and bristle at the thought of receiving or offering constructive criticism, then they're going to feel out of place. Your group's intention, however, may be just that: to offer one another positive feedback. Such a focus is fine as long as you're clear with one another. Another group of writers with whom I worked (and played) years ago met at a downtown club every Wednesday. We had the intention of supporting what was dynamic in each other's works so we eventually could collaborate with one another to create a performance reading event at the club. Consider, too, whether or not you wish to limit your group to discussing works of a specific genre. Some writers work best in fiction groups versus poetry groups, whereas other writers feel completely at home in learning from and mixing genres. Just be clear.

Second, regardless of the format you choose, be clear about how to offer feedback. In a YAM workshop, we keep our comments focused on the writing's craft and its spirit, not on the writer's personality or on our own personal experiences (which can lead to narcissistic responses). We also aim to be as specific as possible, always sure to move far beyond "I like it" or "That's nice."

Identify as specifically as possible two things: 1) what part of a piece of writing you're commenting on and 2) how the part works or doesn't work for the writing as a whole. For instance, if I say, "Your introduction is good," I've specified what I'm referring to (the introduction), but I haven't been specific as to how it works. I could say, "Your opening sentences' references to water and blood set the themes for what follows later in the story when Benny almost drowns in the river after his head cracks against the rock." Notice how this comment not only is more specific (and thereby helpful to a fellow writer); it's also more factual and less evaluative than simply saying something is "good." Other comments, however, may be more subjective in terms of how certain parts of a work pique your curiosity or make you feel as a reader. So, if a writer's story is rather bland until the third scene on page four, you might say, "The scene in which Albert meets this desperate punk-rock chick really hooked my interest in the story and in Albert. Before then, I didn't feel very connected to Albert. Maybe you could move this scene to appear earlier in the story," which is far more specific, helpful, and certainly more compassionate, if not more truthful to the story, than simply saying, "The first three pages are really boring." Thus your response as a reader will help writers figure out how their work potentially affects readers—one of the greatest values, of course, of writing groups and workshops.

Third, encourage risk in one another. A truly supportive *sat-sanga* lets us question the norm and try out new forms. If you notice a fellow writer always begins a story with the same type of interior monologue, then prompt her to imagine another way of beginning—a third-person observation, an ironic or omniscient description of a whole town, a dog's point of view. The dreariest part of being in a writers' group for too long is that everyone's aesthetic response becomes pat and predictable. A good writers' *sat-sanga* guards against complacency and mediocrity—either in writing or responding to writing.

Fourth, extend your *sat-sanga*'s services beyond the workshop model (which is helpful but limited). Invite one another to offer a fifteen-to-thirty-minute talk on a certain topic relevant to writers. Maybe each of you offers an introductory talk on an author's work. Maybe one of you offers a talk on what you view as "the state of fiction in the United States" or "the role of the writer in the twenty-first century." In other words, grant yourself and others permission to think about what it means to be a writer at this time in history. It need not be a forum to pontificate, but a place to explore ideas. A salon, in essence. Such was the spirit of what some of us created when we developed Dallas's first literary nonprofit organization, WordSpace. The idea is for us to guard against being myopic as writers in looking at our work solely in terms of words, images, sentences, and scenes. Such myopia is like regarding Yoga solely with reference to the poses.

Share information. Writers want to know about new publications or old publications that they've never heard of but perhaps should read. As we each keep abreast of what's happening in publishing and should be supporting small presses, we can in turn suggest to each other books and journals and magazines to read.

You may only need, though, a *sat-sanga* of two or three. One good writing friend, a writing mentor, coach, or teacher, can provide regular feedback and guidance. Some mentors and coaches also can ask the right questions—if not the tough questions—to help you move your project along. Cultivate a relationship with someone whom you trust. (The same dictate, incidentally, always followed when I sought a Yoga teacher.) Know the person's background. Know his or her motives for working with you. Sense in the first or second session whether or not the relationship will work and if you each will get from the relationship what you need. Otherwise, you're wasting your time, and writers don't have time to waste.

Myla Goldberg's editor of *Bee Season* wanted to change the ending. The main character should win the spelling bee, the editor thought. At first, Goldberg thought the editor was nuts. "That's the whole point," she thought, "the character has to lose." But rather than throwing out the advice altogether, Goldberg instead very wisely discerned what the rest of the novel lacked that did not make the current ending satisfying. She went back to her manuscript, rewrote several section and scenes, and re-submitted the novel. The character still lost the contest. "Perfect," the editor said in essence.

"Most advise is useful," Goldberg said at The Literary Writer's Conference at New York's New School, "if it comes from someone whose point of view you respect and who has your interest in heart." The author of the novel that went on to become a bestseller and film summed up well the essence of seeking connection as a writer.

A few final caveats about working with groups: Overly critical people can squelch your fire. Overly sympathetic people can fan your hot ego. Also, guard against depending too much upon your allies. Meeting with them and talking about your project can substitute for the actual, regular work that needs to be accomplished: writing.

Which is to say that most writers, like it or not, are happiest and most productive in a *sat-sanga* of one. It is in solitude, after all, when we can best listen to those crazy, multifarious voices, when we can best heed those random images and characters that call for our attention, when we can step across the threshold, out of the familiar house, and into the woods where, perhaps, after a long trek of faith in the dark, we'll find a clearing, we'll find the center of our life that then will guide us back home and to the page.

CHAPTER TWENTY-SIX

A CALL TO TEACHERS OF CREATIVE WRITING

DURING THE PAST THIRTY YEARS, some of us teachers have learned that creative writing *can* be taught. Most of us have found especially useful either some variation of the generation-driven freewrite model, the benign support-centered Amherst model, or the critique-centered Iowa workshop model. All three, in some moderation, are useful. Still, as teachers of an enterprise that is more than the sum of narrative arcs, sequenced scenes, and well-wrought stanzas, we owe it both to our students and to writing itself to consider other ways to approach teaching creative writing during the next thirty years.

I have invested my adult life as a teacher. I can think of few sweeter professional rewards than the exchange that happens between student and teacher. Throughout much of my twenties while teaching creative writing at the secondary and college level, though, I often felt as if I were missing something in teaching "the how" of writing. We would discuss just as readily a student's clunky sentences, abstract phrases, flat characters, and trite endings as we might a student's elegant sentences, concrete images, complex characters, and satisfying yet surprising endings. I could unravel a story's or poem's fragile form and suggest a pattern to rebuild it. We read model poems and stories. We critiqued students' manuscripts in workshops. Still, something in the how of craft, the whole of creativity, and the fullness of consciousness seemed lacking in what we did within four cinder block walls.

If you teach creative writing, you might feel similarly. You also might be wondering how to integrate ideas gleaned from this book into your own classes and workshops. I offer the following suggestions based not only on twenty years of teaching; these ideas also stem from my own wrestling with how to teach with some degree of innovation within an institution and how to convey seemingly obtuse and oft-misunderstood Yoga practices and principles to groups of otherwise skeptical yet curious writers and students.

Teachers and professors of creative writing are not therapists. Don't get confused about your role.

That's Madison Smartt Bell's wise advice in his introduction "Unconscious Mind" from his book *Narrative Design: Working with Imagination, Craft, and Form,* a thoughtful and beautiful eludicidation of form and craft in writing fiction. Bell taught for two semesters at the Iowa Writer's Workshop, known for its workshop method of teaching that has been the template for numerous other MFA program workshops during the past 20 years. Bell draws heavily from the then-current brain science of hemispheric-dominance to explore his ideas about teaching creative writing. Bell's ideas and assumptions about teaching creative writing in 1997 are so insightful and useful for our purposes that they merit summary (although I recommend you read the full introduction yourself).

First, though, I should clarify the findings of brain-hemispheric dominance, in vogue ten, fifteen years ago, that run something like this: Our left hemisphere computes language, logic, algebra, and analysis whereas our right hemisphere dreams, perceives patterns, likes geometry, and senses rhythm. The simplified view basically says that the left analyzes; the right intuits. This reduction led to many dangerous assumptions in teaching: for one, that an otherwise complex human / student personality could be explained away as "left-hemispheric dominant" or "right-hemispheric dominant." I would hear many teachers, privvy to these new trends in education, bemoan, "I'm not a right-hemisphere person. How can I teach differently if I don't think that way?" And on the other side, I still hear people excuse their lack of rational decision-making by saying, "I'm just a right-brain person."

A number of well-intending educators used some version of this brain model to encourage their fellow educators to teach in ways that stimulated both hemispheres. After all, it's no surprise that in most public schools and in most colleges and universities most teachers still teach primarily through lecture and analysis. Why? Typically teachers and professors have a limited amount of time per session – 45 minutes on average – with a large number of students to explore a vast amount of information and skills. Lecture and analysis are efficient. They're the means most of us grew up with. They're the means most students are used to. They're what most administrators and deans understand and support.

Bell is by no means a reductionist. He acknowledges, in essence, that teachers of creative writing and student writers must be of "two minds," so to speak, able to access both critical and unconscious faculties. The first option—opening your students' black box in the classroom—might lead to teachers playing funky music and having students visualize scenes, etcetera, etcetera. The danger, Bell notes, is that teachers are likely to find themselves dealing with complicated, murky emotional stuff that they, as teachers and not therapists, are not trained for. The student's black box is private, Bell says, and should stay that way.

The second option, then, not quite by default, is to teach craft. Yet, most classroom teaching, Bell suggests, is and by necessity should be relegated to activities that develop the critical. Stay out of the student's "black box," what Bell calls that murky unconscious responsible for most rich drafts of fiction that ostensibly dwells in the student's right hemisphere. Instead, keep classroom conversation and activity focused on craft, the essential tool set ostensibly secured in the student's left hemisphere. Bell ably defends the Iowa workshop model with some qualifications. This model goes something like this: 12 to 15 students distribute their photocopied manuscripts to their peers. Each student dutifully reads their peers' manuscripts, making editorial notes and observations in the margins and signing off with a general assessment. Then, when a student's manuscript is "workshopped" (an unfortunate coinage), the student quietly listens while each of the peer writers takes turns commenting and critiquing the manuscript's plot, characterization, form, style, and so forth. Each student, then, leaves such a workshop with a handful of specific critques and, indirectly, has learned as well from participating in the other workshops. This model, Bell admits, is rife with problems. Namely, talented and competetive students also seek to please and, so, dilute their innovative stories to meet the middle. Hence, mediocrity often prevails.

Still, the craft-centered critique workshop remains the best teaching tool, Bell contends.

I agree with almost everything Bell lays out in his introduction with a few exceptions. We don't have only two options, and to have students explore process in class need not lead to group therapy. We also are learning more about the brain, about somatic intelligence, about the embodied mind, and about meditation, each of which has implications for understanding how students of creative writing learn.

It is possible to teach creative writing differently than the standard workshop model. It is possible to integrate some of the ideas posited in this book into a creative writing classroom for teenagers, undergraduates, or MFA students. But to do so might require teachers' self-examination, knowledge in other domains, authentic intention, and flat-out courage.

DON'T TURN OUT THE LIGHTS

If you teach within a system, you teach within a system. Just beware of the limitations any system imposes. A professor, who teaches within one of the nation's most renowned writing programs on the West Coast, has penned numerous writing and rhetoric text books that, while craft-centered, also aid students in mining their "black box" for rich, luminous fodder for writing. For a few years, she also has co-taught with a Yoga teacher a continuing education course that explores how Yoga weaves with writing. When she, in turn, asked some of her undergraduate writing students to move through a simple breathing exercise in class, a student complained to the dean. The dean called in the professor and said, "We're not about that sort of thing here." "That sort of thing" ostensibly meaning to the dean "New Age Quackery," I'm sure. Had the professor inquired if "that sort of thing" meant "trying to help students learn more about how their creative faculties function in accordance with fundamental somatic awareness," I'm sure the dean, to hide his ignorance, would scoff.

If deans don't resist, then undergraduates and graduates themselves do. Award-winning poet Olga Broumas, also Director of Creative Writing at Brandeis University, sometimes leads her undergraduate writing students through breathing exercises. Most of them are so awkward in their bodies, she told me, that any direct reference to the body makes them squirm.

Granted, writing well is difficult, and neither they, nor you, have time for games and trickery.

Be sure your agenda is apparent. Teachers and professors of creative writing should have no other agenda—moral, spiritual, philosophical, existential—than to facilitate students' growth as writers. If such is your aim, frame every method you present (no matter how conventional or unconventional) in those terms: to facilitate students' growth as writers.

Don't turn out the lights. Don't play Indian music. Don't speak in homiles. Don't even be effusive. Be clear, genuine, and knowledgable. And be innovative without being foolish.

START WITH YOURSELF

Of course, you teach mostly from your own experience and expertise. You pay attention to the problems you wrestle with on the page and even getting to the page. You heed how your own imagination, intellect, heckler, and emotions function while writing. And you journey into that space below your neck and shoulders.

Try it out for yourself. You don't have to be a full-fledged yogi or yoga teacher to have your own experiences worth drawing from in the classroom. Over the course of a few weeks, try a few of the breathing and centering TAKE A BREATH exercises recommended in this book's first four chapters.

One novelist and professor of creative writing attended a Yoga As Muse workshop. Two weeks after the workshop, she wrote me to say she had been experimenting simply with setting an intention before she worked on her novel. The simple practice gave her such focus that she started setting an intention each day before she walked into the classroom. She was surprised by how clear she felt while in the midst of teaching. From her experience both as writer and as teacher, she then took her students through a similar simple process of breathing, centering, and setting an intention before working on writing assignments. The process shifted some students' attitude toward writing.

That this professor could speak from her own experience likely made all the difference in how well some of her students received the idea. That experience lends credibility to the teacher and to the process. She also presented the process in the context of her larger educational objectives—to offer students workable ways to learn about their writing process. That this professor is highly rational, intelligent, and knowledgable of her subject area also likely went a long way toward her credibility and toward her students' ability to receive a suggestion that otherwise might be scoffed at.

Bone up on literature outside of literature, too. Start to stock your reading library with a few substantial Yoga books and neuroscience books. I recommend David Coulter's *Anatomy of Hatha Yoga*, Georg Feurstein's *The Yoga Tradition*, and Esther Myers's *Yoga for You* for thorough introductions to Yoga physiology, philosophy, and practice respectively. I also would recommend these highly readable books on neuroscience: Norman Doidge's *The Brain That Changes Itself: Stories of Personal Triumph from the Frontiers of Brain Science* (2007), Oliver Sacks's *Musicophilia: Tales of Music and the Brain* (2007), Jeffrey M. Schwartz and Sharon Begley's *The Mind & the Brain: Neuroplasticity and the Power of Mental Force* (1999), and Sharon Begley's *Train Your Mind, Change Your Brain* an unfortunately glib title for a substantial book that came out in paperback in 2008). These books respectively review stories and studies related to how the mind and habits relate to changes in the brain's neuronal structure for better and worse; how the brain processes music in often odd ways; and how the mind's will can change the brain's neuronal structure and a person's obsessive habits (Would that we all could learn that process.).

In short, teach authentically. Teach from the authority of your own experience, insight, and explorations.

A few words of caution and respect, though: Yoga is an ancient tradition. Its tools should be shared and taught with care. If you teach writing but have not been trained to teach Yoga, then at the very least you need to have a regular Yoga practice and a trusted Yoga teacher. Confer with this Yoga teacher regarding how to safely teach a particular Yoga tool and in what context. As a general rule of thumb, if you are not trained to teach Yoga, avoid teaching any but the most basic of breath harnessing practices. Avoid teaching any breath retention practices until you are trained to do so. But a lack of teacher training should not keep you from beginning to explore more authentic and effective ways of teaching the whole of what it means to be a versatile, self-aware writer.

BREAKING OUT OF THE HEAD: SOMATIC AWARENESS AND MORE

If you wish to introduce some of this book's practices and principles, lay out with your students on the first day of class some assumptions, some of the same assumptions I lay out with readers of this book. For instance, if we accept that mind and body influence one another, then we must accept that the body plays a seminal role in our capacity to imagine, to think, to feel—and to learn. Ask your students what faculties they think they rely on as writers. They will likely include intellect, imagination, will, motivation, passions and emotions, intuition. Ask them how these faculties facilitate their process and their finesse with craft. They likely will have little or no idea how to respond to that question. Let them know that such an inquiry is part of this course on creative writing because part of this course's objective is to help them become more aware of their creative faculties.

Then, draw a figurine of the human body on the board and ask them where in the body these faculties are located. Someone without fail will point to the head, meaning, more than likely, the brain and possibly the mind (terms that are often, incorrectly, interchanged). Ask them if they're sure. Someone surely will bust the head bubble and recognize that the central nervous system extends down the spine and through intricately cellular systems reaches out to the "furthest extremities" of the body. If no one suggests this possibility, lead them to it. So, possibly, you might suggest, the dwelling places of creative faculties cannot be relegated to huts in the head. Possibly, our body's autonomic functionings, our physiological structure, our actions (intentional and unintentional), even perhaps the ways in which we breathe could influence how well and what we imagine, think, feel, intuit, see, hear, and touch.

Throughout a course, introduce Yoga practices and principles as part and parcel of the creative writing fare. Depending on your institution and student body, call what you're doing Yoga or call it somatic awareness or call it awareness of how creative faculties work. One class can address intention and purpose. Another, concentration and immersion. Another, the importance of writing regularly and with perseverance. Another class could address imagination and the importance of convincing detail and precise imagery. Another, intuition and drafting. Yet another could explore the importance of complex characterization and how to embody compassion for a character.

You might begin your teaching journey with this book's first four chapters that, respectively, address intention & purpose, time, perseverance, and concentration. Then, move into specific areas of craft as explored in the second section, and for matters of emotional honesty and complexity use ideas from the third section's chapters.

As a teacher, you also become more resourceful and versatile in helping students one-on-one. A memoirist, poet, and teacher I know told me she has helped numerous students individually just by teaching them a simple yoga tool without necessarily even calling it by name. When she met repeatedly with a graduate student who could not get the momentum to complete her thesis, the professor taught the student SHINING SKULL CLEANSING BREATH (*kapalabhati*)—the rapid-exhalation exercise described in chapter three for perseverance. The student took to the breathing exercise instantly. It cleared her foggy head and tired body and helped her shift a little more energy toward finishing her thesis.

In *The Art of Fiction*, John Gardner defined certain "errors of character" and "errors of the soul" that, mostly, he said, a teacher could only identify but not change in a student. In some cases, he's right. It seems counter-intuitive, for instance, to think that compassion could be taught. Yet, Tibetan Buddhist monks have known for centuries that compassion can be taught. It's not uncommon for such a monk to ask a student, "What is your compassion practice?" *Compassion practice? You either have it or you don't, right?* Everything in the human experience of mind and body is, I venture to say, practice. Creativity, craft, compassion—all largely practice.

I know another professor of creative writing, trained to teach Yoga, who addressed this very matter of compassion with a student. She had noticed that the student, who was writing his memoir, lacked compassion for a character based on the student's father. Gardner might call the quality "undue warmth." Regardless, unsympathetic and flat characters often malign many a memoir and many a novel. The teacher met with the student individually and asked if he were open to exploring how to make this father character more complex. The student hesitated but said he'd try. The teacher simply gave the student a few questions that prompted the student to see, hear, and feel "reality" from the father character's point of view. Then, she suggested the student experiment and spend a day trying, off and on, to experience any given moment—be it in the dorm, at lunch, on a date—from the character's point of view. Even try to feel what it must feel like to inhabit that character's body, she said.

Reluctant at first, the student tried it. Not surprisingly, the student eventually rewrote his whole memoir, much of it all the richer from the shift in embodied perspective. Without ever mentioning Pali (the language of much Buddhism) or Sanskrit, the teacher helped the student embody something utterly essential for most writers, active compassion, or *karuna*. This teacher was clear about her intention—not to "convert" the student into practicing Yoga but to help the student become a more versatile writer, to help the student become the best writer he could possibly be. That's the charge for each of us.

As teachers of creative writing, we are called upon to address matters of craft *and* matters of process. Both involve matters of consciousness. Consciousness involves, at least in part, somatic awareness. Consciousness shapes craft; craft, consciousness. In the classroom, you can deal semi-objectively with students' somatic awareness and awareness of creative faculties. And you can do so in a way without a creative writing class descending into group therapy. MFA Programs and secondary programs can be—and in many cases are—places to support innovative pedagogy based on current findings of how we human beings best learn.

Many of you have the advantage to teach outside of an institution. You lead writing groups, you teach from your homes, or you teach continuing education classes. You're playing a vital role in our culture to facilitate the growth of writers who either cannot afford the time, expense, or energy to devote to a full college program and yet who merit authentic guidance and support.

Regardless of your situation as a teacher, have confidence in your own Yoga practice and writing practice. That confidence will guide your authenticity in the classroom or with your writing group. From that place, you act as an honorable teacher.

CHAPTER TWENTY-SEVEN

YOGA AS MUSE LAB:
MUSES OF THE OTHER ARTS

"In this man Stowitts we have the ancient concept of the true Artist, following with intensity, and fidelity, the constant challenge of his calling. I am reminded of all lonely faithful priests of beauty who have served by their alter, for the joy and faith of the world."

- RUTH ST. DENIS,
dancer on dancer-turned-painter Jay Stowitts

"CREATIVITY IS MY BLOOD," Leslie says. "It is my food." Her nimble hand fidgets with a paintbrush. A mourning dove coos from somewhere beyond our open barn door, and as she glances its way the spring sunlight through the barn wall slats catch her face, and she looks for a moment ten years younger than her fifty-six years. In this barn, she says, she has found some hope since she has moved to the Mid-Hudson Valley. Perhaps, a failed relationship behind her, up here there would be a creative life she could lead. She feels fed, she says.

A small chorus of moans from others in the barn echo the feeding sentiment. Carolyn—a former rock-n-roll bassist-cum-painter-and-yoga teacher—nods. So does Roselyn—an art gallery curator, painter, and novelist. Phillip, a poet and musical composer, and Johaness, a New York City floral designer and abstract painter, smile in agreement.

"It's a challenge," Becky, a dancer and photographer, says, "to keep dancing when my body no longer cooperates and when three teenage kids I've inherited from this marriage definitely don't co-operate. She rubs her legs, then says, "I want to be true, though, to this calling."

A calling. I've never exalted what I do as a writer to that level of reverence. It's what I must do. It's what I can do. Still, I know and regularly meet writers, artists, musicians, and dancers who wrestle with what they deem their callings. How to follow it. How to be faithful. How to have faith—even if you don't otherwise believe in anything else.

During the warm months up here—from May to October—we open our old barn doors to writers, artists, musicians, and dancers. What used to hold hay and a few cows in the 1850s when Walter Osterhoudt settled his farm here; and what held campers from the 1930s to '70s when the farm became Camp Shangri-La for Jewish kids seeking refuge from New York City; and what finally held the debris of a life well-lived until 2006 when my wife Hillary and I bought the place from a widow, this morning holds nine of us—writers, artists, a musician, and a dancer. We each sit on a Yoga mat. Notebooks and pens, canvases and palettes spread around some mats like Yoga props.

We've spent the past two hours or more exploring Yoga As Muse. At the behest of some artist friends who live in Woodstock, I have been wondering for a couple of years about the question, *How can a Yoga As Muse process extend to other creative media?* That question gradually gave birth to the Yoga As Muse Lab.

Yoga yokes, so the yogis say. And, indeed, in this creative lab our mats are our common ground as is our desire to embody a creative life and to deepen our respective artistic process. Our muses meet on the mat.

A YOGA AS MUSE LAB

In a Yoga As Muse Lab, we gather to experiment. On most mornings, we follow a similar process. We begin with a topic, a creative conundrum, or theme that crosses all creative endeavors. We might explore songs of desire as they come out on the page or the canvas, or through an instrument, dance move, or photograph. In the conversation about desire, I might play an Indian *raga*, an intricate, complex musical form whose rhythms correlate with seasons, moods, and time of day. *Raga* translates as "song" and "desire." Or we might explore time. The how and why of time. How time shapes space. How time plays out on the canvas or musical composition. How the past is present. We might listen to a piece by Phillip Glass to hear how repetition and time mix it up, and to hear how an electric guitar clashing with an eliding violin weaves sounds of the past into the present's texture.

After this creative dialogue, we engage Yoga to explore this theme. The muse comes to the mat through our setting a creative intention and moving through a sequence of poses, breathwork, and inner focus. Sometimes, we each will glide through the same sequence as I cue or goad their imaginations. At other times, we each agree to set an intention and intuitively follow our own process. Roselyn might close her eyes while in Warrior II to sense the presence of a past image. Phillip might slow down his breath to hear a musical phrase that keeps coming up in each pose.

Just as the muse comes onto the mat, so Yoga extends to the act of creating. As Carolyn paints, she's also harnessing her breath so as not to get caught in common perceptual loops. Johannes pays more attention, too, to unconscious signals while his eyes hover on the canvas. These experiments usually are less about expressing as they are about experimenting, exploring, expanding.

The outdoors often comes in, too. Since this barn's doors open onto woodlands that wrap around our large pond, several artists continue their process through a walk. They heed how their sense organs' engagement with the world of, say, shag hickory bark and dragonfly wings triggers their intuition—a mindful way to extend their Yoga off the mat and their artistic process off the page and canvas.

Then we share. We avoid letting the group descend into group therapy although we do discuss much of what seems to be stirring within our own faculties.

This particular morning, I have suggested we each follow a line. We will each refrain from knowing too much about where we are going, I suggest, and instead tend to the very line of words or crooked line of black oil or musical line that wants to be played out. I had feared they might think me daft; if they did, they didn't say so. We each set our creative intentions, follow our Yoga sequence, and create. Becky's in the corner quietly trying out new steps and then pauses seemingly to sense "where next?" Phillip scribbles a line then closes his eyes and lifts his arms up and down behind him, his chest opening, and then returns to writing the next musical line.

After two hours of such exploration, we circle and talk. Roselyn says the process took her out of her typical mode of trying to "represent" something in the natural world with paint. Instead, she simply focused on a single line's elegance that had reference to nothing but itself and to other lines. Yoga shifted something, she says, in her perception. Leslie has been struggling to write prose with the same passion she feels for paint. "I need to feel the ink as paint," she says. This morning she watched her mind get caught up in words trying to make meaning and freeze her imagination. When those mental loops tripped her up, she focused on a phrase on the page, moved into Downward Facing Dog, closed her eyes, and followed the seemingly random associations that surfaced with that phrase. The process freed her up.

Then Becky stands up, lifts her left leg like a crane, pauses, swirls in a half circle, counterpoints her weight to one leg, and whirls in the opposite direction. The movement takes all of twelve seconds. "That phrase," she says, "has been haunting me for months. I've finally found a way to articulate it." *Phrase*, I think. I had never heard a dancer use the term that way. Dancers are haunted by phrases in ways that writers are. Yoga instigates a process to become more aware of what haunts us, I think, of what apparitions loom on our consciousness's margins. Despite our different artistic processes and materials, Yoga gives us a common tongue.

Yoga also alters how a group of artists and writers converse. When in college, I would slip away to the art library, flip through large picture books of Picasso to sense a life lived with gusto and inevitably hover around the black-and-white photographs of smoking, well-dressed artists and writers, dead serious expressions, gathered around a café table. I would fantasize of sitting at the same round table with the poet Appolonaire, the Cubist painter Francis Picabia, the filmmaker, playwright, and poet Jean Cocteau, and the dancer Isadora Duncan. We would rap and debate and inspire one another, I would imagine, until dawn or until one of our uncontainable personalities would push everyone else away and out of the café. My outings with my fellow writers and artists in college didn't quite compare, but the flavor of brawling and good ol' rapporte was there.

Serious artists attend this Yoga As Muse Lab, yet no ego dominates or pontificates. No one claims her medium the superior art form. No one stakes out aesthetic territory. The Yoga As Muse Lab is an embodied artist's salon without the intellectual posturing. Yoga opens artists. It opens them to becoming aware of their own faculties and process. It opens the pathways among body, mind, and imagination explored throughout this book. And it opens their empathy for fellow artists.

THE SCULPTOR TAKES HER BODY WITH HER

Shaped forms line the walls of Nancy Azara's barn-studio. Pieces of cedar bark rub up against shreds of gold-laced paper. From wood shards, carved forms emerge. From these carved forms, images take shape again in the imagination. One form suggests a hand silhouette, another a torso's profile. Mostly, though, Nancy's works present moods and sinewy impressions of what the mind might brew in visual and textural forms. To look at one of her works is to gaze into a mirror from the inside-out.

Nancy and I met a few years ago in a Yoga studio in Woodstock. The abstract painter and sculptor has practiced Yoga since 1974— almost as long as she has been an artist. Once a formidable force in New York City's feminist art scene during the 1970s as the founder of the New York Feminist Art Institute, Nancy now lives a quieter life divided between the city and the Catskill Mountains.

Her strong, elegant face rounds like a barred owl, and her eyes, alert yet soft, watch me gaze on her work.

"Since I am a wood carver," she tells me, "I have for years developed a rapport with each tree, limb, log, or plank when I work on it." One piece, about 12' x 12', has 12 panels of wood, three across, four down. One panel's carving suggests a heart or an ovum or an acorn with vibrating lines around it. Beside it, three salmon-hued arms reach up. The material, the forms, the laquered and gilded panels, these elements make up what Janet Koplos in *Art in America* called Nancy's "signature vocabulary." Indeed, she's developed a whole language, a way of conversing. "This listening and embracing has for me an affinity with the experience of Yoga," she says, "probably because it accesses the same place inside."

She agrees that Yoga opens us. "I like the openness that happens in my mind and the visions which I get when I am practicing Yoga," she says and smiles, "the access to another dimension that it gives me. This becomes a strong influence in my art work."

I mention the sense of how what we call inside and outside converse as I gaze on her work. That conversation, she says, is similar to what happens to her when practicing Yoga postures. "I experience the postures both from the outside as well as the inside. The poses are so beautiful, and primitive, really elemental, and very ancient, not necessarily in a historical way although that is the case, but rather in some essential human way. This is the same language that I try to use in my sculpture."

Art emerges from a dialogue of consciousness, the body, techniques, and material. Such was one tenet of the philosopher and psychologist Maurice Merleau-Ponty who, more than any other contemporary philosopher, aimed to dissolve the Cartesian body-mind distinction. Physical action, not thinking, becomes the seminal mode for how human beings learn—a near-inversion of Descartes' *cogito ergo sum*. Consciousness, he writes, is less about "I think that" than it is, "I can."[1] Artists became Merleau-Ponty's primary focus for much of his last incomplete work. After interviewing several artists, Merleau-Ponty quoted poet Paul Valery in agreement: "The painter takes his body with him... we cannot imagine how a mind would paint."[2]

Indeed.

"For as long as I can remember," Nancy has written in a recent anthology of essays, *Painting, Sculpture, and the Spiritual Dimension*, "I have been looking for a way to give shape and form to spirit, a way to touch the nature of the divine." She has found the way.

I've come to Nancy's barn-studio in part because I recently bought one of her collages and need some framing ideas. Nancy has obliged by showing me some of her framed collages and what she thinks works best: top-mounted, white rubbed ash, slightly squared.

But I realize that Nancy's way with art playfully dissolves frames. What I mean is this: As I listen to Nancy describe her artistic process and her way with Yoga, I become more aware of being surrounded by her sculptures in this barn, itself made of cedar and oak and itself surrounded by the same raw stuff from which her art comes. It seems almost an illusion to distinguish too clearly among artistic material, natural material, and artist's body. In this dialogue, it's all Yoga.

CHOREOGRAPHING THE SPIRITUAL LIFE

Dancer Andra Corvino describes Yoga as "spirituality in motion. It is the same feeling of doing a beautiful double turn in attitude and how that feels—you just want to keep recreating it....That's our lot, to try to get all those moments connected that way."[3] In this way Yoga links most intimately with the experience of dance.

Corvino's comments come from a thesis completed in 2007 by dancer and Yoga practicioner Solvieg Santillano, of Wesleyan University, as part of her M.A. in Liberal Studies. Her thesis title says it all: "The Effects of Hatha Yoga on Contemporary Dance: Pitfalls, Practices, and Possibilities." Santillano describes her own experiences with Yoga in a way that I have heard echoed among dancers, writers, and artists. After an ambitious run with dancing, she found herself a middle-aged mother with a less predictable body than when in her 20s. Once she developed her own Yoga practice, under her teacher's guidance, she quickly felt more balance, "strength and stamina in my dancing, and also the stirring of a new calm and creativity that began to surface from within."[4]

Santillano describes her Yoga practice as an "anchor" in her dancer's life amidst the rest of life's unpredictability—loss, disappointment, continuous stress. Her description reminds me of the dancer Becky in my barn as she described the three teenagers who suddenly dominate her daily life. *How to stay true to her calling when all of these other demands are calling, too?* This facet of Yoga is the residue of a practice—what Yoga does for the dancer, artist, the musician, the writer when not directly in the act of creating and when not on the mat or zafu. Yoga, unlike aerobics, weight-lifting, or even many martial arts, provides a full toolbelt to navigate all of that other "stuff" that some of us writers and artists (wrongly, I think) blame as destroying our creativity—namely, the rest of life.

Writer William Styron summed up the matter well. When interviewed by the *Paris Review* in the 1950s, he was asked if his generation of writers had more angst than previous ones since they had to contend with two world wars, the holocaust, Hiroshima. No, he said. His generation of writers had to contend with the same basic stuff that all generations of writers must deal with—what a friend of his calls "the fleas of life." The fleas of life are what artists and writers (and yogis) often try to escape from—love and loss, spouses, children, ailing parents, jobs, a leaking roof, a broken ankle.

How to link the fleas of life with the immersion of creating? Well, they likely cannot be linked in the sense that most of us will not experience creative immersion while an infant vomits on us in an airplane. Still, Hatha-Yoga's essential emphasis on movement and of linking one movement to the next suggests, at the very least, a metaphor for a way of living as much of each day with creative awareness, a way of living to which many of us aspire. It is a curious dance worth engaging.

THE NEXT WAVE OF YOGA RESEARCH: CREATIVITY

Santillano's study is one of many graduate theses and dissertations related to embodied creativity appearing more frequently. This graduate work along with our informal Yoga As Muse Labs might mark the beginning of a new trend among yoga researchers: creativity.

I have started to gather data among small groups of graduate writing students at Western Connecticut State University's MFA in Professional Writing program. Most of these students have as much to contend with in life as, if not more than, the rest of us not in college. Most of these students—aged from 24 to 56—in this low-residency program have part-time or full-time jobs, have families, or have raised families. This "crowded-life" syndrome made them a particularly ripe study group.

I met with each group during the program's residency workshop week. Most of this week's offerings—though intellectually stimulating—is usually of the sedentary writer fare: Sit and listen to a writer read, sit and listen to a writer-professor lecture, sit and discuss a manuscript, sit and discuss issues with writing. We writers sit and talk and listen. A lot. So, no surprise that a handful of these students—and a couple of faculty members—were hungry for movement. I taught the group a simple sequence and ways to integrate the sequence into writing, and then I met with each participant individually to review the sequence, to discuss the study's goals, and to give them supplementary material to help them remember the sequence. Two to three times a week over three months, these graduate writing students integrated a simple sequence of setting an intention, moving through specified Hatha-Yoga postures, and practicing breathwork as a 10-minute prelude to their writing sessions. Judging from these students' pre-study and end-program questionnaires as well as their report journals, Yoga aided them in three key ways: heightened focus and efficiency while writing, increased self-awareness of mental and imaginative patterns that either sabotage or abet writing, and less anxiety while writing.

These graduate students practiced Yoga by themselves. This component is essential. They didn't go to Yoga studios. They didn't have a teacher calling the shots. Each writer learned a simple form and practiced it of her or his own volition. For sedentary writers with next to no Yoga experience, that is no small feat.

Another preliminary study completed in 2006 examines a Yoga lifestyle's effects on musicians' performance anxiety. The study stemmed from the interests of Stephen Cope, psychologist and senior Yoga teacher at the Kripalu Instititute. Kripalu, tucked on idyllic acreage in Lenox, Massachusetts, was the United States' first full Yoga ashram. Since the 1990s, Cope has helped the institute transform itself into a full-range residential retreat center that attracts among the world's most committed and talented teachers of Yoga, meditation, the martial arts, and creative arts. Cope directs Kripalu's Institute for Extraordinary Living. He also, not coincidentally, is a trained classical pianist and has danced professionally both in ballet and modern dance.

Cope has been working with Sat Bir S. Khalsa of Harvard's Medical School to design studies that will assess to what extent a yoga lifestyle can benefit musicians both in enhancing process and, specifically, in ameliorating performance anxiety. The first study gathered subjects from the summer fellowship program of the Boston Symphony Orchestra's academy for advanced musical study, the Tanglewood Music Center. The summer program extends for eight weeks during which talented professional musicians work with internationally renowned musicians. For the yoga lifestyle study, a group of ten fellows stayed at Kripalu, and, after completing pre-study questionnaires regarding moods and music, the fellows followed a regular Yoga practice led by a senior Kripalu teacher. A group of ten fellows, not participating in Yoga during the two-month program, functioned as the study's control group. The Kripalu teachers monitored and reported any issues or problems that arose in the two months as the fellows were trained and counseled as well in how to engage breathing practices when performance anxiety surfaced.

The study examined performance anxiety preceding or during the fellows' musical practices, group performances, and solo performances. Over two months, the most notable difference between the fellows practicing Yoga and those who didn't was in solo performance. Whereas the control group's anxiety rating barely budged before and after the two months, the musicians engaged in Yoga felt remarkably less anxiety preceding their solo performance.

Cope and Khalsa are planning more studies.

THE LAB YOU LIVE IN

Across artistic disciplines, the Yoga As Muse process is similar in the Yoga As Muse Lab:

- Focus on a creative challenge or theme.
- Set a creative intention.
- Engage a sequence of Yoga's tools as part of the artistic process.
- Bring a yogic awareness to the artistic act.

You modify for your own body, your own project and process, your own situation on any given morning or midnight. Test things out for yourself.

Yoga facilitates not only the generation of ideas and insights. It also carries artists through their challenges for transforming a "mistake" into a working part of a composition and through what must be an especially odd moment for painters and sculptors— when to say, "It's done. For now. Enough." So, too, with musicians. They know that art is not only about the splendors of receiving new melodies, phrases, or lines. The process also involves a lot of tinkering, letting go, throwing away, disappointments, and quiet victories.

If you're an artist or musician or dancer, the first four chapters of this book apply – intention, time, persistence, concentration. So, too, the chapters on presence and wonder. For better or worse, fear visits everyone, even the sages, so all muses might benefit from the chapter on the inner heckler.

You don't need a barn for a laboratory. You embody a breathing lab with all kinds of tubes and vessels, the very laboratory that those spiritual empiricists, yogis, have used for centuries. It's dark in there, but something's calling. Are you listening?

For an hour (or has it been two?), I've been stacking sticks outdoors. The impulse overcame me to break branches from the limbs fallen in our woods and make from them some simple structure—dare I call it a 'sculpture'? The sticks from apple, pin oak, poplar, and sugar maple might create a visual lure that could draw visitors more deeply into the scraggly woods and perhaps cause them to pause and take in the individual wood among the collective woods. We see so little sometimes.

Whether the stack of sticks levies any dim effect on anyone—and even whether or not the stack endures the winter storms—I don't care, really. The pleasure has been in finding the right limbs thick and dry and dead enough, in negotiating gravity's inevitable pull, in immersing this fragile mind and these feckless fingers in some tangible enterprise.

So it goes. You stack, and you stack some more, don't you? An impulse lures you into the woods, and before you know it you're stacking words and sentences dead into dusk. You look up and realize you're not quite sure where you are or how long you've been here. Perhaps you build a boat. Or a book made of leaves. Or a life that will not be sentenced to death. At times you do this thing for no other sake but for the sticks themselves, but you're grateful for the material, and you're grateful for these fingers. Enough, you say, enough, put your tools away, and return home.

Glossary of key terms

This list provides definitions of terms related to yoga, writing, and neuroscience that are pertinent to this book.

Abhinivesha ("will to live"), a mode of clinging to certainties. Considered in the Yoga-Sutra as a primary cause of suffering and affliction, it's fueled by fear. It can hinder a writer from taking creative risks.

Ahimsā ("without harm" "nonviolence"), the first ethical practice that Patanjali defines in the first of eight limbs of yoga; an all-encompassing practice that encourages yogis to think, speak, eat, and act without harm to others or to oneself; aids in a writer's capacity to render believable dialogue.

Ajnā-cakra ("command center"), also called the third eye center, located roughly between the eyebrows and is activated by the pituitary and pineal glands. Responsible for our faculties of vision, imagination, and sensory knowledge, it's a vital area for writers to stimulate. .

Alpha waves, brain waves that have 8–13 oscillations per second. Slower than beta waves, these waves are detected in people involved in creative activity, concentration, yoga, and meditation.

Anāhata cakra ("unstruck center"), the heart center; vital for extending compassion to the self, others, and difficult characters.

Anaphora, a sentence pattern in which a writer or speaker repeats the same word or words at the beginning of successive clauses or sentences. .

Anjali-mudrā ("oblations seal"), a hand gesture enacted by placing both hands, palms together, fingers up, at the heart. A common gesture of communicating the best in another person with the best in oneself. By bringing together left and right, it also signifies unifying all dualities.

Antarā kumbhaka is suspension of breath after a full inhalation, useful for stimulating physical energy and brain activity.

Antarā kumbhaka sama vrtti is suspension of the breath after the inhalation with even counts of inhalation, exhalation, and retention.

Antar-jnana ("inner knowledge"), like sahaja-jnana ("inborn knowledge"), intuition. An essential faculty to cultivate for drafting, writing with truthfulness, and re-visioning.

Antar-trataka ("inner gazing"), a Hatha-Yoga method used to deepen concentration and contemplation.

Antithesis, a sentence pattern in which a writer poses a concept's opposing idea, usually in a grammatically parallel form.

Āsana, the term most commonly used for a yoga pose. It also translates to "situation" and "one's relationship to the earth." Patanjali defines it as that pose which is both alert and relaxed, strong and soft.

Avalokiteshvara ("One Who Hears the World's Cries"), an androgynous deity who sprouted a thousand arms and hands with eyes in the palms to reach out to all who suffer—a potent image for writers who wish to extend compassion to their subjects.

Bahya kumbhaka, suspending the breath after a full exhalation. By calming the sympathetic nervous system, this practice helps writers quiet the inner Heckler and deepen their ability to hear language's cadences.

Beta waves, brain waves that have 13–36 waves per second—more than twice as fast as alpha waves.

Bhagavad-Gita ("The Blessed One's Song"), a text that recounts the dialogue between Arjuna and Krishna on how Yoga aids in overcoming fear and doubt. Arjuna is the protagonist and warrior of The Bhagavad-Gita. In this context, the story elucidates the fear-ridden writer's plight.

Bhakti **yoga,** devotional yoga characterized by chanting.

Bhavana ("visualization"), an essential limb of Tantra-Yoga in which the practitioner develops the inner eye and shapes to the interior self by visualization

Bhaya ("fear"), one of a yogi's primary afflictions. In this context, we understand the nature of fear as it inhibits writers' creativity.

Bhranti-darshana ("delusion"), a primary hindrance to yogis' ability to progress on their path, for the writer is attaching oneself to one's writing.

Bija-mantra ("seed syllable"), a word with a sonic vibration that stimulates specific energy centers. OM, HAM, YAM, and RAM are seed syllables believed to stimulate the third eye, throat, heart, and stomach regions respectively.

Cakra ("wheel"), a center of energy located in the subtle body and correlating loosely to centers in the physical body.

Causal body (ānandamaya-kosha, bliss body), the innermost sheath believed to house our capacity for bliss or ecstasy.

Causal imagination, the part of the imagination that houses imagery intimating union and bliss.

Dharana ("concentration"), the sixth of Patanjali's eight-limb yoga system. .

Dhyana ("meditation"), the seventh of Patanjali's eight-limb system. In meditation, a writer's thoughts begin to cease distinguishing between self and the object of concentration.

Dukha ("suffering")

Dukha hridaya ("suffering heart"), a gesture in which the arms cross and the hands hold opposite forearms, and the chin comes to the chest. The upper back is rounded. This pose, in emotional gesture and physical sensation, counters even-hearted pose and open-hearted mountain pose.

Dvesha-yoga ("yoga of hatred"), a rare practice drawn from a story in the *Bhagavata-Purana* and is based on the idea that one can learn to fear the divine by first hating the divine; from this intense near-feverish concentration, the practitioner ends up loving the divine.

Ekagrata ("one-pointedness"), a practice of centering, for a sustained period, one's attention on a single concept or object. It is a writer's ideal state of body-mind-imagination when no external or internal distractions draw one away from the desk or page.

Epistrophe, a sentence pattern that repeats a word or words at the ends of successive clauses or sentences.

Form for writers is the shape a piece of writing assumes. Ideally, it relates integrally to content, message, and intention. (See rūpa)

Ganesha, an elephant-headed god who, among other attributes, signifies auspicious beginnings. Also the scribe of yoga, he can remind writers that they embody the ability to remove obstacles.

Hatha-Yoga ("forceful yoga"), a term generally applied to all yoga practices and traditions in which the body is a vehicle of self-realization rather than something that should be negated or transcended.

Hatha-Yoga *Pradipika* ("Light on Forceful Yoga"), a seminal fourteenth-century yoga manual.

Hridaya tadāsana ("open-hearted mountain pose), a pose designed to stimulate the heart center and a writer's compassion. .

Hypnagogic state, the state of mind and imagination in which a person, while awake, experiences intense imagery surfacing from memory or from the subtle imagination. It can be induced by calming the sympathetic nervous system, increasing cerebral blood flow, and slowing down the brain's waves to alpha and theta wave lengths.

Ida-nādī ("comfort channel"), a channel of energy connected with the left nostril, the body's left side, the parasympathetic nervous system, and the right hemisphere. When stimulated, it can arouse the unconscious and imagination. Chapter 8.

Imagery, language that creates sensory impressions in a reader's imagination. It is a foundational trait of an embodied writing style—a way of writing that affects readers on a physiological as well as imaginative and emotional level.

Jāgrat ("waking reality"), daily consciousness and awareness. A yogi or a writer can practice being awake while dreaming (hence, lucid dreaming, which can lead to lucid writing).

Jālandhara-bandha ("throat lock"), a lock enacted by bringing the chin to the collarbone notch. Believed to help keep vital energy in the brain region, it also helps writers stimulate the throat or communication center to write with truthfulness..

Jīva-ātman, the individuated self, the personality that lives as a separate entity in this world.

Jīvan-mukta, the self that achieves liberation while in this body and world.

Jnāna-indriya, the "cognitive senses" believed to be essential for the yogi to harness for advanced practice. Similarly, writers can learn to heighten and harness their senses.

Kaimura, described in the Shiva-Sutras as a "proclivity toward play."

Kapāla-bhāti-kriya ("Shining skull cleansing"), a cleansing practice enacted by passively inhaling and forcefully exhaling. Its work on the abdominal muscles and the immediate rush of oxygenated blood to the brain makes it an essential practice for writers wanting concentration and perseverance.

Karma ("action"), the belief that both a person's actions and a person's intention for acting will have moral consequences in the future or in a future life.

Karunā, a Pali word meaning "active compassion."

Kosha ("sheath"), our bodies' different layers. In most schools of yoga, it's believed that human beings have a physical, subtle (made up of three sub-sheaths), and causal body.

Krodha ("anger"), described in some ancient yoga texts as a primary gateway to mental, physical, and spiritual hell. In this context, it becomes a powerful force that can be converted into authentic writing.

Maitrīyāsana ("Friendship Pose"), also translated here as Writers Pose because it is a pose in which a yogi sits in a chair—a writer's most common "pose" or situation.

Manipura cakra ("treasure-city center"), the solar plexus, the center of energy located approximately in the upper pelvis, the stomach region, and below the rib cage. Associated with willfulness and action, it's a vital center for writers needing perseverance.

Mantra, expressing a thought or an intention by sound.

Marjarāsana ("Cat pose") is a foundational pose in which a yogi is on hands and knees, wrists beneath the shoulders and knees beneath the hips.

Metaphor, a direct comparison of the familiar to the unfamiliar, the invisible to the visible, the physical to the metaphysical.

Mūla-bandha ("root lock"), a practice of sealing energy in the upper body by contracting the perineum. Its stimulation of the pudendal nerves is believed to help vital organs function properly. It can help writers concentrate and "root" their thoughts.

Mūlādhāra cakra ("root center"), a center of energy located generally near the perineum and when balanced can induce calmness, groundedness, and focus.

Nādī shodhana ("Alternate Nostril Breathing"), a breath practice performed by inhaling and exhaling through one nostril at a time. .

Nādī ("energy conduit"), not unlike an acupuncture meridian, a channel of energy. Some yoga texts claim we have seventy thousand nadis in our bodies that each contain vital energy.

OM, the universe's essential sound. Pronounced "AUM," the first sound correlates to the lower part of the spine as well as to the waking world (*jagrat*); the second sound to the cervical spine and the dream world (*svapna*); the third sound to the third eye center and the sleeping world (*nidra*). When embodied together, the yogi experiences the fourth world (*turiya*), bliss, or joy-filled amazement (*vismaya*).

Parallelism, a patterned sentence in which parts of speech, phrases, or clauses are grammatically the same.

Particularity, rendering a subject's attributes so uniquely as to make it at once believable and memorable.

Patanjali, the author of Yoga-Sutra (circa probably 200 c.e. although some scholars have attributed them to 200 b.c.e.).

Physical imagination, that part of our imagination that receives and stores images and ideas from our cognitive senses; responsible in part for memory and the recollection of images. Āsanas and other yoga tools help stimulate this imagination.

Pingalā-nādi ("tawny current"), complementary to the ida-nadi as it is connected to the right nostril, the body's right side, the brain's left side, and the sympathetic nervous system. When stimulated, it heats the body and boosts adrenaline.

Prāna ("life force"), that force which makes breath possible and which animates all life outside and inside of sentient beings.

Prānāyāma, harnessing the life force through breath work.

Pratyahara ("sensory withdrawal"), the active reduction of responding to sensory stimulation in order to heighten control of one's faculties. Helpful for writers who need to develop intuition for re-visioning.

Proprioception, awareness of the body's proprioceptors, specialized receptors that receive signals related to tendons, muscles, and joints. This awareness increases writers' presence by helping them pay attention to their body's interior world.

Ritam ("universal truth").

Rūpa ("form") also translates to body, physical beauty, and the manifestation of the divine; thus, the term reminds yogis of a yoga pose's beautiful, if not divine quality.

samādhi ("bliss"), the eighth of Patanjali's eight-limb yoga system characterized by the individuated self's complete union with one's realized self, which is part and parcel of all animate and sentient life in the universe. A Tantra view is that bliss is embodied by harnessing the energy and faculties of this physical body while living with joy in this physical world—not by negating this body or this world.

Sama vrtti prānāyāma (Even-length breathing), a form of breath control in which one inhales and exhales the same length. Retention of breath for the same length after a full inhalation or exhalation can be added.

Samprajnāta samādhi ("supported bliss"), the practice of concentrated gazing and meditation with a physical object.

Samshaya ("doubt"), the state of having two conflicting drives. A primary obstacle to yogis and writers.

Samskāra ("subtle impressions"), impressions made on our subconscious, our subtle body, and our subtle imagination. When left unconscious, they can dictate our thoughts and actions.

Satire, writing that criticizes human behavior, figures, groups of people, or institutions; characterized by the intention to reveal truth and stylistically characterized by wit, irony, and clever use of language.

Satya ("worldly truth"), the ability to speak and to act with certainty and yet without harm to others. (See "truthfulness")

Satyagraha ("firm in one's truth"), Gandhi's practice of political resistance, dis tinguished from passive resistance.

Savāsana ("lying release/corpse pose"), a supine pose in which one rests on one's back, palms up.

Sensuousness, the quality of writing that stimulates readers' inner senses.

Shimbava, the practice of gazing upward and between the eyebrows to help stimulate the third eye center.

Shiva-Sutra, a "revealed" text from the ninth century. An essential text for Kashmir Shaivism (a school of yoga), these seventy-seven aphorisms provide guidelines for reaching bliss in this body and world.

Shraddhā, "faith" and "confidence," fully embodied. This essential trait helps writers counter fear and doubt.

Subtle body, a sheath of the human body composed of the vital breath body, emotional body, and intellectual body. One way to understand how energy, emotions, and intellect are "embodied" or directly influenced by, yet still distinct from, the physical body.

Subtle imagination, part of the imagination that houses and releases random images from the unconscious body; often filters images with emotions.

Svādhyāya ("moving into one's self"), self-study that involves both studying classic texts to understand the great teachings that precede one's path as well as studying the inner workings of one's own mind. This study applies to yogis as well as to writers.

Svapna ("dream reality"), the state of dreaming while asleep or while awake. A vital state of awareness for writers wishing to access their unconscious consciously.

Syntax is the word order of a sentence.

Tādāsana ("mountain pose/standing pose"), a fundamental standing pose from which many other poses derive.

Tantra-Yoga, a wide-reaching term that applies to diverse schools of philosophy including Buddhism, Shaktism, and Shaivism. What most Tantrikas share is a belief that the body is a vehicle for liberation.

Tapas ("heat"), "self-discipline," the burning enthusiasm that helps one manifest an intention, "voluntary self-challenge." An essential quality for writers who wish to persevere.

Truthfulness, that quality of writing that indisputably rings to the reader as right, honest, and real if not disconcerting. It typically addresses a subject's complexities.

Uddīyāna bandha ("soaring lock"), an essential means to maintain vital energy in the torso and to stimulate physical energy in the body by drawing in and up the abdomen after a full exhalation. An effective tool for writers to cultivate perseverance.

Ujjayī prānāyāma ("victorious breath"), a form of breath control enacted by contracting the glottis and creating a raspy-sounding breath along the back of the throat.

Upanishads ("to sit near one's teacher"), a set of "revealed" texts that set forth the philosophy of the individuated self's relationship to the universe.

Upaya ("skillful means"), all of the tools and practices that yoga and other disciplines afford one for transformation.

Vāc ("voice"), the goddess of sacred speech. Applies to how the sounds that emanate from any voice and alphabet are divinely connected to the universe's primal sounds of creation.

Vāc-maya-tapas ("disciplined speech"), the practice of refraining from unnecessary and wasteful talk.

Vaikhari ("crude sound"), the basest level of audible sound. It is an essential yet superficial level of speech and communication.

Vedanta, a far-reaching philosophy of nondualism that is reflected in the Vedas and especially in the Upanishads.

Vinyasa ("flow" "linking tool"), a way of connecting one situation to the next with mindful intention.

Vishuddi cakra ("purity wheel"), the energy center located in the throat area; associated with truthfulness and clear communication.

Vismayo, "joy-filled amazement" experienced when one can engage wakefulness, dreaming, and sleeping as one reality.

Viveka ("discernment"), a critical faculty to help a yogi distinguish what elements of life help versus hinder one's progress; for writers, this analytical and clearheaded faculty is essential when revising to distinguish what parts of writing need to stay, be changed, or omitted.

Yoga, derived from the root yuj meaning "to yoke, to harness," applies generally to endeavors aimed at harnessing the mind's fluctuations; extends in this book to endeavors, practices, and tools aimed also at harnessing intellect, emotion, and imagination.

ENDNOTES

PREFACE TO SECOND EDITION

1. Joan Acocella. Introduction. *Twenty-Eight Artists and Two Saints.* Pantheon Books: New York, 2007. xii

INTRODUCTION: Remember Your Body

1. Margaret Atwood, Negotiating with the Dead:A Writer on Writing (Cambridge University Press, 2002): xxiv.

CHAPTER ONE: Putting on the Robe: Exploring Your Intentions for Writing

1. Bonnie Myotai Treace, Sensei, "Priest's Robe and Sound of a Bell: Gateless Gate, Case #16," Dharma Talk, Zen Mountain Monastery, Mt. Tremper, New York (7 July 2002).
2. M. P. Kilgard and M. M. Merzenich. 1998. "Cortical map reorganizaation enabled by nucleus basalis activity." Science, 279 (5357): 1714-18. Jeffrey Schwartz, M. D., also recounts much of the research in this area within the context of his pioneering efforts to help OCD patients with mindfulness-based practices. *The Mind & the Brain: Neuroplasticity and the Power of Mental Force.* (with Sharon Begley). HarperCollins: NY, 2002.
3. Vanda Scaravelli, *Awakening the Spine* (HarperSanFrancisco, 1991): 106. Scaravelli, one of my teacher's teachers before she died a few years ago, wrote this remarkable book when she was in her eighties. I have much gratitude for Scaravelli's liberating and authentic approach to practicing yoga.
4. Jhumpa Lahiri, interview with Matthew Solan, *Poets & Writers* (Sept.– Oct. 2003): 37.
5. Sindiwe Magona, "Clawing at Stones," *The Spirit of Writing: Classic and Contemporary Essays Celebrating the Writing Life,* ed. Mark Robert Waldman (New York: Tarcher/Putnam, 2001).
6. Jean Bernstein, "How and Why," *The Essayist at Work: Profiles of Creative Nonfiction Writers,* ed. Lee Gutkind. (Portsmouth, NH: Heinemann, 1998): 215.
7. Ellen Gilchrist, "Like a Flower of Feathers or a Winged Branch," *The Essayist at Work: Profiles of Creative Nonfiction Writers,* Ed. Lee Gutkind (Portsmouth, NH: Heinemann, 1998): 110.

CHAPTER TWO: Show Up & Shape Time

1. This teaching of *vinyasa* is the heart of Krishnamacharya and his son Sri T.K.V. Desikachar's practice. Krishnamacharya was the direct teacher not only of his son, who has developed the *Viniyoga* of yoga, but also of the two earliest and most influential yogis in the West, B.K.S. Iyengar and Sri K. Pattabi Jois, who developed the physical *Ashtanga* Yoga system. Pattabi Jois in turn inspired David

Life and Sharon Gannon to develop their innovative and spiritually grounded form of *vinyasa* called *Jivamukti Yoga*.

2. John Daido Loori, *The Eight Gates of Zen: Spiritual Training in an American Zen Monastery* (Mt. Tremper, NY: Dharma Communications, 1992): 172.

CHAPTER THREE: Stroke Your Writer's Fire

1. Georg Feurstein, *The Yoga Tradition: Its History, Literature, Philosophy, and Practice* (Prescott, AZ: Hohm Press, 1998): 87–90, and Georg Feurstein, "Heating Up Your Practice," *Yoga International*, Jan. 2003: 28.

2. In this book I'm less interested in yoga's mystical or esoteric dimensions. I mention these energy centers and channels because after just a few years of deliberate practice, I began to experience ways to harness and direct my energy in ways that improved my clarity and my writing process. This book will share with you very practical ways to do likewise without feeling as if you're trying to levitate. Some yogis, I should note, dispute the idea that energy centers correlate to anything in our physical body. Shyam Sundar Goswami's *Layayoga: An Advanced Method of Concentration* (1980) is one such text. Although daunting, it's considered to be one of the most comprehensive texts on understanding the subtle body. For those of you, however, interested in one of the other, more comprehensive studies of these energy centers and channels and how they may correlate to the physical body's anatomy, I recommend you read Hiroshi Motoyama, *Theories of the Chakras: Bridge to Higher Consciousness* (Wheaton, IL: The Theosophical Publishing House, 1981). I'm particularly indebted to Motoyama's thorough empirical, scholarly, and personal insight. Readers also may find of value and interest the following studies:

• Arpita, "Physiological and Psychological Effects of Hatha Yoga: A Review of the Literature," *The Journal of The International Association of Yoga Therapists*, 1(1990): 1–28.

• Vinod D. Desmukh, "Neurophysiological interpretation of ida, pingala and sushumna," *Holistic Science and Human Values* 2 (1995): 68ff. Reprinted from *Neurology India*: 1991.

3. B.K.S. Iyengar, *Light on Yoga* (*Yoga Dipika*) (Harper Collins: India, 1999): 425.

CHAPTER FOUR: Ride The Wave of Concentration

1. Patanjali defines *dharana* as the sixth limb of yoga—an advanced state that leads to meditation and bliss, the seventh and eighth limbs respectively. Shyam Sundar Goswami elucidates the extensive practices of *dharana* common among some schools of yoga in his *Layayoga: An Advanced Method of Concentration* (London: Routledge & Kegan Paul, 1980).

2. Richard Restak. *The New Brain: How the Modern Age is Rewiring Your Mind.* (New York: Rodale, 2003): 58.

3. Ibid.

4. B. K. Anand, G. S. Chhina, and B. Singh, "Some Aspects of EEG Studies in Yogis," *EEG and Clinical Neurophysiology* 13 (1961):452–456; B. Timmons, J. Salamy, J. Kamiya, and D. Girton, "Abdominal, Thoracic Respiratory Movements and Levels of Arousal," *Psychonomic Science* 27 (1972):173–5. See Herbert Benson,

M.D., and William Proctor. *The Breakout Principle* (New York: Scribner's, 2003) for recent research on how breath awareness releases nitric oxide, a key brain chemical that heightens creativity.

5. Swami Buddhananda, *Moola Bandha: The Master Key.* (Yoga Publications Trust: Bihar, India, 2000): 1.

CHAPTER FIVE: From Pea to Garden: Consciousness & Craft

1. William James. *The Varieties of Religious Experience.* Random House, 2002. 422

2. George Lakoff and Mark Johnson. *Philosophy in the Flesh: The Embodied Mind and its Challenges to Western Thought.* (Basic Books: New York, 1999): 13.

CHAPTER SIX: The Art of First Drafts

1. Joel Agee. "A Lie That Tells the Truth: Memoir and the art of memory." Harper's November 2007: 55

2. Kent Haruf, "To See Your Story Clearly, Start by Pulling the Wool Over Your Eyes," *Writers [on Writing]*: Collected Essays from *The New York Times* (New York: Henry Holt and Co., 2001): 87.

CHAPTER SEVEN: Unspoken Words, Unstruck Sounds: To Throw an Authentic Voice

1. Seamus Heaney, Introduction, *Beowulf: A New Verse Translation* (New York: W. W. Norton & Co., 2000): xxiii.

CHAPTER EIGHT: Presence & The Writer's Resevoir of Images

1. Barbara Kingston, *The Poisonwood Bible* (New York: HarperPerennial, 1998): 13.

2. George Lakoff and Mark Johnson, *Philosophy in the Flesh: The Embodied Mind and its Challenge to Western Thought* (New York: Basic Books, 1999): 25, 26. George Lakoff and Mark Johnson make a compelling case for the ways our bodies influence how we construct ideas and concepts such as love, courage, and truth. Even our experience of color, they contend, our experience of blue phlox and of red poppies, doesn't come solely from any objective quality of a thing outside of human beings but comes from how human beings' physical circuitry interprets the ways light hits the surfaces of the outside world. "[C]olor is created jointly by our biology and the world," they write. "[T]he qualities of things as we can experience and comprehend them depend crucially on our neural makeup, our bodily interactions with them, and our purposes and interests. For real human beings, the only realism is an embodied realism."

CHAPTER NINE: TheGenuius of Wonder

1. In more than one interview, Baker has noted that he doesn't fret about readers' wondering how much of his characters are "him." One novel he said is "87

percent myself." Another novel he said stemmed from remembering how, when in fourth grade, he wished he could stop time so he could read the chalkboard while the teacher stood still. Then, he imagined, with time stopped, he could take off the teacher's clothes. From that boyhood fantasy, a novel was born.

2. Swami Lakshmanjoo, *Shiva-Sutra: The Supreme Awakening* (Universal Shaiva Fellowship, 2002). The Kashmiri adept Vasugupta composed this text in the early ninth century. I am indebted to Swami Kahsmanjoo's commentaries on the *Shiva-Sutra*.

3. The play between waking and dreaming, the outer and inner, is the heart, too, of a practice called Tibetan Dream Yoga and Nidra Yoga (Sleep Yoga). These types of yoga include practices of lucid dreaming to heighten awareness about the nature of reality and self, to increase control of circumstances, and thereby to recognize the boundless possibilities of existence.

4. Green, Elmer and Alyce Green, *Beyond Biofeedback* (New York: Delacourt, 1977); K. C. Khare and S. K. Nigam, "A Study of Electroencephalogram in Meditators," *Indian Journal of Physiological Pharmacology* 44.2 (2000): 173–8.

5. Gladys Cardiff, "Combing," *To Frighten a Storm*, reprinted in *The Gift of Tongues*, ed. Sam Hamill (Port Townsend, WA: Copper Canyon Press 1996): 41.

CHAPTER TEN: Rain & the Brain: Embodied Metaphors and Symbols

1. George Lakoff and Mark Johnson. *Philosophy in the Flesh: The Embodied Mind and its Challenge to Western Thought* (New York: Basic Books, 1999).

2. Ibid. See especially Chapter Three, "The Embodied Mind," Chapter Four, "Primary Metaphor and Subjective Experience," and Chapter Five, "The Anatomy of Complex Metaphor."

3. This shift from a changing body to an altered worldview is precisely what author and Kundalini Yoga practitioner Terry Wolverton of Los Angeles described to me as having happened to her. Her whole outlook on life's possibilities and on other human beings has changed so subtly yet significantly that, of course, her writing's point of view has changed as well. My experience within two or three years of consistent yoga practice affecting my writing reflects Wolverton's.

4. Mitti Mohan, "Nostril Dominance (Svara) and Bilateral Volar Galvanic Skin Resistance," *International Journal of Yoga Therapy* 9 (1999): 33–40.

5. Annie Dillard, *Holy the Firm* (New York: Harper & Row, 1977): 17–18.

6. Henry David Thoreau, *Walden* (Penguin: New York, 1983): 354.

CHAPTER ELEVEN: Bliss in a Toothbrush: Writing Into Things

1. Although different schools of yoga define *samādhi* differently and far more complexly than what I'm offering here, I'm of the view that bliss need not be overly mystified, lest it lead our thoughts away from the grandeur of this world; as writers we need ways to be at once in and out of this world.

2. Charles Baxter. "Talking Forks: Fiction and the Inner Life of Objects." *Burning Down the House: Essays on Fiction.*(Minnesota: Graywolf Press, 1997): 79-108

3. Nicholson Baker, *The Mezzanine* (New York: Random House, 1986): 49–50.

4. Herbert Benson, M.D., of Harvard University reviews his own team's studies as well as those of other scientists in *The Breakout Principle* (New York: Scribner, 2003).

CHAPTER TWELVE: Listening to the Sunrise: Music in Poetry & Prose

1. James Joyce, *A Portrait of the Artist as a Young Man* (New York: Viking Press 1969): 7.

2. William Gass. "The Music of Prose." *Finding a Form*. (New York: Knopf, 1996): 314.

3. William Faulkner, "The Bear," *Three Famous Short Novels* (New York: Vintage 1961): 194.

4. Suzanne Britt, "That Lean and Hungry Look," *Newsweek* (9 October 1978).

5. Annie Dillard, *Pilgrim at Tinker Creek* (New York: HarperCollins Perennial Classics, 1999): 79.

CHAPTER THIRTEEN: The Kiss of Syntax, Rhythm, & Kirtan

1. Seamus Heaney, "Introduction," *Beowulf* (New York: W. W. Norton & Co., 2000): xxiii.

2. George Lakoff and Mark Johnson, *Philosophy in the Flesh: The Embodied Mind and its Challenge to Western Thought* (New York: Basic Books, 1999): 13.

3. Don DeLillo, *The Body Artist* (New York: Simon & Schuster, 2001): 12.

4. Dianne Ackerman, *A Natural History of the Senses* (New York: Random House Vintage Books, 1990): 109.

5. Rick Moody, *Purple America* (Boston: Little, Brown & Co., 1997): 3, 7.

6. Maxine Kumin, "Morning Swim," Our Ground Time Here Will Be Brief (New York: Viking Books, 1981).

7. Annie Dillard, *Pilgrim at Tinker Creek* (New York: HarperCollins Perennial Classics, 1999): 3.

CHAPTER FOURTEEN: Non-Violence & the Art of Dialogue as Revelation

1. Jack Hitt, Act V, Episode 218, Dir. Ira Glass. This American Life, WBEZ, Chicago, 9 August 2002.

2. Ibid.

3. Charles Baxter, "The Cliff," *Harmony of the World* (Columbia, MO: University of Missouri Press, 1984).

4. John Cheever, "Reunion," *The Stories of John Cheever* (New York: Alfred A. Knopf, 1962).

5. Nathaniel Hawthorne, *The Scarlet Letter* (New York: Bantam, 1986).

CHAPTER FIFTEEN: When The Inner Heckler Calls

1. I am indebted to Thomas Moore's interpretation of this myth in his book *Soul Mates: A Guide for Cultivating Depth and Sacredness in Everyday Life* (New

York: Harper Perennial, 1994) in the context of the spirit and soul of relationships.

2. J. Mager, Vijayendra Pratap, Barbara Levitt, John Hanifin, George Brainard, "The Influence of Classical Yoga Practices on Plasma Cortisol Levels." ENDO 2003, Philadelphia, PA, June 2003. The Endocrine Society Web site: http://www. endo-society.org/pubrelations/pressreleases/archives/2003/yoga_endo.cfm (19 September 2003).

3. Andre Dubus, "Witness," *Meditations from a Movable Chair* (New York: Random House Vintage, 1999).

4. Stephen Mitchell, translator. *Bhagavad Gita* (New York: Harmony Books, 2000): 55.

CHAPTER SIXTEEN: Dogs, Lovers, and Other Things That Bite: Writing the Truth

1. B.K.S. Iyengar, *Light on the Yoga Sutras of Patanjali* (New York: HarperCollins, 1993): 142.

2. Ibid.

3. Roy J. Mathews, *The True Path: Western Science and the Quest for Yoga* (Cambridge, MA: Perseus Publishing, 2001): 47–49.

4. Ibid, 57–59. I am indebted to Mathews for his information and for his thorough argument of how the brain experiences truth as expressed in the Vedas and Upanishads.

5. Mohandas K. Gandhi, *Autobiography: The Story of My Experiments with Truth* (New York: Dover Publications, 1983): 284.

CHAPTER SEVENTEEN: Web of Contradictions: Writing the Self in Memoir, Fiction, & Poetry

1. Nancy Mairs, *Remembering the Bone House: An Erotics of Time and Space* (Boston: Beacon Press, 1995): xiii.

2. F. Scott Fitzgerald, *The Crack-Up*, ed. Malcolm Cowley (New York: New Directions Press, 1945).

3. Adrienne Rich, "Integrity," *A Wild Patience Has Taken Me This Far* (New York: Norton, 1981).

CHAPTER EIGHTEEN: Stories of Scars and Deep Memories: Writing Beyond Trauma

1. Trent Masinki. "The Path of Creation." *Poets & Writers*.November/December 2007

2. Ibid.

CHAPTER NINETEEN: Compassion for Your Characters— the Good, the Bad, and the Downright Depraved

1. I am grateful to Joseph Chilton Pearce's description of the heart in relation to the HeartMath Institute's research in his book *The Biology of Transcendence: A Blueprint of the Human Spirit* (Rochester, Vermont: Park Street Press, 2002).

2. Rosellen Brown, "Characters' Weaknesses Build Fiction's Strengths," *Writers [on Writing]: Collected Essays from The New York Times* (Henry Holt and Co: New York, 2001).

CHAPTER TWENTY: Be Careful What You Hate: From Anger to Satire

1. "I'll Try Anything with a Detached Air of Superiority," *The Onion*, Vol. 38, No. 41, 2002 Rptd. in *The Best American Nonrequired Reading* 2003 (Boston: Houghton Mifflin Co., 2003): 222, 223.

CHAPTER TWENTY-ONE: Eating Leaves and Other Ways to Re-Vision for Form

1. Paul Heilker, *The Essay: Theory and Pedagogy for an Active Form* (Urbana: NCTE, 1996): 169.
2. John Cheever, "Reunion," *The Stories of John Cheever* (New York: Alfred A. Knopf, 1962).
3. Gary Soto, *A Summer Life* (New York: Bantam Doubleday Dell Books, 1990).

CHAPTER TWENTY-FOUR: For Writers Who Already Practice Yoga

1. See particularly Chapter Nine of H. David Coulter's exceptional text *The Anatomy of Hatha Yoga: A Manual for Students, Teachers, and Practitioners* (Pennsylvania: Body and Breath, 2001).

CHAPTER TWENTY-SEVEN: Yoga As Muse Lab: Muses of the Other Arts

1. Merleau-Ponty. *The Phenomenology of Perception.* (London: Routledge, 1945; reprinted 2006): 159.
2. Merleau-Ponty. "Eye and Mind." *The Primacy of Perception.* (Northwestern University, 1964): 255.
3. Solvieg Santillano. "The Effects of Hatha Yoga on Contemporary Dance: Pitfalls, Practices, and Possibilities." Weslyean U, 2007 . 107
4. Ibid. 148

ABOUT THE AUTHOR

A writing coach, poet, freelance writer, and editor, **Jeff Davis** founded the Yoga as Muse for Authentic Writing workshops and has taught writing for twenty years, assisting students of all ages and from all walks of life. His poetry, fiction, essays, and articles appear in publications throughout the United States. He is on faculty at Western Connecticut State University's MFA in Professional Writing Program, and his work has taken him to numerous locales, including The University of New Mexico's Taos Writers Conference; The Cape Cod Writer's Conference; The Writer's Lab in Skyros, Greece; the Block Island Poetry Project; and New York City's Om Yoga Center. He has Yoga teacher certification in two Yoga traditions and has studied Yoga, meditation, philosophy, and therapy in-depth with Sri T.K.V. Desikachar and his family of teachers in South India. He lives between the Catskill Mountains and Shawangunk Ridge in upstate New York with his wife Hillary where they are restoring a small farm with permaculture principles and have co-founded WEN Barn & Gardens.

NOTES

Notes

NOTES

Notes

NOTES

Notes

NOTES